Airway maintenance with cervical spine protection
- **Protect spinal cord**
- Assess airway for patency. If patient can speak airway is ok for now.
- Consider foreign body, facial, tracheal/laryngeal fractures.
- Perform jaw thrust, consider naso-/oropharyngeal airway.
- If patient unable to maintain airway integrity secure a definitive airway.

Breathing and ventilation
- Administer high-flow O_2 using a non-rebreathing reservoir.
- Inspect for chest wall expansion, symmetry, respiratory rate, wounds. Palpate, percuss, auscultate. Tracheal deviation, s/c emphysema.
- Identify and treat life-threatening conditions: tension pneumothorax, open pneumothorax, flail chest, massive haemothorax.

Circulation with haemorrhage control
- Look for signs of shock (p.116), cardiac tamponade (p.128).
- ↓BP usually due to blood loss; bleeding into chest, abdomen, retroperitoneum, any fracture.
- Control external bleeding with pressure.
- Wide bore IV access, send blood for XM, FBC, clotting, U&E.
- Commence bolus of warmed Ringer's lactate solution; unmatched, type specific blood only for immediate life threatening blood loss.
- Consider surgical control of bleeding (laparotomy, thoracotomy).

Disability
- Perform a rapid CNS evaluation. **AVPU** (**A**lert, responds to **V**oice, responds only to **P**ain, **U**nresponsive to all), Glasgow Coma Scale.
- After excluding hypoxia and hypovolaemia, consider changes in level of consciousness to be due to head injury.

Exposure/Environment control
- Undress patient for thorough examination: prevent hypothermia by covering with warming device and use warm intravenous fluids.

Adjuncts to Primary Survey
- Monitoring—noninvasive BP, ECG, pulse oximetry.
- Urinary catheter (after ruling out urethral injury).
- Diagnostic studies—x-rays (lateral cervical spine, AP chest, and AP pelvis), US scan, CT scan, diagnostic peritoneal lavage.

Secondary survey:

Begin only after primary survey is complete and resuscitation is continuing successfully. Take history—AMPLE (**A**llergy, **M**edication, **P**ast medical history, **L**ast meal, **E**vents). Perform a head to toe physical examination. Continue reassessment of all vital signs. Perform specialized diagnostic tests.

Conversions

$1\ kPa = 7.3\ mmHg = 10\ cmH_2O$

Reference ranges

Laboratory blood tests

Haematology

Haemoglobin	Male 14-18g/dl, Female 12-16g/dl
Haematocrit	Male 40-50%. Female 37-47%
MCV	Male 80-94fl, Female 81-99fl
White cell count	$4-11 \times 10^3$ cells/µl
	Neutrophils 50-70% ($2-7.5 \times 10^3$cells/µl)
	Eosinophils 1-3% (100-300/µl)
	Basophils 0.4-1% (40-100/µl)
Platelets	$150-450 \times 10^3$/µl

Coagulation

Prothrombin time (PT)	27-38s
Activated Partial Thromboplastin Time (APTT)	11-13.5s
International normalized ratio (INR)	1.0

Biochemistry (serum) / Liver function tests

Biochemistry (serum)		Liver function tests	
Sodium	136-145mmol/l	ALP	30-135U/l
Potassium	3.5-5.1mmol/l	ALT	7-40U/l
Creatinine	70-120µmol/l		
Urea	<7.5mmol/L	Bilirubin	2-17µmol/L
Chloride	95-106mmol/l	gGT	
Bicarbonate	22-39mmol/l	Albumin	30-44g/L
Calcium	2.2-2.6mmol/l	Total protein	63-83g/L
Creatinine clearance	90-120mL/min		

Arterial blood gases

PaO_2	>10.5kPa	75mmHg
$Pa\ CO_2$	4.7-6.0kPa	35-54mmHg
pH	7.35 – 7.45	
H^+	35 – 45 mmol/l	
Base Excess	-2 - +2 mmol/l	
$HCO_3$4.7-5.7kPa	24-30mmol/l	
SaO_2	>95%	
30-40%		

Pulmonary function tests (marked variation with age, height, and sex)

FVC = Forced vital capacity	3.5 – 5 L
FEV_1 = Forced expiratory volume in 1 second	>2.0L
FEV_1 / FVC	70-80%
PEFR = Peak expiratory flow rate	450-600l/min

Oxford Specialist Handbooks published and forthcoming

Oxford Specialist Handbooks

Perioperative Medicine

SECOND EDITION

Managing surgical patients with medical problems

Joanna Chikwe

Consultant Cardiothoracic Surgeon
Mount Sinai Medical Center
New York, USA

Axel Walther

Specialist Registrar in Medical Oncology
and Clinical Research Fellow
Cancer Research UK

Philip Jones

Consultant Intensivist and Cardiothoracic Anaesthetist
St Bartholomew's Hospital
London, UK

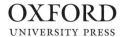

OXFORD
UNIVERSITY PRESS

OXFORD
UNIVERSITY PRESS

Great Clarendon Street, Oxford OX2 6DP

Oxford University Press is a department of the University of Oxford.
It furthers the University's objective of excellence in research, scholarship,
and education by publishing worldwide in

Oxford New York

Auckland Cape Town Dar es Salaam Hong Kong Karachi
Kuala Lumpur Madrid Melbourne Mexico City Nairobi
New Delhi Shanghai Taipei Toronto

With offices in

Argentina Austria Brazil Chile Czech Republic France Greece
Guatemala Hungary Italy Japan Poland Portugal Singapore
South Korea Switzerland Thailand Turkey Ukraine Vietnam

Oxford is a registered trade mark of Oxford University Press
in the UK and in certain other countries

Published in the United States
by Oxford University Press Inc., New York

British Library Cataloguing in Publication Data
Data available

Library of Congress Cataloging-in-Publication-Data
Data available

Typeset by Cepha Imaging Private Ltd., Bangalore, India
Printed in Italy
on acid-free paper by
L. E. G. O. S. p. A. — Lavis TN

ISBN 978–0–19–953335–0

10 9 8 7 6 5 4 3 2 1

Preface

73-year-old Mrs Khan starts complaining of chest pain and looking a bit grey three days after her total hip replacement. Although many medical handbooks will help you once you've decided she's having an acute MI, we would recommend this one. Because this one is written for surgical patients with medical problems and Mrs Khan may be having a massive PE. Or be bleeding into her thigh. Or gut. Or she may just be in septic shock. Or fast AF. Or any combination of these. This book will help you diagnose and treat these conditions in surgical patients, help you avoid the complications in the first place, and, if Mrs Khan does need an emergency laparotomy, it will give you practical advice so you know how much blood to cross-match, whether to talk to ICU, what to tell her relatives, how to look after her when she's back on the ward, and when she might go home.

This is a concise, practical text that gives junior doctors the guidance that they need to cope with medical problems in surgical patients early in pre-assessment clinic, the night before surgery, and out-of-hours on the wards postoperatively. It brings together a didactic, practical approach to problems with up-to-date guidelines based on current recommendations.

It is aimed at a wide readership—clinicians running pre-assessment clinics or responsible for assessing emergency and elective surgical admissions, members of the hospital-at-night team, and students interested in learning more about the practical management of patients.

JC
AW
PJ

Contents

Detailed contents

Acknowledgements

In addition to the great working platform provided by the first iteration of this book, we would like to record the large debt we owe to previous Oxford Handbooks, particularly the *Oxford Handbook of Clinical Surgery* 3rd edition, the *Oxford Handbook of Clinical Medicine* 7th edition, and the *Oxford Handbook for the Foundation Programme*, which were packed full of great ideas and writing. In several cases where it didn't seem possible or useful to express things differently we have used topics with minimal changes.

We would like to record our heartfelt thanks to Dr Mattias Powlowski at the Institute of Physiology at the University of Munster, Germany for his work as co-author on Chapter 1. We thank the Resuscitation Council UK for permission to reproduce the ALS algorithm from their 2005 guidelines on the inside cover.

Finally, we would like to thank the staff at Oxford University Press for their help, support, and encouragement from beginning to end.

Symbols and abbreviations

📖	cross reference
↑	increased
↓	decreased
♂	male
♀	female
☜	controversial
⚠	warning
+ve	positive
−ve	negative
AA	Alcoholics Anonymous
AAA	abdominal aortic aneurysm
AB	amyloid beta
ABC	Airway Breathing Circulation
ABG	arterial blood gas
ACS	acute coronary syndrome
ACTH	Adrenocorticotrophic stimulating hormone
AD	Alzheimer's disease
ADL	activity of daily living
A&E	accident and emergency
AED	anti-epileptic drug
AF	atrial fibrillation
αFP	alpha-Fetoprotein
ALD	alcoholic liver disease
ALI	acute lung injury
ALT	alkaline phosphatase
ALP	alanine aminotransferase
AMI	Acute MI
AMT	abbreviated mental test
APO E	apolipoprotein E
AP	abdominoperineal
APC	antigen presenting cell
APP	amyloid precursor protein
APTR	activated partial thromboplastin time ratio
APTT	activated partial thromboplastin time.
AR	aortic regurgitation
ARDS	acute respiratory distress syndrome

ARF	acute renal failure
AS	aortic stenosis
ASB	assisted spontaneous breathing
AST	aspartate transaminase
AVR	aortic valve replacement
AVM	arteriovenous malformation
AXR	abdominal X-ray
BAL	broncho-alveolar lavage
BBVs	blood borne viruses
bd	twice a day
BE	base excess
BiPAP	biphasic positive pressure ventilation
BMT	bone marrow transplant
BP	blood pressure
BS	breath sounds
BUN	blood urea nitrogen
CABG	coronary artery bypass graft
CBD	common bile duct
CBT	cognitive behaviour therapy
CBW	current body water
CHF	congestive heart failure
CCU	Coronary Care Unit
CDT	carbohydrate deficient transferium
CEA	carcinoembryonic antigen or carotid endarterectomy
CES-D	Centre for Epidemiological Studies: Depression Scale
CHEI	cholinesterase inhibitor
CKMB	creatine kinase (muscle brain)
CNS	central nervous system
CO	carbon monoxide
COHb	carboxyhaemoglobin
COPD	chronic obstructive pulmonary disease
CPAP	continuous positive airway pressure
CPK	creatinine phosphokinase
CPN	community psychiatric nurse
CPX	cardio-pulmonary exercise (testing)
Cr	creatinine
CRP	C-reactive protein
CSU	catheter specimen of urine

CT	computed tomography
CTZ	chemoreceptor trigger zone
CVA	cerebrovascular accident
CVS	cardiovascular system
CXR	chest X-ray
DCM	dilated cardiomyopathy
DHS	dynamic hip screw
DIC	disseminated intravascular coagulation
DKA	diabetic ketoacidosis
DM	diabetes mellitus
DVT	deep vein thrombosis
DWML	deep white matter lesion
ECG	electrocardiogram
Echo	echocardiogram
ECT	electroconvulsive therapy
EEG	electroencephalogram
EPO	erythropoietin
ESM	ejection systolic murmur
ESR	erythrocyte sedimentation rate
ESS	endoscopic sinus surgery
EtOH	ethanol
5-HT	5-hydroxy tryptamine
FBC	full blood count
fem-pop	femoral-poplited
fem-distal	femoral-distal
FDP	fibrim degradation product
FEV_1	forced expiratory volume (in 1 second)
FFP	fresh frozen plasma
FiO_2	fraction of inspired oxygen
f/u	follow-up
FVC	forced vital capacity
GA	generalized anaesthesia
γGT	gamma glutamyl transferase
GBS	Guillain–Barré syndrome
GCS	Glasgow coma scale
GI	gastrointestinal
GORD	gatro-oesophagial reflux disease
GP	general practitioner
G-CSF	granulocyte colony stimulating factor
GTN	glyceryl trinitrate

GVHD	graft-versus-host disease
H	home
HAART	highly active anti-retroviral therapy
HCG	human chorionic gonadotropin
HDL	high density lipoprotein
HGV	heavy goods vehicle
Hep	hepatitis
HIT	heparin induced thrombocytopaenia
HITT	heparin induced thrombocytopaenia and thrombosis
HIV	human immunodeficiency virus
HOCM	hypertrophic obstructive cardiomyopathy
HONK	hyperosmolar non-ketotic coma
HRT	hormone replacement therapy
Hx	history
Hz	Hertz
IBD	inflammatory bowel disease
ICD	internal cardioverter defibrillator
ICH	intracranial haemorrhage
ICP	intracranial pressure
IF	intrinsic factor
IHD	ischaemic heart disease
IM	intramuscular
INH	inhaled
INR	international normalized ratio
IQ	intelligence quotient
ISC	intermittent self-catheterization
IU	international units
IV	intravenous
IVDU	intravenous drug user
JVP	jugular venous pressure
LA	local anaesthesia
LBO	large bowel obstruction
LDH	lactate dehydrogenase
LDL	low density lipoprotein
LFT	liver function test
LMWH	low molecular weight heparin
LRTI	lower respiratory tract infection
LVF	left ventricular failure
MACE	major adverse cardiac events

MAOI	monoamine oxidase inhibitor
µ	micro
MCA	mental capacity act
MCI	mild cognitive impairment
MC&S	microscopy, culture, and sensitivity
mcg	microgram
MCV	mean cell volume
µmol	micromoles
MDRD	modification for diet in renal disease
MET	metabolic equivalent
mg	milligrams
MG	myasthenia gravis
MI	myocardial infarction
MIBG	meta-iodo-benzyl-guanidine
ml	millilitres
mmol	millimoles
MMSE	mini mental state examination
MMV	mandatory minute ventilation
MND	motor neurone disease
MR	mitral regurgitation
MRA	magnetic resonance angiography
MRI	magnetic resonance imaging
MS	mitral stenosis or multiple sclerosis
MSU	mid-stream urine
MVR	mitral valve replacement
NBW	normal body water
NCA	nurse controlled analgesia
NEB	nebulized
NFT	neurofibrillary tangle
NG	nasogastric
NGT	nasogastric tube
NHS	National Health Service
NICE	National Institute for Health and Clinical Excellence
NIPPV	non-invasive intermittent positive pressure ventilation
NMDA	N-methyl D aspartic acid
NOF	neck of femur
NPO	nil per os (nil by mouth)
NSAID	non-steroidal anti-inflammatory drug
NSTEMI	non ST elevation MI

OCD	obsessive compulsive disorder
OGD	oesophago-gastro-duodenoscopy
ORIF	open reduction with internal fixation
OSA	obstructive sleep apnoea
PCA	patient controlled analgesia
PCI	percutaneous coronary intervention
PD	peritoneal dialysis
PEEP	positive end-expiratory pressure
PEFR	peak expiratory flow rate
PEG	percutaneous endoscopic gastrostomy
PEP	post-exposure prophylaxis
PET	positron emission tomography
PF	platelet factor
PFT	pulmonary function test
PICC	peripherally inserted central catheter
plts	platelets
PMHx	past medical history
PND	paroxysmal nocturnal dyspnoea
PO	by mouth (*per os*)
POD	post-operative day
POW	Prisoner of war
PPI	proton pump inhibitor
PR	by rectum (*per rectum*)
PSA	prostate-specific antigen
PSS	progressive systemic sclerosis
PT	prothrombin time.
PTH	parathyroid hormone
PTSD	post-traumatic stress disorder
PV	vaginal *(per vagina)*
PVD	peripheral vascular disease
QALY	quality adjusted life year
QT_c	corrected QT interval
RBC	red blood cell
RCT	randomized controlled trial
REM	rapid eye movement
RTA	road traffic accident
RTI	respiratory tract infection
SALT	speech and language therapist
SBO	small bowel obstruction
SC	subcutaneous
SIADH	syndrome of inappropriate anti-diuretic hormone

SIMV	synchronized intermittent mandatory ventilation
SIRS	systemic inflammatory response syndrome
SLE	systemic lupus erythematosus
SNRI	serotonin noradrenaline reuptake inhibitor
SOA	swelling of ankles
SPECT	single photon emission computerized tomography
SSRI	selective serotonin and noradrenaline reuptake inhibitor
stat	immediately
STEMI	ST elevation myocardial infarction
T_3	tri-iodothyronine
T_4	thyroxine
TCA	tricyclic antidepressants
tds	three times a day
TFT	thyroid function test
THA	tetrahydroaminoacridine
TIA	transient ischaemic attack
TIPSS	transjugular intrahepatic porto-systemic shunt
TOE	transoesophageal echocardiogram
TPN	total parenteral nutrition
TTE	transthoracic echocardiogram
TTO	discharge prescription (to take out)
TTP	thrombotic thrombocytopaenic purpura
TURP	transurethral resection of prostate
UA	unstable angina or urinalysis
u/o	under observation
U&E	urea and electrolytes
URTI	upper respiratory tract infection
US	ultrasound
UTI	urinary tract infection
VC	volume control
VDRL	veneral disease research laboratory
VF	ventricular fibrillation
VS	volume support
VT	ventricular tachycardia
VTE	venous thromboembolism
vWD	von Willebrand disease
WBC	white blood cell
WCC	white cell count
XR	X-ray

Investigations

Table 1.1 Summary of recommendations for preoperative testing

Test	Indications
No tests required for healthy adults <80 years undergoing minor surgery	
CXR	Patients >60 years, or with unexplained breathlessness, or undergoing major cardiovascular or thoracic surgery
ECG	Patients >60 years, or with respiratory, renal, or cardiovascular morbidity undergoing all except very minor surgery
FBC	Patients >60 years, or with renal failure, or undergoing major surgery, or clinical suspicion of anaemia or sepsis
U&E	Patients >60 years, or with renal dysfunction, or severe cardiovascular morbidity, or undergoing major surgery
Glucose	Patients >60 years, or suspected diabetes
LFTs	Previous or suspected liver dysfunction, ↑EtOH, malnutrition, biliary surgery
Clotting	Patients on anticoagulation, or with bleeding history, or undergoing cardiovascular surgery
Sickle	Patients with African, Afro-Caribbean, East Mediterranean, Cypriot descent
Pregnancy	♀ of child-bearing age
ABGs	Severe respiratory disease undergoing major surgery (📖 p. 172)
PFTs	Severe respiratory disease undergoing major surgery (📖 p. 176)
Echo	Ejection systolic murmur, signs of cardiac failure (📖 p. 114)

Guidelines

Key to recommendations

- Each recommendation falls into one of three categories:
  - NO: test not recommended.
  - **YES**: test recommended.
  - ▨: the value of carrying out this test is not known, and may depend on specific patient characteristics.

Keys to surgery grades and American Society of Anesthesiologists (ASA) patient grades

Table 1.2 Surgery grades

Grade	Example
1 (minor)	Excision of skin lesion, drainage of breast abscess
2 (intermediate)	Primary repair of inguinal hernia, excision of varicose veins, tonsillectomy/adenotonsillectomy, knee arthroscopy
3 (major)	Total abdominal hysterectomy, endoscopic resection of prostate, lumbar discectomy, thyroidectomy
4 (major+)	Total joint replacement, lung operation, colonic resection, radical neck resection
Neurosurgery	Evacuation of subdural haematoma
Cardiovascular surgery	Coronary artery bypass grafting, repair of abdominal aortic aneurysm

Key facts: These are adapted from the 2003 NICE publication *Preoperative tests.*

Table 1.3 ASA patient fitness grades

ASA grade	Description
1	'Normal healthy patient' i.e. without any clinically important comorbidity and without clinically significant past/previous medical history
2	'A patient with mild systemic disease' no functional limitation
3	'A patient with severe systemic disease' and definite functional limitation
4	'A patient with severe systemic disease that is a constant threat to life'

Key facts: These are adapted from the 2003 NICE publication *Preoperative tests.*

Consent

- Valid consent should be obtained before ordering tests: patients should have enough information about risks, benefits, alternatives, and implications of a +ve result to be able to make an informed decision.
- Should discuss which tests are recommended, what they involve, and rationale: abnormal results should be discussed in full with patients.

Table 1.4 Examples of ASA grades 2–4 comorbidity for cardiovascular, respiratory, and renal disease

	ASA grade 2	ASA grade 3	ASA grade 4
Cardiovascular disease			
Angina	Uses GTN 2–3 times a month	Uses GTN 2–3 times a week or limiting angina	Acute MI
Exercise	Not limited	Limited activity	Very limited activity
Hypertension	Well controlled with single agent	Very symptomatic, requiring multiple antihypertensives	Systolic BP >200mmHg
Diabetes	Well controlled, no complications	Very symptomatic, complications (claudication, renal dysfunction)	DKA
Previous CABG	Not directly relevant—depends on current signs and symptoms		
Respiratory disease			
COPD	Productive cough, wheeze well controlled by inhalers, occasional URTI	Breathless on climbing stairs/ carrying shopping) wheezy much of time, several URTI per year	Acute infective exacerbation of severe COPD
Asthma	Well controlled by medication, not limiting life-style	Poorly controlled, limits lifestyle, on high dose of steroids, frequent hospital admissions	Acute asthma attack not responding to nebulizers
Renal disease			
	Cr >100µmol/L but <200µmol/L, some dietary restrictions	Cr >200µmol/L, on regular dialysis	Acute renal failure with ↑K$^+$, pulmonary oedema, ↓pH

COPD chronic obstructive airways disease; Cr creatinine; GTN glyceryl trinitrate, DKA diabetic ketoacidosis; MI myocardial infarction

Key facts: These are adapted from the 2003 NICE publication *Preoperative tests*.

Routine preoperative tests

Key facts
- The aim is to identify, avoid, or plan for the adverse outcomes listed.
- Most tests are low yield in young patients, and most abnormal findings will not change management in minor surgery.
- Often little good evidence for these tests: recommendations are based on consensus statements such as NICE guidelines (📖 p. 2).
- Generally, tests required are determined by patient fitness and background, and severity of surgery. If you can think why a test is useful, order it.

Table 1.5 Summary of indications for common preoperative blood tests

Test	Indicated	Not indicated	Rationale for testing
FBC	Patients >60 years, or with renal failure, or undergoing major surgery, or clinical suspicion of anaemia or sepsis	Minor surgery	Identify anaemia (📖 p. 100), sepsis (📖 p. 90), thrombocytopaenia (📖 p. 32), neutropaenia (📖 p. 330)
U&E	Patients >60 years, or with renal dysfunction, or severe cardiovascular morbidity, or undergoing major surgery, or on cardiovascular meds/steroids	Minor or intermediate surgery in adults <60 years	Identify renal dysfunction (📖 p. 220), ↑↓Na$^+$ (📖 p. 228 to p. 230), ↑↓K$^+$ (📖 pp. 232–234)
Glucose	Patients >60 years, or suspected diabetes	Not routinely indicated	Screen for diabetes (📖 p. 274)
LFTs	Suspected liver dysfunction, ↑EtOH, biliary surgery	Not routinely indicated	Confirm malnutrition (📖 p. 244), detect liver dysfunction (📖 p. 264) including alcoholic hepatitis (📖 p. 264)
Clotting	Patients on anticoagulation, or with bleeding history, or undergoing cardiovascular surgery, or Hx of liver disease	Not routinely indicated	Identify coagulopathy (📖 p. 68)

Table 1.5 Summary of indications for common preoperative blood tests (continued)

Test	Indicated	Not indicated	Rationale for testing
Sickle	Patients with African, Afro-Caribbean, East Mediterranean, Cypriot descent	Patients with documented sickle cell status, most Caucasians	Detect sickle cell disease (📖 p. 14)
Pregnancy	♀ of child-bearing age	Pre-menstrual girls, ♀ >50 years	Identify pregnancy (📖 p. 14)

Key facts: These are adapted from the 2003 NICE publication *Preoperative tests*.

Table 1.6 Indications for other pre-op investigations and main rationale

Test	Indicated	Not indicated	Rationale for testing
ECG	Patients >60 years, or with respiratory, renal, or cardiovascular morbidity undergoing all except very minor surgery	Minor surgery, young ASA 1 patients	Identify IHD (📖 p. 118), AF (📖 p. 136), heart block (📖 p. 135) and establish a baseline for post-op comparison
CXR	Patients >60 years, or with unexplained breathlessness, or undergoing major cardiovascular or thoracic surgery	Minor surgery, young ASA 1 patients	Rule out LRTI or chest infection (📖 p. 192), screening for malignancy in elderly
ABGs	Severe respiratory disease undergoing major surgery (📖 p. 172)	Not routinely indicated	Quantify comorbidity in high risk patient
PFTs	Severe respiratory disease undergoing major surgery (📖 p. 176)	Not routinely indicated	Quantify comorbidity in high risk patient
Echo	Any new murmur, all ejection systolic unless echo within last 6/12, signs of cardiac failure (📖 p. 124)	Not routinely indicated	Identify AS (📖 p. 148), LVF (📖 p. 124)

* ABGs + PFTs do not identify the high risk patients. They are done on patients that HxαEx[b] has already identified as being high risk.

Key facts: These are adapted from the 2003 NICE publication *Preoperative tests*.

Normal healthy adults

Table 1.7 Minor surgery* in ASA 1 adults

Test	Age (years)			
	16 to <40	40 to <60	60 to <80	>80
CXR	NO	NO	NO	NO
ECG	NO			YES
FBC	NO	NO		
Clotting	NO	NO	NO	NO
U&E	NO	NO		
Glu	NO	NO	NO	NO
LFTs	NO	NO	NO	NO
UA				
ABGs	NO	NO	NO	NO
PFTs	NO	NO	NO	NO

*E.g. excision of skin lesion, incision, and drainage

Key facts: These are adapted from the 2003 NICE publication *Preoperative tests*.

Table 1.8 Intermediate* surgery in ASA 1 adults

Test	Age (years)			
	16 to <40	40 to <60	60 to <80	>80
CXR	NO	NO	NO	NO
ECG	NO			YES
FBC	NO		YES	YES
Clotting	NO	NO	NO	NO
U&E	NO	NO		
Glu	NO			
LFTs	NO	NO	NO	NO
UA				
ABGs	NO	NO	NO	NO
PFTs	NO	NO	NO	NO

*E.g. inguinal hernia repair, varicose veins removal

Key facts: These are adapted from the 2003 NICE publication Preoperative tests.

NO: test not recommended; YES: test recommended; : the value of carrying out this test is not known, and may depend on specific patient characteristic

Table 1.9 Major surgery* in ASA 1 adults

Test	Age (years)			
	16 to <40	40 to <60	60 to <80	>80
CXR	NO	NO		
ECG	NO		YES	YES
FBC	YES	YES	YES	YES
Clotting	NO	NO	NO	NO
U&E			YES	YES
Glu				
LFTs	NO	NO	NO	NO
UA				
ABGs	NO	NO	NO	NO
PFTs	NO	NO	NO	NO

*E.g. total abdominal hysterectomy, endoscopic resection of prostate, lumbar discectomy, thyroidectomy

Key facts: These are adapted from the 2003 NICE publication *Preoperative tests*.

Table 1.10 Major+ surgery* in ASA 1 adults

Test	Age (years)			
	16 to <40	40 to <60	60 to <80	>80
CXR	NO	NO		
ECG	NO		YES	YES
FBC	YES	YES	YES	YES
Clotting	NO	NO	NO	NO
U&E	YES	YES	YES	YES
Glu				
LFTs	NO	NO	NO	NO
UA				
ABGs	NO	NO	NO	NO
PFTs	NO	NO	NO	NO

*E.g. total joint replacement, lung operation, colonic resection, radical neck resection

Key facts: These are adapted from the 2003 NICE publication *Preoperative tests*.

NO: test not recommended; YES: test recommended; : the value of carrying out this test is not known, and may depend on specific patient characteristic

Adults with mild comorbidity

Table 1.11 Minor surgery* in adults with mild comorbidity

Test	16 to <40	40 to <60	60 to <80	>80
		Age (years)		
CXR	NO	If respiratory/cardiovascular comorbidity		
ECG	YES in patients with cardiovascular comorbidity			
FBC				
Clotting	NO	NO	NO	NO
U&E	Maybe in patients with renal comorbidity			
	Maybe indicated in patients with CVS comorbidity or >60			
Glu	NO	NO	NO	NO
LFTs	NO	NO	NO	NO
UA				
ABGs	May be indicated in patients with respiratory comorbidity			
PFTs	NO	NO	NO	NO

*E.g. excision of skin lesion, incision, and drainage

Key facts: These are adapted from the 2003 NICE publication *Preoperative tests.*

Table 1.12 Intermediate surgery* in adults with mild comorbidity

Test	16 to <40	40 to <60	60 to <80	>80
		Age (years)		
CXR	May be useful in patients with respiratory/cardiovascular comorbidity, otherwise not indicated if patient <60			
ECG	YES in patients with cardiovascular comorbidity, patients >60 with renal comorbidity			
FBC				
Clotting	NO	NO	NO	NO
U&E	YES in patients with renal comorbidity, or >60 with CVS comorbidity.			
Glu	NO	NO	NO	NO
LFTs	NO	NO	NO	NO
UA				
ABGs	May be useful in patients with respiratory comorbidity			
PFTs	NO	NO	NO	NO

*E.g. inguinal hernia repair, varicose veins removal

Key facts: These are adapted from the 2003 NICE publication *Preoperative tests.*

NO: test not recommended; YES : test recommended; : the value of carrying out this test is not known, and may depend on specific patient characteristic

Table 1.13 Major surgery* in adults with mild comorbidity

Test	Age (years)			
	16 to <40	40 to <60	60 to <80	>80
CXR	May be useful in patients with respiratory/cardiovascular comorbidity, or >60 years, otherwise not indicated			
ECG	YES in patients with cardiovascular comorbidity, patients >60 with renal comorbidity			
FBC	YES	YES	YES	YES
Clotting	May be	May be	May be	May be
U&E	YES in patients with ASA 2 renal comorbidity, or >60 with ASA 2 CVS comorbidity.			
Glu	NO	NO	NO	NO
LFTs	NO	NO	NO	NO
UA				
ABGs	May be useful in patients with respiratory comorbidity			
PFTs	NO	NO	NO	NO

*E.g. total abdominal hysterectomy, endoscopic resection of prostate, lumbar discectomy, thyroidectomy

Key facts: These are adapted from the 2003 NICE publication *Preoperative tests*.

Table 1.14 Major+ surgery* in adults with mild comorbidity

Test	Age (years)			
	16 to <40	40 to <60	60 to <80	>80
CXR				
ECG	YES	YES	YES	YES
FBC	YES	YES	YES	YES
Clotting				
U&E	YES	YES	YES	YES
Glu	May be useful in patients with renal comorbidity, otherwise NOT indicated			
LFTs	NO	NO	NO	NO
UA				
ABGs	May be	May be	May be	May be
PFTs	May be indicated in patients with respiratory disease, otherwise NOT indicated			

* E.g. total joint replacement, lung operation, colonic resection, radical neck resection

Key facts: These are adapted from the 2003 NICE publication *Preoperative tests*.

NO: test not recommended; YES: test recommended; : the value of carrying out this test is not known, and may depend on specific patient characteristic

Adults with major comorbidity

Table 1.15 Minor surgery* in adults with severe comorbidity

Test	Age (years)			
	16 to <40	40 to <60	60 to <80	>80
CXR				
ECG	YES in patients with cardiovascular comorbidity			
FBC	YES in patients with renal comorbidity			
Clotting	May be useful in patients with ASA 3 renal, otherwise NOT indicated			
U&E	YES	YES	YES	YES
Glu	May be useful in patients with ASA 3 renal, otherwise NOT indicated			
LFTs	NO	NO	NO	NO
UA				
ABGs				
PFTs	NO	NO	NO	NO

*E.g. excision of skin lesion, incision, and drainage

Key facts: These are adapted from the 2003 NICE publication *Preoperative tests*.

Table 1.16 Intermediate surgery* in adults with severe comorbidity

Test	Age (years)			
	16 to <40	40 to <60	60 to <80	>80
CXR				
ECG	YES in patients with cardiovascular comorbidity, or any patient >60			
FBC	YES in patients with renal comorbidity, or respiratory disease >80			
Clotting	Only in patients with ASA 3 renal, otherwise NOT indicated			
U&E	YES	YES	YES	YES
Glu	May be useful in patients with ASA 3 renal, otherwise NOT indicated			
LFTs	NO	NO	NO	NO
UA				
ABGs				
PFTs	May be useful in patients with ASA 3 respiratory disease, otherwise NOT indicated			

*E.g. inguinal hernia repair, varicose veins removal

Key facts: These are adapted from the 2003 NICE publication *Preoperative tests*.

NO: test not recommended; YES: test recommended; : the value of carrying out this test is not known, and may depend on specific patient characteristic

Table 1.17 Major surgery* in adults with severe comorbidity

Test	16 to <40	40 to <60	60 to <80	>80
CXR				
ECG	YES in patients with cardiovascular comorbidity, or any patient >60			
FBC	YES in patients with renal comorbidity, or respiratory disease >80			
Clotting	Only in patients with ASA 3 renal, also ASA 3 cardiovascular otherwise NOT indicated			
U&E	YES	YES	YES	YES
Glu	May be useful in patients with ASA 3 renal, also ASA 3 respiratory otherwise NOT indicated			
LFTs	NO	NO	NO	NO
UA				
ABGs				
PFTs	May be useful in patients with ASA 3 respiratory disease, otherwise NOT indicated			

*E.g. total abdominal hysterectomy, endoscopic resection of prostate, lumbar discectomy, thyroidectomy

Key facts: These are adapted from the 2003 NICE publication *Preoperative tests*.

Table 1.18 Major+ surgery* in adults with severe comorbidity

Test	16 to <40	40 to <60	60 to <80	>80
CXR			YES if cardiovascular comorbidity	
ECG	YES	YES	YES	YES
FBC	YES	YES	YES	YES
Clotting				
U&E	YES	YES	YES	YES
Glu	May be useful in patients with ASA 2 renal or respiratory comorbidity, otherwise NOT indicated			
LFTs	NO	NO	NO	NO
UA				
ABGs	NO	NO	NO	Maybe
PFTs	May be indicated in patients with ASA 3 respiratory disease, otherwise NOT indicated			

*E.g. total joint replacement, lung operation, colonic resection, radical neck resection

Key facts: These are adapted from the 2003 NICE publication *Preoperative tests*.

NO: test not recommended; **YES**: test recommended; ░: the value of carrying out this test is not known, and may depend on specific patient characteristic

Cardiovascular and neurosurgery

Table 1.19 Cardiovascular surgery* in ASA 1 children <16 years

Test	Age (years)			
	<1	1 to <5	5 to <12	12 to 16
CXR	YES	YES	YES	YES
ECG	YES	YES	YES	YES
FBC	YES	YES	YES	YES
Clotting				
U&E	YES	YES	YES	YES
Glu	NO	NO	NO	NO
UA				

Key facts: These are adapted from the 2003 NICE publication *Preoperative tests*.

Table 1.20 Cardiovascular surgery* in adults

Test	Age (years)			
	16 to <40	40 to <60	60 to <80	>80
CXR	YES	YES	YES	YES
ECG	YES	YES	YES	YES
FBC	YES	YES	YES	YES
Clotting	May be	May be	May be	May be
U&E	YES	YES	YES	YES
Glu	May be	May be	May be	May be
LFTs	YES	YES	YES	YES
UA				
ABGs	May be useful in patients with respiratory disease, otherwise NOT indicated			
PFTs				

*E.g. CABG, AAA repair

Key facts: These are adapted from the 2003 NICE publication *Preoperative tests*.

NO: test not recommended; YES: test recommended; ▢: the value of carrying out this test is not known, and may depend on specific patient characteristic

Table 1.21 Neurosurgery in ASA 1 children < 16 years

	Age (years)			
Test	<1	1 to <5	5 to <12	12 to 16
CXR	NO	NO	NO	NO
ECG	NO	NO	NO	NO
FBC				
Clotting				
U&E	YES	YES	YES	YES
Glu	NO	NO	NO	NO
UA				

Key facts: These are adapted from the 2003 NICE publication *Preoperative tests*.

Table 1.22 Neurosurgery in adults

	Age (years)			
Test	16 to <40	40 to <60	60 to <80	>80
CXR	NO	NO	May be	May be
ECG	Maybe		YES	YES
FBC	Maybe		YES	YES
Clotting	Maybe	May be	May be	May be
May be	YES	YES	YES	YES
Glu	NO			
LFTs	NO	NO	NO	NO
UA				
ABGs	NO	NO	NO	NO
PFTs	NO	NO	NO	NO

Key facts: These are adapted from the 2003 NICE publication *Preoperative tests*.

NO: test not recommended; **YES**: test recommended; ▨: the value of carrying out this test is not known, and may depend on specific patient characteristic

Other preoperative tests

Sickle cell (Table 1.23)

- These patients should be tested prior to anaesthesia if there is any uncertainty about whether they have the sickle cell gene, especially:
  - Patients with no previous surgical history.
  - Patients with a +ve family history.
- Patients should ideally be offered genetic counselling before and after screening so that they can give informed consent.
- Document the result in the patient's medical record.

Table 1.23 Testing for sickle cell preoperatively

Ethnic group	Sickle cell test
African and Afro-Caribbean origin	YES
Eastern Mediterranean origin	YES
Middle East and Asian origin	YES
Cypriot origin	YES

Pregnancy test (Table 1.24)

- The need to test for pregnancy depends on the risk presented by the anaesthetic and surgery to the fetus: all ♀ of child-bearing age should be asked whether or not there is any chance that they are pregnant before surgery, or undergoing XRs or CT scans.
- ♀ should be advised of the risks of surgery or XRs to the fetus.
- If there is any doubt a pregnancy test should be carried out.

Table 1.24 Pregnancy testing

Woman of child-bearing age	Pregnancy test
With history of last menstrual period within 2 weeks	
Who says it is not possible for her to be pregnant	
Who says it is possible that she may be pregnant	YES

Echo and stress testing (Table 1.25)

Table 1.25 Indications for echo or stress testing (📖 see also p. 114)

Indication	Rationale	TTE / stress test
Dyspnoea of unknown origin	Evaluate LV function	YES for intermediate or major surgery
>3 cardiac risk factors and poor functional capacity	Evaluate LV function and identify IHD	YES for intermediate or major surgery
Symptoms and ESM	Identify critical AS	YES for intermediate or major surgery

Cross-match and group & save (Table 1.26)

Table 1.26 Suggested XM (check local protocols)

Category	Procedure	G&S/XM
G&S takes 5min, emergency XM takes 15min		
General surgery	Oesophagectomy, oesophagogastrectomy, liver resection, pancreatic surgery, rectum AP/anterior resection,	2U
	Gastrectomy, cholecystectomy, small bowel resection, colectomy, laparotomy, mastectomy, splenectomy, thyroidectomy,	G&S
Vascular surgery	Emergency aortic reconstruction	6U, FFP, plts
	Elective aortic reconstruction	2U
	Carotid endarterectomy, distal reconstruction, axillo-femoral bypass, amputation	G&S
Urology	Cystectomy	4U
	Nephrectomy	3U
	Open prostatectomy	2U
	TURP, re-implantation of ureter	G&S
Transplant	Renal	2U
Cardiothoracic	Re-op CABG/valve	4U, FFP, plts
	Thoracotomy, CABG, mitral valve replacement (MVR)/aortic valve replacement (AVR)	2U
	Mediastinoscopy	G&S
Trauma	Major RTA	4U
ENT/plastic surgery	Major head/neck reconstruction	2U
	Free flaps	2U
	Breast reduction	G&S
Orthopaedic surgery	Total hip replacement/revision	2U
	Total knee replacement	G&S
	Total shoulder replacement	G&S
	Major spinal stabilisation	2–4U
Maxillofacial	Bimaxillary osteotomy	2U

Arterial blood gases and pulmonary function tests (Table 1.27)

Table 1.27 Indications for ABGs and/or PFTs (📕 see also p. 172)

Indication	Rationale	ABG/PFTs
Lung resection	Predict post-op lung capacity	PFTs on all patients
ASA grade 3 respiratory disease (📕 p. 10)	Risk assessment, establish baseline, is ICU bed indicated?	ABG, PFTs

A–Z of laboratory investigations

A

ACTH (Table 1.28)

ACTH stimulation test: used to diagnose adrenal insufficiency (📖 p. 280). Tetracosactide® 0.25mg IM or IV given with blood collected at 0, 30min for cortisol. Normal response cortisol increase to >50mmol/L.

Table 1.28 ACTH testing 8am: < 80mg/L

Indication	Increased	Decreased
Endocrine Malignancy	Addison's disease, ecotopic ACTH e.g. small cell lung cancer, thymic tumrs	Adrenal adenoma or carcinoma, pituitary insufficiency

ALT, AST, and ALP (Table 1.29)

- INR, PT, and APTT may also be elevated in hepatic dysfunction.
- ALP can be fractionated to differentiate between bone and liver.

Table 1.29 AST (8–20U/L), ALT (8–20U/L)

Indication	Increased	Decreased
ALT: evaluate liver function	Hepatitis, liver mets, biliary obstruction, liver congestion (ALT<AST),	
AST: liver and cardiac function	AMI, hepatitis, muscle trauma, pancreatitis, intestinal injury, post CABG/cardiac cath, brain damage	Severe diabetic ketoacidosis, liver disease
ALP: liver and bone disease	Hyperparathyroidism, Paget's disease, osteoblastic bone tumours, osteomalacia, rickets, pregnancy, biliary obstruction	Malnutrition

Acid fast bacilli

Histological stain used to identify *Mycobacterium* (tuberculosis, avium much less common) in urine, sputum, pus etc.

Albumin (Table 1.30)

Table 1.30 Albumin 35–50g/L

Indication	Increased	Decreased
Nutrition Oedema		Malnutrition, (📖 p. 244) nephrotic syndrome (📖 p. 226) cystic fibrosis, multiple myeloma, Hodgkin's disease, leukaemia, protein losing enteropathy, IBD (📖 p. 270),

Acid phosphatase (Table 1.31)

- Collection of enzymes catalyzing the hydrolysis of phosphate from a variety of substrates.
- It is found in liver, erythrocytes, platelets, bone marrow, prostate.
- Today assays for acid phosphatase are rarely used. For its main indication monitoring patients with prostate cancer, it has been replaced by PSA, which is more sensitive and specific.

Table 1.31 Acid phosphatase <3.0ng/mL or <0.8IU/L

Indication	Increased	Decreased
Prostate Bone	Carcinoma of the prostate, prostatic surgery or trauma, excessive platelet destruction (ITP), rarely in bone disease	

Aldosterone (Table 1.32)

Table 1.32 Aldosterone serum (only early AM: depending on body position—supine: 3–10ng/dL, upright: 5–30ng/dL)

Indication	Increased	Decreased
Endocrine	Hyperaldosteronism (1° or 2°)	Adrenal insufficiency, panhypopituitarism

Alpha-fetoprotein (αFP) (Table 1.33)

Serum αFP serves as a screening test for neural tube defects, fetal death, or other abnormalities in pregnancy. It is usually done between 16–20 weeks of gestation.

Table 1.33 AFP <25ng/mL

Indication	Increased
Malignancy	Hepatoma, germ cell tumours of the gonads (testicular tumour, embryonal carcinoma, malignant teratoma)
Pregnancy	During pregnancy (in mother's serum): neural tube defects and other anomalies

Amylase (Table 1.34)
- Consists of pancreatic and salivary isoenzyme, small enough to pass through glomerular membrane and can be found in the urine.
- In acute pancreatitis amylase levels rise within hours after onset for 2 days, but specificity for acute pancreatitis is <50%

Table 1.34 Amylase 25–125U/L

Indication	Increased	Decreased
Pancreas	Acute pancreatitis, pancreatic duct obstruction, alcohol ingestion, mumps, parotiditis, cholecystitis, peptic ulcers, intestinal obstruction, mesenteric thrombosis, after upper abdominal surgery, renal failure,	Pancreatic destruction (chronic pancreatitis, cystic fibrosis), liver damage (hepatitis, cirrhosis)

B

B12 (vitamin) (Table 1.35)
- Use Schilling test to diagnose pernicious anemia: vitamin B12 absorption is ↓ when given without intrinsic factor (IF), whereas it is normal when administered with IF at the same time.
- The clinical triad of vitamin B12 deficiency: heamatologic-, neurologic-, GI dysfunction.
- Assuming a previously healthy diet, strict avoidance of foods containing B12 for a period of 3 years is required for complete exhaustion of B12-body-storage

Table 1.35 Vitamin B12 140–700pg/mL

Indication	Increased	Decreased
Anaemia malnutrition	Leukemia, polycythaemia vera	Inadequate intake (malnutrition) or defective absorption (pernicious anemia, after gastrectomy, malabsorption, bacterial overgrowth in blind loop syndrome)

Bilirubin (Table 1.36)
- When serum bilirubin levels exceed 30µmol/L icterus becomes evident by a yellow discoloration of the sclera. When levels rise even higher jaundice will be visible.
- Direct bilirubin is conjugated (after passage through hepatocytes), indirect bilirubin is unconjugated.
- Indirect bilirubin = total bilirubin – direct bilirubin.

Table 1.36 Total bilirubin: 3–17µmol/L; direct bilirubin: <3µmol/L; indirect bilirubin: <14µmol/L

Indication	Increased	Decreased
Total: liver and bile duct	Liver damage, biliary obstruction, haemolysis, fasting	
Direct: liver and bile duct	Billiary obstruction, drug induced cholestasis, Dubin–Johnson and Rotor's syndrome	
Indirect: liver and haemolysis	Any type of haemolytic anaemia, neonatal jaundice, Gilbert's disease, Crigler–Najjar syndrome	

Bleeding time (Table 1.37)
- Bleeding time is ↑ in disorders affecting 1° hemostasis, It is not ↑ in coagulopathies, since they usually impair 2° hemostasis only. vWD is an exception as it prolongs both 1° and 2° hemostasis.
- Several techniques have been described to determine bleeding time. Pitfalls occur in all of them and there is no role for the bleeding time as a routine preoperative screening test.

Table 1.37 Duke, Ivy <6min, template <10min

Indication	Increased	Decreased
Coagulation	Thrombocytopenia, thrombocytopathy, TTP, vascular hemorrhagic diathesis, aspirin, vWD	

Blood urea nitrogen (Table 1.38)
- Urea is an endproduct of protein metabolism.
- In order to determine renal function calculation of BUN/serum creatinine ratio can be useful. It typically is ↓ in acute tubular necrosis and low protein intake. It is ↑ due to renal hypoperfusion, glomerular disease, obstructive uropathy, or high protein intake

Table 1.38 BUN/urea 2.5–7.0 mmol/L (7–18mg/dL)*

Indication	Increased	Decreased
Kidney	Renal failure, dehydration, high protein intake, sepsis, acute MI, GI bleeding, drugs	Starvation or protein malnutrition, liver failure, pregnancy, infancy, overhydration, phenothiazines

C

Calcitonin (Table 1.39)

Calcitonin is produced in the C-cells of the thyroid. It is mainly used as a mode of recurrence of medullary carcinoma of thyroid.

Table 1.39 Calcitonin $\male$: <159ng/L, $\female$ <114ng/L

Indication	Increased	Decreased
Thyroid	Thyroid medullary carcinoma, paraneoplastic or reactive hypercalcaemia, CRF, Zollinger–Ellison syndrome (hypergastrinaemia), pernicious anemia	

Calcium (Table 1.40)

Serum calcium is divided into an ionized fraction (50%) and a fraction that is bound to proteins (mainly albumin). When interpreting calcium results differentiate between total calcium and ionized calcium. Values for total calcium need to be corrected according to the following equation if protein levels are not within normal limits:

$$\text{Corrected } Ca^{++} = \text{measured } Ca^{++} + (40 - \text{albumin [g/L]}) \times 0.02$$

Table 1.40 Calcium 2.12–2.65mmol/L

Indication	Increased (📖 p. 236)	Decreased (📖 p. 238)
Electrolytes	1° hyperparathyroidism, malignancy, vitamin D excess, osteoporosis, immobilization, sarcoidosis, multiple myeloma, CRF, thiazides	Hypoparathyroidism, pseudohypoparathyroidism, insufficient vitamin D, CRF (phosphate retention), renal tubular acidosis, hypoalbuanaemia

Calcium, urine (Table 1.41)

Table 1.41 Urine calcium 100–300mg/24 hours

Indication	Increased	Decreased
Urinalysis	Hyperparathyroidism, hyperthyroidism, hypervitaminosis D, distal renal tubular acidosis type I, sarcoidosis, immobilization, malignancy,	Thiazides, hypothyroidism, renal failure, steatorrhoea, rickets, osteomalacia

Carboxyhaemoglobin (Table 1.42)

Carbon monoxide (CO) binds haemoglobin 250 times more avidly compared to O_2, therefore even small amounts can result in significant levels of COHb.

Table 1.42 Carboxy-Hb—smokers: <6%; non-smokers <2%; toxic: >15%

Indication	Increased	Decreased
Haemoglobinopathies	Smokers, smoke inhalation, CO inhalation (e.g. automobile exhaust)	

Carcinoembryonic antigen (CEA) (Table 1.43)

- CEA has its main indication in monitoring colorectal carcinoma. If elevated pre-op, should normalise after radical surgery, and then be used to monitor remission.
- Pre-op CEA levels are also correlated with prognosis, 220mg/L suggesting poorer prognosis.

Table 1.43 Non-smoker: 3.0mg/L; smoker: 5.0mg/L

Indication	Increased	Decreased
Malignancy	Carcinoma (colon, lung, pancreas, stomach, breast, ovaries), non-neoplastic liver disease, IBD, smokers	

Catecholamines, serum (Table 1.44)

Ensure stress-free environment, at least 20min without physical activity. No alcohol, nicotine, tea, coffee, chocolate, citrus fruits, bananas for at least 12h.

Table 1.44 Supine: epinephrine <110 pg/mL, norepinephrine <750pg/mL, dopamine <30pg/mL

Indication	Increased	Decreased
Hypertension	Phaeochromocytoma, neural crest tumours (neuroblastoma), anxiety	

Chloride (Table 1.45)

- Chloride is quantitatively the most important extracellular anion. Although abnormalities in serum chloride itself are of little concern, both hyper- and hypochloraemia warrant investigation of the underlying disorder.

Table 1.45 Chloride 96–110mmol/L

Indication	Increased	Decreased
Electrolytes	GI bicarbonate loss with metabolic acidosis (diarrhoea), renal tubular acidosis, hypoaldosteronism, respiratory alkalosis, hyponatraemia with sodium losses in excess of chloride, bromism, administration of: ammonium chloride, amino acids (hyperalimentation), saline azetazolamides	GI chloride losses (vomiting, nasogastric suction), anion-gap metabolic acidosis, compensated respiratory acidosis, metabolic alkalosis, hyperaldosteronism, hyponatraemia

Cholesterol (Table 1.46)

Samples should be taken after a prolonged (16 h) fast.

Table 1.46 Cholesterol: <5.0 mmol/L

Indication	Increased	Decreased
Lipid status	Idiopathic hypercholesterolaemia, biliary obstruction, nephrosis, hypothyroidism, diabetes mellitus, hyperlipoproteinaemia (type IIb, III, IV), dietary intake	Liver disease, hyperthyroidism, malnutrition, cancer, chronic anaemia, steroid therapy

Cold agglutinins (Table 1.47)

- The serum cold agglutinin assay is a simple and inexpensive procedure used by some physicians for the diagnosis of *M. pneumonia* infection.
- The presence of cold agglutinins is not specific for *M. pneumonia*: Sensitivity (with titres ≥1:32) is 50–90%. The higher the cold agglutinin titre the more likely *M. pneumonia*. infection.

Table 1.47 Cold agglutinins titre of <1:32

Indication	Increased	Decreased
Pneumonia	Atypical pneumonia (mycoplasmal pneumonia), viral infections (mononucleosis, measles, mumps), cirrhosis, some parasites	

Coombs' test (Table 1.48a and b)

Direct Coombs' test

- Uses patient's erythrocytes, tests for presence of antibody on the patient's cells.

Table 1.48a Direct Coombs

Indication	Positive	Negative
haemolytic anaemia	autoimmune haemolytic anaemia (leukaemia, lymphoma, collagen–vascular diseases), haemolytic transfusion reaction, some drug sensitizations (methyldopa, levodopa, cephalothin), haemolytic disease of the newborn (erythroblastosis felalis)	normal

Indirect Coombs' test

- uses serum that contains antibody, usually from the patient.

Table 1.48b Indirect Coombs

Indication	Positive	Negative
haemolytic anaemia	immunization from previous transfusion, incompatible blood due to improper crossmatching	normal

Cortisol (Table 1.48)

In healthy individuals cortisol levels change with a circadian rhythm. These diurnal variations are blunted in conditions with sustained cortisol excess such as Cushing's disease.

Table 1.48 Cortisol 8am: 450–700mmol/L; midnight: 80–280 mmol/L

Indication	Increased	Decreased
Endocrine Malignancy	Adrenal adenoma, adrenal carcinoma, Cushing's disease, non-pituitary ACTH producing tumour, steroid therapy, oral contraceptives	Addison's disease, congenital adrenal hyperplasia, Waterhouse–Friedrichsen syndrome

Creatinine (phospho)kinase (CPK or CK) (Table 1.49)

Table 1.49 CPK 25–145mU/mL

Indication	Increased
Acute coronary syndrome	Muscle damage (acute MI, myocarditis, muscular dystrophy, muscle trauma, after surgery) brain infarction, defibrillation, cardiac catheterization, rhabdomyolysis, polymyositis

Creatinine serum (Table 1.50)

- Creatinine is a byproduct of muscle metabolism, derived from break-down of muscle creatine and creatine phosphate
- Only when ≥50% of nephrons are destroyed does creatinine level ↑.
- In order to detect more subtle reduction in glomerular function (creatinine blind window) use either creatinine clearance or the MDRD-formula to calculate an estimated GFR

Table 1.50 Creatinine ♂: 73–126 µmol/L, ♀: 55–102 µmol/L

Indication	Increased
Kidney	Renal failure, acromegaly, ingestion of meat, aminoglycosides, and other nephrotoxic drugs

Creatinine urine

- Total creatinine ♂: 160–220 µmol/kg/24h, ♀: 110–180/kg/24h.
- For urine creatinine, see Table 1.51.

Creatinine clearance (Table 1.51)

Table 1.51 Creatinine clearance ♂: 97–137mL/min; ♀: 88–128 mL/min

Indication	Increased	Decreased
Kidney	Pregnancy	Decreases with age, see causes for increase in serum creatinine

CRP (Table 1.52)
- High sensitivity for the detection of acute and chronic inflammation.
- No organ/disease specificity.

Table 1.52 CRP <3mg/L

Indication	Increased	Decreased
Infection	Infection, acute pancreatitis, rheumatic disease (classically not SLE), chronic inflammatory disease, malignancy, acute MI, pregnant, OCP	

D

Dexamethasone suppression test
Normal cortisol: 450–700nmol/L at 8am, 80–280nmol/L at midnight (📖 see also p. 286).

Dexamethasone is given at low (1mg) and high dose (8mg), and cortisol levels are measured. A normal result is a decrease in cortisol with the low dose test.
- Cushing's syndrome due to pituitary ACTH secreting tumours is suggested by no change in cortisol with the low dose test, but a decrease with the high dose test. If there is no change in cortisol with either the low or high dose test, then other causes of Cushings syndrome, e.g. ectopic ACTH secreting tumours and adrenal Cushings are the likely causes: these can be differentiated by measuring ACTH levels.

E

Erythrocyte Sedimentation rate (ESR) (Table 1.52a)
- ESR is a very non-specific test.

Table 1.52a Westergren scale: ♂: <15–20mm/h; ♀: <25–30mm/h

Indication	Increased	Decreased
Inflammation	Infection, inflammation, rheumatic fever, endocarditis, neoplasm, acute MI	Dehydration, sickle cell anaemia, polyerthaemia, high WBC cadrexia

Ethanol (Table 1.53)

- No prior disinfection of the site of blood withdrawal.
- Determination of ethanol levels is useful only in acute alcohol consumption (for chronic alcoholism: Carbohydrate-deficient transferin CDT).
- The UK legal limit for drivers is 80gm EtOH per 100mL blood (0.08%), breath alcohol 35mcg per 100mls, or 107mg per 100mls urine.

Table 1.53 Ethanol <0.01% (<10mg of alcohol per 100mls blood) (CDT <6%)

Indication	Increased	Decreased
Alcohol	Alcohol consumption	

F

Ferritin (Table 1.54)

Ferritin is the most sensitive and earliest sign in iron deficiency before RBCs or the serum-iron itself show any change.

Table 1.54 Ferritin ♂: 15–200mcg/L, ♀: 12–150mcg/L

Indication	Increased	Decreased
Anaemia	Anaemias (haemolytic, pernicious, thalassaemia, megaloblastic), metastatic carcinoma, leukaemias, lymphomas, hepatic disease, iron overload (haemochromatosis), acute and chronic inflammation, CRF, hyperthyroidism, polycythaemia	Iron deficiency, IBD, GI surgery, pregnancy

Fibrin degradation products (FDP) (Table 1.55)

Frequently elevated after surgery (due to tissue destruction) which may mask thrombosis and its complications.

Table 1.55 FDP <10mcg/mL

Indication	Increased	Decreased
Thrombosis	Thrombosis, DVT, pulmonary embolism, MI, after surgery, DIC, liver cirrhosis, HUS	

Fibrinogen (Table 1.56)

- Fibrinogen belongs to the acute-phase proteins.
- Persistent high values (>500mg/dL) are independent risk factors for cardiovascular and cerebrovascular events.

Table 1.56 Fibrinogen 1.5–4.5g/L

Indication	Increased	Decreased
Coagulation	Infection, neoplasia, after surgery, burns, uraemia	Liver damage, DIC, surgery, neoplastic and haematological conditions with hyperfibrinolysis, acute severe bleeding, asparaginase therapy

Folic Acid (Table 1.57)
- Without exogenous intake of folic acid, stores in the liver are sufficient for a period of 3 months.
- The most common cause of folic acid deficiency is a folate-poor diet. Folic acid is found in green leafy vegetables, citrus fruits, animal products, liver.

Table 1.57 Folic Acid 2.0–21ng/mL

Indication	Increased	Decreased
Anaemia malnutrition	Folic acid administration	Inadequate intake (malnutrition, alcoholism), malabsorption (disorders involving the whole small bowel: coeliac disease, widespread Crohn's disease), requirements (haemolytic anaemias, rapidly dividing tumours), impaired folate metabolism due to chemotherapy (e.g. methotrexate)

G

Gastrin (Table 1.58)
- Gastrin levels follow a circadian rhythm, with highest values during the day and especially during meals.
- Gastrin is a hormone secreted by the G cells of the pyloric mucosa, stimulating the secretion of gastric hydrochloric acid.
- Use gastrin stimulation test to differentiate between Zollinger–Ellison syndrome and other causes of hypergastrinaemia.

Table 1.58 Gastrin ♂ <100pg/mL, ♀ <75mg/mL

Indication	Increased	Decreased
Endocrine	Zollinger–Ellison syndrome, pyloric stenosis, pernicious anaemia, atrophic gastritis, ulcerative colitis, renal insufficiency, steroid and calcium administration, insulin	Vagotomy, atropine, hypothyroidism

Glucose (Table 1.59)

Table 1.59 Glucose fasting: 3.5–5.5mmol/L

Indication	Increased	Decreased
Endocrine	Diabetes mellitus, Cushing's syndrome, acromegaly, ↑epinephrine, ACTH administration, acute pancreatitis, pancreatic glucagonoma	Exogenous insulin, oral hypoglycaemics, factitious hypoglycaemia, malnutrition, pancreatic-, hepatic-, endocrine disorders (pancreatitis, islet cell tumour, after gastrectomy

Gram stain
- Technique: spread thin layer of specimen onto glass slide, allow to dry, apply Gentian violet (15–20s), apply Iodine (15–20s), apply alcohol (few seconds only), rinse with water, counterstain with Safranin (15–20s).
- Results: Gram-+ve: dark blue; Gram--ve: red.
- 📖 See p. 87 for influence of Gram stain on likely organism and choice of antibiotic.

Gamma-glutamyl transferase (γGT) (Table 1.60)
γGT is located in the cell membrane of nearly all cells and tissues. The γGT measured in the serum originates in large parts from the liver, but also from the prostate explaining why levels in ♂ are usually slightly higher than in ♀.

Table 1.60 γGT ♂: <28U/L; ♀: <18U/L

Indication	Increased
Liver	Cirrhosis, hepatitis, cholestasis, malignancy (liver, pancreas, prostate, kidney), renal disease, alcoholism, drugs (aminoglycosides, statins, phenytoin, phenobarbital, warfarin)

H

Haptoglobin (Table 1.61)
- Haptoglobin belongs to the acute-phase proteins and travels with the a2-fraction in electrophoresis.

Table 1.61 Haptoglobin 26–185mg/mL

Indication	Increased	Decreased
Liver	Obstructive liver disease, acute	Intravascular haemolysis
Anaemia	inflammatory reactions, necrosis, tumours	(any type), liver damage

Haematocrit (Table 1.62)

Table 1.62 Hk ♂: 40–54%, ♀: 37–47%

Indication	Increased	Decreased
Anaemia	Polycythaemia vera, 2° polycythemia, high altitudes, vigorous exercise, smoking, haemoconcentration	Anaemia Artefact in drip arm

Haemoglobin (Table 1.63)

Table 1.63 Hb ♂: 14–18g/dL, ♀: 12–16g/dL

Indication	Increased	Decreased
Anaemia	Dehydration, polycythaemia, high altitudes, COPD, CHF	Anaemias, kidney disease, overhydration, malignancy

Hepatitis

- HBsAg: hepatitis surface antigen.
- Anti-HBc: antibody to hepatitis B core antigen; early indicator of infection.
- Anti-HBc IgM: IgM antibody to hepatitis B core antigen.
- HBeAg: hepatitis B e antigen; when present indicates high degree of infectivity.
- Anti-HBe: antibody to hepatitis B antigen; presence associated with resolution of infection.
- Anti-HBs: antibody to hepatitis B surface antigen; typically indicates immunity and clinical recovery.
- Anti-HAV: total antibody to hepatitis A virus; confirms previous exposure to hepatitis A virus.
- Anti-HAV IgM: IgM antibody to hepatitis A virus; indicative of recent infection with hepatitis A virus.

High density lipoprotein cholesterol (HDL-C) (Table 1.64)

- ↓ HDL-Cholesterol is an independent risk factor for CAD.

Table 1.64 HDL 0.9–1.9mmol/L

Indication	Increased	Decreased
Lipid status	Oestrogen (♀)	♂, obesity, diabetes mellitus, uraemia, liver disease, Tangier's disease

HIV antibody

- In a healthy person HIV antibodies are –ve. They are usually determined as a screening test for HIV infection.
- The antibody levels rise within 3–12 weeks after exposure and are detected by ELISA method. +ve tests need to be confirmed by Western immunoblot.

Human chorionic gonadotropin (HCG) (Table 1.65)

Table 1.65 β-HCG (<3mIU/mL)

Indication	Increased	Decreased
	Pregnancy, testicular tumours, throphoblastic disease (hydatidiform mole, choriocarcinoma)	

5-HIAA (5-hydroxyindoleacetic) (Table 1.66)

5-HIAA is the main serotonine metabolite (monoaminoxidase).

Table 1.66 5-HIAA 2–8mg/24h urine

Indication	Increased	Decreased
	Carcinoid tumours, epilepsy, coeliac disease	

I

Iron (Table 1.67)
- Iron levels change dramatically throughout the day due to an underlying circadian rhythm.
- ↓ iron levels alone are not helpful for the investigation of iron deficiency. Ferritin is a much more sensitive and specific parameter.

Table 1.67 ♂: 65–175mcg/dL, ♀: 50–170mcg/dL

Indication	Increased	Decreased
Anaemia	Haemochromatosis, haemosiderosis, excess destruction or ↓ production of erythrocytes, liver necrosis, porphyria	Iron deficiency anaemia, chronic blood loss (e.g. menorrhagia, GI bleeding), nephrosis with loss of iron binding protein, chronic infections or neoplastic disease

Total iron binding capacity (TIBC) (Table 1.68)
TIBC measures the maximum amount of iron that can bind to transferrin.

Table 1.68 TIBC 250–450mcg/dL

Indication	Increased	Decreased
Iron	Iron deficiency anaemia, chronic blood loss, polycythaemia	Age, haemochromatosis, renal failure, cirrhosis, rheumatoid arthritis, infections, cancer of the GI tract

L

Lactate dehydrogenase (Table 1.69)

Table 1.69 LDH 45–100U/L

Indication	Increased	Decreased
Acute coronary syndrome Skeletal muscle	Acute MI, cardiac surgery, prosthetic valve, haemolysis, hepatitis, pernicious anaemia, malignant tumours, sepsis, sarcoid, acute pancreatitis, renal infarction, CCF trauma, CPR pulmonary embolism	

Lactate (Table 1.70)

Table 1.70 Lactate 0.5–2.2mmol/L

Indication	Increased	Decreased
Acidosis	Lactic acidosis due to hypoxia, haemorrhage, circulatory collapse, sepsis, cirrhosis, exercise shock	McArdle's disease (glycogenosis type V), reduced lactate production, high LDH values

Lipase (Table 1.71)

- Lipase catalyzes the hydrolysis of trigycerides into β-monoglycerides and free fatty acids.
- Like amylase it rises within a few hours after onset of acute pancreatitis for approximately 2 days, the clinical specificity is only 60%.

Table 1.71 Lipase 10–150U/L

Indication	Increased
Pancreas	Acute pancreatitis, pancreatic duct obstruction, fat embolus syndrome

M

Magnesium (Table 1.72)

Magnesium acts as an activator in all ATP-dependent reactions and is a physiological antagonist of calcium. In hypomagnesaemia cell-membrane permeability for sodium-, potassium-, and calcium ions increase leading to an intracellular influx of calcium and hypocalcaemia.

Table 1.72 Magnesium 0.8–1.1mmol/L

Indication	Increased	Decreased
Electrolytes	Renal failure, hypothyroidism, Addison's disease, diabetic coma, severe dehydration, exogenous administration	Malabsorption, steatorrhoea, alcoholism and cirrhosis, hyperthyroidism, aldosteronism, diuretics, acute pancreatitis, hypo-, hyperparathyroidism, hyperalimentation, chronic dialysis, renal tubular acidosis

Metanephrines, urine (Table 1.73)

Urinary metanephrines can be falsely elevated due to drug-therapy with phenobarbital or hydrocortisone.

Table 1.73 Urine metanephrines 2 mg/24h urine collection

Indication	Increased	Decreased
Hypertension	Pheochromocytoma, neural crest tumours (neuroblastoma)	

Myoglobin, urine (Table 1.74)

- Myoglobin is a found in all skeletal muscle and in myocardial tissue. Both forms are indistinguishable.
- It is an O_2-binding protein that serves as a reserve for O_2 and facilitates movement of O_2 within muscle cells.
- In acute MI myoglobin has the earliest diagnostic window compared to other biochemical markers for MI.

Table 1.74 Myoglobin <0.3mg/L

Indication	Increased	Decreased
Acute coronary syndrome	Acute MI, surgery, muscle injury, delirium tremens, renal failure, seizures	

Mean cell volume (Table 1.75)

Determination of the MCV is always the first step in the evaluation of anaemia in order to classify as micro-, normo-, or macrocytic.

Table 1.75 MCV ♂: 80–94fL; ♀: 81–99fL

Indication	Increased	Decreased
Anaemia	Vitamin B12 or folic acid deficiency, alcohol excess, liver disease, reticulocytosis, cytotoxics, myelodysplastic syndromes, marrow infiltration, hypothyroidism, antifolate drugs (e.g. phenytoin)	Iron-deficiency anaemia, thalassaemia, sideroblastic anaemia chronic disease (can be monocytic)

N

Nitrogen balance

- Nitrogen balance +4 to +20g/d, urinary nitrogen 12–24g/24h.
- Nitrogen balance = 24h protein intake(g)/6.25 – 24h urine nitrogen + 4.
- Most often used in the assessment of patients on hyperalimentation, a +ve nitrogen balance is usually the goal.

O

Oestrogen receptors

- Oestrogen receptors are determined on fresh surgical specimens.
- The presence of the receptors is associated with longer disease-free interval and survival from breast cancer, and a patient is more likely to respond to endocrine therapy.

Osmolality, serum (Table 1.76)

Serum osmolality = $2 \times [Na^+] + [urea] + [glucose]$.

Table 1.76 Serum osmolality 278–298mosm/kg

Indication	Increased	Decreased
Kidney	Hyperglycaemia, alcohol, ↑sodium (water loss) nephrogenic diabetes insipidus	Low serum sodium (diuretics), Addison's disease, SIADH, iatrogenic (poor fluid balance)

Osmolality, urine
- Spot urine: 50–1400 mosm/kg, after 12h of fluid restriction: >850mosm/kg.
- The loss of the ability to concentrate urine, especially during fluid restriction, is an early indicator of impaired renal function.

P

Parathyroid hormone (Table 1.77)

Table 1.77 PTH 1–8 pmol/L

Indication	Increased	Decreased
Endocrine	Primary, secondary, tertiary hyperparathyroidism, pseudohypoparathyroidism	Hypercalcaemia not due to hyperparathyroidism, hypoparathyroidism

Partial thromboplastin time (Table 1.78)
Falsely elevated in prolonged use of tourniquet.

Table 1.78 PTT 27–38s

Indication	Increased	Decreased
Coagulation	Heparin, any defect in the intrinsic clotting system (incl. factors: I, II, V, VIII, IX, X, XI, XII)	

Phosphate (Table 1.79)

Table 1.79 Phosphorus 0.8–1.45 mmol/L

Indication	Increased	Decreased
Endocrine	Hypoparathyroidism, excess Vit. D, 2° renal failure, bone disease, Addison's disease, childhood	Hyperparathyroidism, alcoholism, diabetes, gout, salicylate poisoning, IV steroid, hypokalaemia, hypomagnesaemia, diuretics, vit. D deficiency, phosphate-binding antacids

Platelets (Table 1.80)
In conditions where platelet numbers are normal, but function is impaired, determine bleeding time, platelet function, and thromboelastograms to evaluate haemostasis.

Table 1.80 Platelets 150–450000/μL

Indication	Increased	Decreased
Coagulation	Sudden exercise, after any trauma including surgery (esp. after splenectomy), acute haemorrhage, haematological disorders, cancer	Major haemorrhage, sepsis, ITP, TTP, bone marrow suppression (chemotherapy, neoplastic infiltration, radiation), aplastic anaemia, hypersplenism, infectious mononucleosis, other viral infections, pre-eclampsia, eclampsia, HIT

Potassium (Table 1.81)

Falsely elevated in prolonged use of tourniquet.

Table 1.81 Potassium 3.5–5.0mmol/L

Indication	Increased (📖 p. 234)	Decreased (📖 p. 232)
Electrolytes	Renal failure, Addison's disease, acidosis, spironolactone, triamterene, dehydration, haemolysis, massive tissue damage, excess intake	Diuretics, vomiting, nasogastric suction, villous adenoma, diarrhoea, Zollinger–Ellison syndrome, chronic pyelonephritis, renal tubular acidosis, metabolic alkalosis, 1° aldosteronism, Cushing's syndrome

Prostatic specific antigen (Table 1.82)

- Higher in black and older men.
- PSA levels >10ng/dL almost always represent prostate carcinoma. Values between 4–10ng/dL are associated with BPH and prostate carcinoma.
- Useful parameter in the follow-up of patients after prostatectomy.

Table 1.82 PSA ♂: 4.0ng/mL; after radical prostatectomy: 0.2ng/mL

Indication	Increased	Decreased
Prostate	BPH, prostate carcinoma, prostatitis	After prostatectomy

Protein, serum (Table 1.83)

Table 1.83 Protein 60–80 g/L

Indication	Increased	Decreased
Liver Malignancy	Multiple myeloma, macroglobulinaemia, sarcoidosis	Malnutrition, IBD, leukaemia, Hodgkin's disease, any cause of ↓ albumin (📖 p. 16)

Protein, urine (Table 1.84)

- Urine protein levels can be falsely elevated in gross haematuria.

Table 1.84 Urine protein

Indication	Increased
Kidney Malignancy	Nephrotic syndrome, glomerulonephritis, lupus nephritis, amyloidosis, venous congestion of kidney (renal vein thrombosis, CHF), multiple myeloma, pre-eclampsia, interstitial renal disease, malignant hypertension

Prothrombin Time (Table 1.85)

- Falsely elevated in prolonged use of tourniquet.

Table 1.85 PT 11.5–13.5sec

Indication	Increased
Coagulation	Any defect in the extrinsic clotting system (factors: I, II, V, VII, X), Vitamin K deficiency, fat malabsorption, liver disease, DIC

R

Red blood cell count (Table 1.86)

Table 1.86 RBC ♂: 4.7–6.1 × 10⁶; ♀: 4.2–5.4 × 10⁶

Indication	Increased	Decreased
Anaemia	Polycythaemia vera, haemoconcentration, high altitude, cor pulmonale, cardiovascular disease	Haemorrhage, anaemia, chronic infection, leukaemia, myeloma, excessive IV fluid, chronic renal failure, pregnancy, overhydration

Red blood cell morphology

- Anisocytosis: irregular RBC size (microcytes, macrocytes).
- Burr cells (acanthocytes): severe liver disease, high levels of bile, fatty acids, or toxins.
- Helmet cells (schistocytes): microangiopathic haemolysis, haemolytic transfusion reaction, other severe anaemias.
- Howell–Jolly bodies: after splenectomy.
- Nucleated RBCs: severe bone marrow stress (haemorrhage, haemolysis, etc.), neoplastic bone marrow infiltration, extramedullary haematopoiesis.
- Poikilocytosis: irregular RBC shape (sickle, burr).
- Polychromasia: the appearance of a bluish-gray red cell on routine Wright's stain suggests reticulocytes.
- Sickling: sickle cell disease, trait.
- Spherocytes: hereditary spherocytosis, immune or microangiopathic haemolysis.
- Target cells: thalassemia, haemoglobinopathies (e.g. sickle cell disease) obstructive jaundice, any hypochromic anaemia, after splenectomy.

Reticulocyte count (Table 1.87)

If haematocrit is abnormal, correct RC

Corrected count = RC(in %) × haematocrit/45

Table 1.87 RC 0.5–1.5%

Indication	Increased	Decreased
Haematology Infection	Haemolysis, acute haemorrhage, therapeutic response to treatment of anaemia	Bone marrow depression (marrow aplasia, infiltration, chemotherapy, aplastic anaemia)

Rheumatoid arthritis latex test (rheumatoid factor) (Table 1.88)

- Screening test to detect antibodies found in 70–80% of patients with RA (in 70–80%).
- Low specificity: found in most patients with mixed cryoglobulinaemia (usually caused by Hep C) and other conditions (below).

Table 1.88 RA <1:40

Indication	Increased	Decreased
Rheumatoid arthritis	RA, SLE, syphilis, chronic inflammation, SBE, sarcoidosis, hepatitis, renal disease	

S

Sodium (Table 1.89)

Table 1.89 Sodium 135–145mmol/L

Indication	Increased (📖 p. 230)	Decreased (📖 p. 228)
Electrolytes	Excess water loss (sweating, diarrhoea), diuresis (diabetes mellitus, diabetes insipidus, drugs)	CHF, renal failure, cirrhosis, sodium depletion (vomiting, diarrhoea, diuretics), adrenal cortical insufficiency, SIADH, hypokalaemia

Stool for occult blood (Haemoccult test)

+ve in any GI-tract ulcerated lesion (ulcer, carcinoma, polyp), large doses of vitamin C (>500mg/d), swallowed blood (e.g. after ENT/Mac-fax/surgery), ingestion of rare meat. 📖 See differential diagnosis of GI-bleeding, p. 260.

T

T3 (triiodothyronin) and T4 (thyroxin) (Table 1.90)

- Nearly all of T3 and T4 is bound to proteins (e.g. TBG, albumin), changes in the concentrations of these proteins have a big impact on total T3 and T4 concentrations. However they do not alter free hormone concentration

Table 1.90 T3 1.6–3.0nmol/L

Indication	Increased	Decreased
Thyroid	Hyperthyroidism, thyrotoxicosis, oral oestrogen, pregnancy, exogenous T4	Malnutrition, severe illness or trauma

T4 (thyroxin) (Table 1.91)

📖 for comments see TSH, p. 37

Table 1.91 T4 65–140nmol/L

Indication	Increased	Decreased
Thyroid	Hyperthyroidism, exogenous T4, oestrogens, pregnancy	Hypothyroidism, malnutrition, anterior pituitary hypofunction, strenuous exercise, renal failure severe illness

Thyroglobulin (Table 1.92)

- Thyroglobulin is useful in the follow-up of differentiated papillary and follicular thyroid carcinoma. Persistent elevation indicates residual or recurrent disease.
- It is a protein produced exclusively in the thyroid and contains the tyrosine residues that serve as the basis for thyroid hormone production.

Table 1.92 Thyroglobulin <50ng/mL

Indication	Increased	Decreased
Thyroid	Differentiated thyroid carcinomas (papillary, follicular), Graves' disease, non-toxic goitre	Hypothyroidism, testosterone, steroids, phenytoin

Thrombin time (Table 1.93)

- TT is useful in ruling out the presence of heparin in a patient sample: a prolonged TT that corrects within addition of protamine is diagnostic of heparin.

Table 1.93 TT 10–14s

Indication	Increased
Coagulation	Heparin, DIC, fibrin-/fibrinogen degradation products, fibrinogen deficiency, dysfibrinogenemia, antithrombin–antibodies, uraemia, some patients with lupus anticoagulants

TORCH

Infections which present a prenatal danger to an unborn child are summarized as the TORCH-complex, the battery test is based on serologic evidence of exposure to toxoplasmosis, rubella, cytomegaly, and herpes virus.

- (T)oxoplasmosis.
- (O)ther infectous microorganisms: varicella, measles, mumps, coxsackie, hepatitis, HIV, parvo-virus-B19, papillomavirus, EBV, lues, syphillis, gonoccus, chlamydia, borrelia, β-haemolytic streptococci.
- (R)ubella.
- (C)ytomegalovirus.
- (H)erpes simplex.

The battery test is based on serologic evidence of exposure to toxoplasmosis, rubella, cytomegaly, and herpes virus.

Transferrin (Table 1.94)

Transferrin is an anti-acute-phase protein and is therefore reduced in any acute inflammatory process.

Table 1.94 Transferrin 2.4–4.9 g/L

Indication	Increased	Decreased
Iron	Iron deficiency, pregnancy	Acute inflammatory reaction, tumours, haemochromatosis, haemoglobinopathy

Triglycerides (Table 1.95)

Samples shouldbe taken after prolonged (16h) fast.

Table 1.95 0.5–2.0mmol/L vary with age

Indication	Increased	Decreased
Lipid status	Hyperlipoproteinaemias, hypothyroidism, liver diseases, alcoholism, pancreatitis, acute MI, nephrotic syndrome, familial increase	Malnutrition, congenital abetalipoproteinaemia

Troponin (Table 1.96)

- Troponin levels rise 3–6h after beginning of infarction. It peaks at 12–24h and is elevated for ≥1 week.
- If the troponin level is normal ≥6h after the onset of chest pain and if ECG is normal, the risk is of missing an MI is extremely low (<0.5%)

Table 1.96 Troponin <0.4mcg/L

Indication	Increased
Acute coronary syndrome	Acute or subacute MI, unstable angina (microinfarctions)

Thyroid stimulating hormone (TSH) (Table 1.97)

- TSH is a very sensitive marker for subclinical hypo-/hyperthyroidism, it remains the screening test of choice. Free thyroid hormones only need to be determined in cases when TSH is abnormal.

Table 1.97 TSH <5mU/L

Indication	Increased	Decreased
Thyroid	1° hypothyroidism, very rarely in TSH-secreting tumours of the pituitary gland	Hyperthyroidism, 2° excess exogenous T4, anterior pituary hypofunction

U

Urea
📖 See Blood Urea Nitrogen

Uric acid (Table 1.98)

Table 1.98 Uric acid ♂: 440μmol/L; ♀: 340μmol/L

Indication	Increased	Decreased
Kidney Metabolism	Gout, renal failure, destruction of large amounts of nucleoproteins (leukaemia, neoplasia, anaemia, chemotherapy, pregnancy), diuretics, hypothyroidism, parathyroid disease	Uricosuric drugs (salicylates, probenecid, allopurinol), Wilson's disease, Fanconi syndrome

Urinalysis (Table 1.99)
- Macroscopic appearance, pH, density, dipstick analysis and microscopy.
- Appearance:
  - Normal: yellow, clear, straw-coloured.
  - Pink/red: blood, haemoglobin, myoglobin, food colouring, beets.
  - Orange: pyridium, bile pigments, rifamicin
  - Brown/black: myoglobin, bile pigments, melanin, iron, sickle cell crisis.
  - Cloudy: UTI with pyuria, blood, myoglobin, chyluria, mucus, phosphate salts (in alkalic urine), urates (in acidic urine), hyperoxaluria.
  - Foamy: proteinuria, bile salts.
- Microscopy: search for RBCs, WBCs, epithelial cells, parasites, yeast, spermatozoa, crystals, contaminants, mucus, casts.

Table 1.99 Dipstick analysis, pH, and density:

pH	Acidic:	Basic:
	High protein diet, mandelamine other medications, acidosis, ketoacidosis (starvation), COPD, diarrhoea, dehydration	UTI, renal tubular acidosis, diet (high vegetable, milk), bicarbonate or acetazolamide therapy, vomiting, metabolic alkalosis, CRF

Table 1.99 Dipstick analysis, pH, and density: (*continued*)

Specific density	↑: Volume depletion, CHF, adrenal insufficiency, diabetes mellitus, inappropriate ADH, ↑proteins (nephrosis), excretion of radiographic contrast media, artifact	↓: Diabetes insipidus, pyelonephritis, glomerulonephritis, water load with normal renal function
Bilirubin	+ve dipstick: Cholestasis, hepatitis, cirrhosis, CHF with hepatic congestion, congenital hyperbilirubinaemia	−ve = normal
Haemoglobin	+ve dipstick: Stones, trauma, tumours, prostatic hypertrophy Note: a dipstick +ve for haemoglobin, in the absence of RBCs indicates free haemoglobin (trauma, transfusion reaction, haemolysis)	−ve = normal
Glucose	+ve dipstick: Diabetes mellitus, other endocrine disorders (phaeochromocytoma, hyperthyroidism, Cushing's syndrome, hyperadrenalism), stress states (burns, sepsis), pancreatitis, renal tubular disease, iatrogenic causes (steroids, thiazides), false +ve results with vitamin C ingestion	−ve = normal
Ketones	+ve dipstick: Starvation, high fat diet, DKA, vomiting, diarrhoea, hyperthyroidism, pregnancy, febrile states	−ve = normal
Nitrite	+ve dipstick: Bacterial infection Note: only +ve in infection caused by microorganism with the ability to reduce nitrate (e.g. *E. coli, Klebsiella, Proteus, Staphylococcus, Pseudomonas*)	−ve = normal
Leucocyte esterase	+ve dipstick: Bacterial infection Note: screening test for the presence of WBCs	−ve = normal
Urobilinogen	+ve dipstick: Cholestasis, antibiotic suppression of gut flora	−ve = normal

Urinary electrolytes (Table 1.100)

Spot urines are of limited value because of large variations in daily fluid and salt intake. Results are uninterpretable if a diuretic has been given.

Table 1.100 Urinary electrolytes

Indication	Increased	Decreased
Sodium	Acute tubular necrosis, adrenal insufficiency, renal salt wasting	Volume depletion, hyponatraemia, prerenal azotaemia, hepatorenal syndrome, oedematous state
Potassium	Renal potassium wasting, diuretics, brisk urinary output	Hypokalaemia, potassium depletion, extrarenal loss
Chloride	Chloride sensitive metabolic acidosis (GI losses, diuretic induced)	Chloride resistant metabolic alkalosis (Cushing's syndrome, hyperaldosteronism, exogenous steroids, alkali ingestion)

V

Vanillylmandelic acid, urine (Table 1.101)

VMA is false +ve when administering methyldopa, chocolate or vanilla.

Table 1.101 16–48 µmol/24h

Indication	Increased	Decreased
2° HTN	Phaeochromocytoma, neural crest tumours (neuroblastoma, ganglioneuroma)	

Veneral disease research laboratory (VDRL test)

- Test searches for antilipoidal antibodies. Their presence indicates inflammatory cell destruction in the acute phase of syphilis.
- Useful test for the follow-up management after successful therapy or after spontaneous healing
- If +ve the result needs to be confirmed.

W

White blood cell count, total (Table 1.102)

The total WBC consists of neutrophils, eosinophils, basophils, lympho-cytes and monocytes.

- Neutrophils: 2.0–7.5 × 10^9/L (40–70% of WBC)
- Eosinophils: 0.04–0.44 × 10^9/L (1–6% of WBC)
- Basophils: 0.0–0.1 × 10^9/L (0–1% of WBC)
- Lymphocytes: 1:3–3.5 × 10^9/L (20–45% of WBC)
- Monocytes: 0.2–0.8 × 10^9/L (2–10% of WBC)

Table 1.102 WBC 4000–11000 cells/μL

Indication	Increased	Decreased
Blood	Infections, leukaemia, leukaemoid reactions, tissue necrosis, post-splenectomy, exercise, fever, pain, anaesthesia	Overwhelming bacterial infection, certain viral infections (influenza, hepatitis, mononucleosis), aplastic anaemia, reactive arthritis, SLE, MDS, bone marrow depression (due to drugs, radiation, infiltrative tumour) pernicious anaemia, hypersplenism

Neutrophils increase in response to bacterial infection, inflammatory disease and bone marrow disorders. Eosinophils increase in response to allergic disorders, inflammation of the skin and parasitic disorders. Basophils increase in response to leukaemia, chronic inflammation, and hypersensitivity.

Lymphocytes increase in response to viral infecton, leukaemia. They are decreased in the late stages of HIV infection.

Monocytes increase in response to infection, inflammation and malig-nancy.

Perioperative care

Duties of a doctor

The GMC lists the duties of a doctor in its document *Good Medical Practice*. The duties can be thought of under four headings (the 4 C's):

1. Competency
- Keep your professional knowledge and skills up to date.
- Recognize the limits of your professional competence.
  - Perform an adequate assessment of the patient's conditions, based on the history and symptoms and, if necessary, an examination.
  - Arrange investigations or treatment where necessary.
  - Take suitable and prompt action when necessary.
  - Refer the patient to another practitioner, when indicated.
  - Be willing to consult colleagues.
  - Keep clear, accurate, legible, and contemporaneous patient records which report the relevant clinical findings, the decisions made, the information given to patients, and any drugs or other treatment prescribed.
  - Keep colleagues well informed when sharing the care of patients.
  - Provide the necessary care to alleviate pain and distress whether or not curative treatment is possible.
  - Prescribe drugs or treatment, including repeat prescriptions, only where you have adequate knowledge of the patient's health and medical needs. You must not give or recommend to patients any investigation or treatment which you know is not in their best interests, nor withhold appropriate treatments or referral.
  - Report adverse drug reactions as required under the relevant reporting scheme, and co-operate with requests for information from organizations monitoring the public health.
  - Take part in regular and systematic medical and clinical audit, recording data honestly, and respond to the results of audit to improve your practice, for example by undertaking further training.

2. Communication
- Treat every patient politely and considerately.
- Respect patients' dignity and privacy.
- Listen to patients and respect their views.
- Give patients information in a way they can understand.

3. Correctness (or probity)
- Make the care of your patient your first concern.
- Respect the rights of patients to be involved in decisions.
- Be honest and trustworthy.
- Respect and protect confidential information (📖 see p. 45).
- Make sure your personal beliefs do not prejudice your patients' care.
- Act quickly to protect patients from risk if you have good reason to believe that you or a colleague may not be fit to practice.
- Avoid abusing your position as a doctor.
- Work with colleagues in the ways that best serve patients' interests.
- In an emergency, wherever it may arise, you must offer anyone at risk the assistance you could reasonably be expected to provide.

4. Confidentiality

Patients have a right to expect that information about them will be held in confidence by their doctors. Confidentiality is central to trust between doctors and patients. Without assurances about confidentiality, patients may be reluctant to give doctors the information they need in order to provide good care. The GMC states that if you are asked to provide information about patients you must:

- Inform patients about the disclosure, or check that they have already received information about it.
- Anonymise data where unidentifiable data will serve the purpose (this includes your surgical logbook).
- Keep disclosures to the minimum necessary.
- Keep up to date with and observe the requirements of statute and common law, including data protection legislation.

Daily practice

- When you are responsible for personal information about patients you must make sure that it is effectively protected against improper disclosure at all times (e.g. password-protected electronic files).
- Many improper disclosures are unintentional: you should not discuss patients where you can be overheard, or leave patients' records, either on paper or on screen, where they can be seen by other patients, unauthorized health care staff, or the public, and you should take all reasonable steps to ensure your consultations with patients are private.
- Patients have a right to information about the health care services available to them, presented in a way that is easy to follow and use.

Special circumstances

If in any doubt contact your medical defence union for advice.

- You must disclose information to satisfy a specific statutory requirement, such as notification of a known or suspected communicable disease: inform patients about such disclosures, wherever that is practicable, but their consent is not required.
- You must also disclose information if ordered to do so by a judge or presiding officer of a court; you should object if attempts are made to compel you to disclose what appear to you to be irrelevant matters.
- You must not disclose personal information to a third party such as a solicitor, police officer, or officer of a court without the patient's express consent, except when:
  - The patients are not competent to give consent.
  - Reasonable efforts to trace patients are unlikely to be successful.
  - The patient has been, or may be violent; or obtaining consent would undermine the purpose of the disclosure (e.g. disclosures in relation to crime).
  - Action must be taken quickly (for example in the detection or control of outbreaks of some communicable diseases) and there is insufficient time to contact patients.

Communication skills

Communicating with patients and relatives

Privacy and confidentiality

- All personal health information is held under strict legal and ethical obligations of confidentiality which you must uphold (📖 p. 45).
- Additionally always try to maintain a patient's privacy and dignity:
  - Knock on doors and close them after you.
  - Draw the curtains round the bed.
  - Always ask the patient if they want relatives to stay if you are discussing health issues: they may not want information shared.
  - Always say 'I would like to examine you now' before you do so.
  - Always allow (or help) the patient to redress after you have finished examining them, and *before* talking to them.

Communicating effectively and sensitively

- *Ask a nurse to accompany you*: particularly if you are explaining something complex or breaking bad news. They will answer the patients' and relatives' questions after you have left.
- *Know your facts*: are you giving the right diagnosis to the right patient, are you equipped to consent a patient for the surgical procedure?
- *Sit at the same level* as the person to whom you are talking, maintain appropriate eye contact and introduce yourself.
- *Find out what the patient knows* and what they are expecting.
- *Listen*: the patient's own knowledge, state of mind, and ability to grasp concepts will dictate how, and how much, you explain.
- *Tell the truth*: be sensitive to what the patient may not want to know at this stage and you might omit certain facts, but never lie.
- *Avoid jargon*: 'chronic' may simply mean 'longstanding' to you, to most patients it means 'severe', acronyms mean nothing to patients.
- *Avoid vague terms where possible*: describe risk quantitatively 'one in a hundred chance' if this is known, be qualitative if it is not, e.g. 'a small risk', this is particularly true for prognosis.
- *Check the patient understands*, **do not assume** that they do.
- *Help the patient to remember*: use information booklets, draw diagrams, write instructions down, repeat and summarize at intervals.
- *Maintain a professional relationship*: never allow your personal likes, dislikes, and prejudices to influence your clinical skills and decision making.

Breaking bad news

- All of the above applies!
- Understand if a patient wishes to have a relative or friend with them, who may provide emotional support as well as retain information.
- Know what options are available: if a cancer is inoperable, is chemotherapy planned? If an operation is cancelled, when is the new date?
- Do not be afraid to stop to allow the patient time to gather their thoughts and emotions; give them time to ask questions.
- Recommence at a later time if patient overwhelmed by information.
- Do not mistake numbness for calm acceptance, and try not to take anger personally unless the bad news is actually your fault.

Communicating with nurses

- Always be professional and friendly: nurses are colleagues and senior nurses are likely to know more than you.
- Introduce yourself on arrival to staff nurse in charge of ward/patient.
- Establish early on which nurses are experienced: it allows you to gauge what you can reasonably expect from them.
- In theatre, scrub nurses are not the enemy: your inexperience is.
- Try to remember all their names as they will remember yours.
- Do ward work efficiently: recognize how important it is for the smooth running of the ward for your ward-rounds, note-keeping, prescriptions, and discharge letters to be timely and accurate.
- Let the nurses know when you are going for lunch, teaching, or sleep: if they can discuss problems now it will save you being paged later.
- *Do an evening ward round* to check on problem patients and drug requirements: your sleep is less likely to be constantly interrupted.

Communication with hospital doctors

- Don't refer to specialists without asking your consultant or registrar.
- When requesting clinical consultations, write a concise, clear letter in notes to appropriate clinician, include question(s) to be answered.
- When asked to see a patient, go the same day if possible, write your opinion in the case notes stating clearly what you recommend, and always discuss it with the seniors on your own firm.

Communication with general practitioners

The GP has usually looked after your patient for years and will often sort out the complications that occur once the patient is discharged. They often know your consultant well. So think!

- *Telephone the GP* in the case of death of a patient, if you unexpectedly admit a patient, or to help with a difficult discharge.
- *Write useful, legible discharge summaries*: what would *you* want to know if you were going to have to wait 4 weeks for the typed discharge letter to arrive—at an absolute minimum, the date and name of operation, postoperative complications and plan.
- *Keep clinic letters clear and concise*

Radiology and laboratory colleagues

- Know exactly how the investigation will change your management.
- If there is doubt about the correct investigation, ask for advice.
- Complete request forms correctly and include clinical data: it can make a big difference, particularly if you have requested the wrong test.

Administration

- Introduce yourself to your consultant's secretary early, find out how they like things run, and then run things their way: they will usually have more than typing input on your reference.
- Produce GMC, defence union, occupational health, holiday and study leave paperwork with good grace: they are mostly legal requirements and being rude won't change that.

Box 2.1 Right patient, right operation, right SITE and SIDE

Write name, DOB, number, operation, side (which you should mark on patient in permanent ink), **no** abbreviations.

Correct site surgery

Key facts

- Surgery performed at the wrong site (wrong patient, wrong organ, wrong side or wrong level) is rare but potentially devastating.
- National recommendations from the Royal College of Surgeons (RCS) and National Patient Safety Agency (NPSA), modelled on work done in the US now cover preoperative marking, verification, and checklists.
- Communication breakdowns, failures of preoperative routines, and the increasing complexity of healthcare systems all contribute to wrong site surgery.

Marking

- Pre-op marking helps reduce wrong site surgery

How to mark

- Ideally on the ward prior to transfer to theatre on the day of surgery
- Before the pre-med is given
- Either the surgeon or a nominated deputy who will be present at surgery should mark the patient
- Check the patient name, date of birth, and planned procedure verbally with the patient themselves and their ID tag, and relevant imaging studies e.g. X-rays
- Check the surgical procedure and site in the patient's notes
- Use an indelible marker pen
- Draw an arrow extending to the incision site
- Draw it in so that it doesn't encroach on the future incision (to avoid tattooing ink into the patient), and so it will be visible after prepping and draping the patient
- The surgical site and patient ID should be checked to ensure a) correct location and b) legibility at every transfer of the patient and immediately before surgery.

Where to mark

- Surgical operations involving side (right / left or anterior / posterior)
- Digits (the arrow should extend on to the correct digit)
- Marking may not be appropriate in the following setting:
  - Emergency surgery which shouldn't be delayed
  - Teeth and mucous membranes
  - Bilateral simultaneous organ surgery
  - When the site of surgery depends on examination under anesthesia or surgical exploration
  - Mid-line incisions for single organs
  - Where the patient refuses to be marked

In theatre

- Final verification should take place before anaesthesia and always before incision.
- Final verification of patient ID, consent, mark, allergies and procedure which should always involve the surgeon, a nurse and anaesthetist.
- Always check and clearly display relevant imaging
- See Fig 2.1 for an example of a standard preoperative verification checklist.

Pre-operative marking verification checklist

Patient's name: Date:

Hospital No. / DOB: Intended procedure:

Addressograph label

	Responsibility	**Signature to confirm check completed**
Check 1 • Check the patient's identify • Check reliable documentation and/or images to ascertain intended surgical site • Mark the intended site with an arrow using an indelible pen	The operating surgeon, or nominated deputy, who will be present in the theatre at the time of the patient's procedure	Signed: Print name:
Check 2 • Prior to leaving ward/day care area the mark is inspected and confirmed against the patient's supporting documentation • Relevant imaging studies accompany patient of are available in operating theatre or suite	Ward or day care staff	Signed: Print name:
Check 3 • In the anaesthetic room and prior to anaesthesia, the mark is inspected and checked against the patient's supporting documentation • Re-check imaging studies accompany patient or are available in operating theatre or suite • The availability of the correct implant (if applicable)	Operating surgeon or a senior member of the team	Signed: Print name:
Check 4 The surgical anaesthetic and theatre term involved in the intended operatre procedure prior to commencement of surger should pause for verbal briefing to confirm: • Pretence of the correct patient • Marking of the correct site • Procedure to be performed	Theatre staff directly involved in the intended operative procedure	Signed: Print name:

• If failure of any preoperative check occurs, the surgeon in charge should assess the situation and either return the patient to the ward/day care area or note and sign a decision to proceed at risk.
• If the patient is returned to the ward/day care area, a patient safety incident report from should be completed in line with local governance procedures.
• A senior member of staff should offer an explanation and apology.
• If surgery is carried out at the incorrect site, a full root cause analysis of events is recommended.

Fig 2.1 Example of a standard pre-operative verification checklist

Consent

Legal aspects

The patient's right to autonomy must be respected, even if their decision results in harm or death. This right is protected by law:

- Only a competent patient can give consent.
- Performing a procedure on a patient without their consent constitutes *battery*; failing to give the patient adequate information to allow them to give informed consent constitutes *negligence*.
- *No adult in the UK can legally consent to surgery on behalf of another adult*: involve relatives, particularly where patients are unable to consent, but their wishes *do not* constitute legal consent.

Obtaining consent

The key to good consenting is good communication (📖 p. 46). It may be necessary to use a translator, and some hospitals will not accept consent gained by using a patient's relatives as translators.

- GMC guidelines state that *'If you are the doctor providing treatment or undertaking an investigation, it is your responsibility to discuss it with the patient and obtain consent'*.
- *The person obtaining consent should be the person either doing the procedure or capable of doing the procedure:* if the surgeon documents a discussion of the procedure, risks, and consent in the notes, then the actual signing of the consent form may be delegated to you.
- Patients may not be put under duress to consent by clinicians, employers, police, etc.
- Declare any potential conflicts of interest.
- The *amount* of information should be sufficient to allow a mentally competent patient to make an informed decision, and varies with the individual, condition, complexity of treatment, and risks involved.
- Don't limit information to avoid distress, but be sympathetic to needs.
- Consent is required for taking photographs for teaching or publication, and taking samples (including resection specimen) for research.

Informed consent

There are five aspects that the patient must understand to give consent:

- *The reason for carrying out the procedure:* illness and its prognosis.
- *What the procedure involves:* where and how long is the scar, what is being removed, what prosthesis will be implanted, will there be drains?
- *The risks of the procedure: specific* to the procedure (e.g. stoma, limb dysfunction) and in *general* (e.g. anaesthesia, bed rest, DVT).
- *The benefits of the procedure:* symptoms/prognosis/diagnosis.
- *Alternatives* including conservative treatment, with pros and cons.

Modes of consent

- *Implied consent:* the patient is presumed to consent to minor procedures, e.g. XRs, phlebotomy, by co-operating with ward procedures.
- *Express written consent:* whenever possible, this should be obtained for all patients undergoing procedures involving an anaesthetic, complex treatments with significant risks and side effects, or as part of research: **written consent is not legal proof that adequate consent was obtained at the time the document was signed**.

- *Express verbal consent:* should be obtained when it is not possible to get written consent and witnessed by an independent healthcare professional, and documented in the notes accordingly, or for simple procedures with minimal risk of harm, e.g. Foley catheter insertion.

Special considerations

Emergencies
When consent cannot be obtained you may provide emergency medical treatment provided it is limited to what is needed to preserve life. However, you must respect any **valid** advance directives which you know about or are drawn to your attention.

Mentally incapable patients
No adult in the UK can legally consent to surgery on behalf of another adult. Assess the patient's competence to make an informed decision. If unable to decide, and provided they comply, treatment may be instigated which is judged to be in their best interest. Otherwise, treatment for the under-lying mental condition may be carried out under the Mental Health Act 1989. Controversial and non-therapeutic treatments (e.g. sterilizations) require court approval.

Advance directive/living wills
Advance statements made by patients before losing the capacity of informed consent must be respected provided the decision is applicable to the present circumstances and there is no reason to believe that they may have changed their minds. The known wishes of the patient should be taken into consideration if a written advance statement is unavailable.

Children
- Over 16s are regarded as young adults, and have capacity to decide.
- Under 16s may give their own consent, if they are judged to understand what is involved.
- Unlike adults, where a competent child refuses treatment, a person with parental responsibility (except in Scotland) or a court may authorize treatment if deemed in the child's best interests.
- If the parents refuse treatment deemed in the child's best interests, you are not bound by this and may seek a ruling from a court.
- Emergency treatment may be instigated without consent in a similar manner to that in adults.

Pregnancy
The right to autonomy applies equally to pregnant women. It includes the right to refuse treatment which is intended to benefit the unborn child.

Planning for elective surgery

📖 Preop investigations are detailed in Chapter 1, p. 3–11.

Key facts

- Elective surgery is non-urgent or non-emergency surgery.
- New/uncontrolled AF (📖 p. 136), uncontrolled ↑BP (📖 p. 152), recent URTI, anticoagulation (📖 p. 61) are often cause for cancellation.
- Usually a consultant surgeon will have explained the intended operation in clinic, and discussed the risks and benefits of surgery.
- It may be days to months until surgery: investigation of medical problems are best dealt with at this stage, including specialist referral.
- Some units operate a pre-admission clinic where significant medical problems can be identified and treatment plans made.

Pre-admission clinic

- Usually run by junior doctors, nursing staff, or physicians' assistants.
- Patients normally attend a few weeks before their operation.
- Perform a full history and examination (📖 see Box 2.2) aiming to:
  - Reassess the surgical problem: this may have resolved or deteriorated, changing the indication or patient's desire for surgery.
  - Assess fitness for GA and surgery (particularly CVS and RS).
  - Identify conditions that may change perioperative management.
- Request preoperative investigations (📖 see Guidelines, p. 2).
- Obtain consent (📖 see p. 50) if not already done in clinic.

Specialist referral

Specialist referrals are sometimes necessary: *always* discuss these with a more senior team member, *always* contact the patient's GP to advise them of any referrals or change in patient management, and be aware that in many PCTs, specialist referrals must be done via the GP.

Preoperative assessment on the ward

Patients already seen in pre-admission

Spend 10min taking a history: focus on changes since patient was last seen, check consent, and review investigations: blood tests, ECG, imaging (*ensure you have all relevant imaging*), check preop adjuncts e.g. bowel prep (📖 p. 60), stopping warfarin (📖 p. 61) have been completed

Patients not seen before in pre-admission

- The aim is to obtain a full history and examination (📖 see Box 2.2).
- Multiple patients often arrive on the ward at a similar time, and need to be seen by an admitting nurse, anaesthetist, and surgeon, so it is important to be organized, efficient, and that you prioritize the patients.
  - Write down as much history as you can from notes/clinic letters (always double-check the salient facts with patient).
  - Patients with difficult problems or requiring many preop tests should be seen first, so there is time to react to new developments.
  - Order investigations while you're waiting for patients (📖 p. 2).
  - Try to delegate phlebotomy, or take history while taking bloods.
- Keep your history and examination focussed (📖 see Box 2.2).
- If elderly or incapacitated start planning convalescence care now.

Box 2.2 Clinical assessment of elective admission

Focused history
- Main condition and planned surgery, including:
  - Presentation.
  - Summarize key investigations by type with dates and results, to ensure that key information is not missing, and check that you have original reports and films, e.g.

CXR 06/08	RUL 2cm mass
CT 06/08	T2N0M0
PET 06/08	No metastatic disease
Histology	Needle Bx NSCLC
Bronch 07/08	Normal mucosa
PFTs 07/08	FEV1 2.4 (78%), FVC 3.2 (89%)

  - Previous treatment (e.g neo-adjuvant therapy, surgery).
  - Any changes in symptoms/Ix since last seen by surgeons.
- Other medical problems: condition, severity, past/current treatment.
- Ask specifically about previous admissions/operations/anaesthetic; exercise tolerance, angina, SOA, MI, palpitations diabetes, DVT; asthma, wheeze, cough, recent cold, dyspnoea, orthopnoea, snoring; dyspepsia/GORD, recent weight loss/gain, change bowel habit, prostatism, CVA, fits, faints.
- Current medication, OCP, allergies, smoking/alcohol/recent travel history.

Focused examination
BP, pulse, temperature, JVP, heart sounds, peripheral oedema and pulses, breath sounds, abdominal palpation for organomegaly/masses/ hernias, orientation in time/place/person, full neuro exam if known neurological problem, or undergoing neurosurgery.

Main preop checklist
- Warfarin, aspirin, clopidogrel stopped (🕮 p.61).
- Bowel-prep completed (🕮 p.60).
- Antibiotics (🕮 p.60) DVT prophylaxis (🕮 p.61), analgesia (🕮 p.78), antiemetics (🕮 p.253), sliding scale 🕮 (p.276), fluids (🕮 p.64), pre-med (🕮 p.56)
- You have seen all relevant investigations (🕮 p.4)
- XM/G&S requested (🕮 p.68).
- Patient marked: stomas, side-specific surgery, plastic surgery, varicose vein surgery.
- Consent correct (procedure, side, within date, signed).
- NBM after midnight.

Planning for emergency surgery

Key facts

Emergencies have a higher mortality and morbidity for several reasons:
- Often associated cardiovascular collapse, renal dysfunction, sepsis.
- True diagnosis often unknown and the planned operation uncertain.
- Time to prepare the patient medically is limited.
- Patients may be elderly or compromised by both the underlying surgical condition and pre-existing medical disease.

Preoperative assessment of emergency patients (Box 2.3)

- Look out for changes in clinical condition: *hypotension* (📖 p. 116), *hypoxia* (📖 p. 172), *and unresponsiveness* (📖 p. 292) *are medical emergencies:* ***GET HELP*** and start emergency resuscitation before further assessment. 📖 ALS/ATLS algorithms are on inside back covers of this book.
- Usually more to gain than lose by treating pain first.

Medical records

Scan the hospital notes and laboratory records for evidence of significant medical disorders.

Examination

Check for problems listed in Table 2.1. At a minimum:
- General inspection: cold and clammy? Drowsy—document GCS.
- BP, pulse (rate *and* rhythm), temperature.
- Heart sounds, JVP, ankle oedema, peripheral pulses.
- Respiratory rate, SaO_2 and FiO_2, breath sounds.
- Abdominal tenderness, masses, hernias, bowel sounds.
- 'Squeeze my hands, wiggle your toes', orientation in person/time.

Investigations

- FBC, U&Es, coagulation screen, G&S (all patients), βHCG in ♀.
- XM 2—6U depending on surgery (📖 p. 68).
- ECG, erect CXR in all patients, other imaging as indicated.
- Urinalysis, BM fingersticks in all patients.

Box 2.3 Focused history

If patient unresponsive talk to paramedics/relatives. Specifically:
- *Pain*: SOCRATES (site, onset, character, radiation, associated symptoms, timing, exacerbating/relieving factors, signs of sepsis).
- *Other symptoms* (e.g. urinary retention/nausea and vomiting/swellings etc) duration, onset, previous episodes, signs of sepsis.
- *Trauma*: speed and direction of impact, damage to other vehicle/ object, restraints, distance thrown, able to weight bear, LOC.
- *Previous surgery and general anaesthetic* and adverse reactions.
- *Medical conditions*/admissions: ask specifically about asthma/diabetes/ DVT/epilepsy in all patients and MI, CVA, COPD in elderly.
- *Current drug history allergies* smoking, alcohol, recreational drugs.
- *Time last ate and drank.*

Table 2.1 Common medical problems in emergency surgical patients

Cardiovascular	Hypovolaemia (📖 p.116), shock (📖 p.116), IHD (📖 p.118), CCF (📖 p.124), arrthymia (📖 p.130), hypertension (📖 p.152)
Respiratory	Hypoxia (📖 p.172), atelectasis and consolidation (📖 p.220), pulmonary oedema (📖 p.182), diaphragmatic splinting (📖 p.198), aspiration (📖 p.220)
Blood	Anaemia (📖 p.100), coagulopathy (📖 p.68)
Renal	Oliguria (📖 p.214), anuria (📖 p.222)
CNS	Coma (📖 p.292), pain (📖 p.78), confusion (📖 p.294)
GI	Nausea/vomiting (📖 p.252), malnutrition (📖 p.244),
Metabolic	Fever/hypothermia (📖 p.90), acidosis (📖 p.174), diabetic emergencies (📖 p.278), electrolyte imbalances (📖 p.228 to p.241)

Resuscitation of emergency surgical patients

1 minute

- Address patient, if consciousness impaired, or respiratory distress:
  - Assess airway, if compromised: *call anaesthetist*.
  - Assess breathing, if no respiratory effort: *call arrest team*.
  - Assess circulation, if no pulse: *call arrest team*.
- 📖 ALS and ATLS protocols are on the inside cover of this book.
- In drowsy/unconscious breathing patient with pulse, place in recovery position, insert Guedel or nasopharyngeal airway, give 6L/min O_2. The resuscitation of comatose patients is described on 📖 p. 293.
- If patient seems well, is sitting up and talking with no obvious signs of distress, proceed with a focused history and exam (Box 2.3).
- *The following patients are at risk of rapid clinical deterioration, and the following management is aimed at patients in these groups:*
  - Hypotension (📖 p. 116), hypoxia (📖 p. 172), sepsis (📖 p. 90).
  - Confusion, or disoriented (📖 p. 294) patients.
  - The very young (📖 p. 104) or very elderly (📖 p. 105).

2–5 minutes

- Sit the patient up and give 2–6L/min O_2 by face mask.
- Attach pulse oximetry, BP cuff, and telemetry for continuous monitoring.
- Get IV access, send blood for FBC, U&Es, LFTs, clotting, G&S, blood cultures, blood glucose, and βHCG in women.
- Start IV fluids: bolus 500mL over 10min if BP <120mmHg systolic, or pulse rate >100bpm, or clinical signs of shock: reassess BP immediately after fluid bolus to determine further resuscitation (📖 p. 116).
- For severe pain: 5mg morphine IV if patient alert (plus antiemetic).

5–10 minutes

- Focused history (Box 2.3) from carers/relatives, clinical exam concentrating on immediate presentation.
- Assess response to fluid bolus: repeat if necessary (📖 p. 116)
- Call senior cover to discuss management early.
- Urethral catheter (📖 p. 360), ABG (📖 174), CVP line (📖 p. 352).
- CXR, abdominal plain film, 12–lead ECG.
- Further management directed by diagnosis/investigation findings.

Day case surgery

Key facts

- Admission, surgery, and discharge on same day.
- It is often preferred by patients, and efficient in terms of hospital bed utilisation and theatre throughput.
- Type of procedure 1° consideration for suitability.

Patient selection

- Careful patient selection avoids cancellations or the need for postoperative admission due to medical problems: 📖 see Table 2.2.
- The patient is selected for day surgery at the surgical outpatients:
  - The procedure is explained and consent obtained (📖 p. 50).
  - Give literature to the patient regarding their planned procedure.
  - Fill in preop anaesthetic questionnaire to make admission to hospital more efficient on the day of surgery. The questionnaire should be reviewed by the anaesthetist either prior to admission or on the day of surgery.
  - Request preop investigations. (📖 Chapter 1)
- Common medical factors leading to cancellation on the day of surgery are acute URTI, uncontrolled hypertension, or fast AF.

Table 2.2 Selection of patients for day surgery

Complexity of surgery	Operations lasting >45min and those associated with a risk of significant postoperative pain, haemorrhage, or prolonged immobility should not be performed as day cases
Health status	Generally fit and healthy (ASA 1 or 2). Patients with significant cardiovascular or respiratory disease, usually or those with gross obesity (BMI >30) are not suitable
Age	Patients generally <70 years: however, *physiological* fitness should be considered, rather than a strictly applied chronological age limit
Transport	All patients must be escorted home by a responsible, informed adult and be adequately supervised during their recovery at home for a minimum of 24h
Social support	Patients must have suitable home conditions with adequate toilet facilities, and a telephone should be readily available for advice in an emergency
Geography	The patient should live within 1h travelling distance from the hospital

Admission for day-case surgery

- Recheck consent and results of preoperative investigations.
- Clinical evaluation should be limited to a check of the following. If the answer to any is yes, further assessment may be required:
  - Has *physical condition* changed in any way since assessment?
  - Have any *new drugs* been prescribed?
  - Any history URTI in the *previous 2 weeks*?
  - Is the patient's *BP* outside the range 100/60–170/100?

- Recommendations for investigations vary according to the age and fitness of the patient (📖 see Table 2.3).
- Sedative premedication is not routine but may benefit the occasional particularly nervous person (temazepam 10–20mg). Patients with symptoms of acid reflux should be treated with omeprazole 40mg po 90min before surgery.

Table 2.3 Preoperative investigations for patients undergoing day surgery

Urinalysis	All patients, check for blood, glucose, protein
ECG	Patients >60 years or when clinically indicated
FBC	If anaemia suspected
U&E	Patients on diuretics or those with possible renal disease
Blood glucose	All diabetic patients, glycosuria
Sickle test	Patients of African/Mediterranean origin uncertain of their sickle status
Pregnancy test	Whenever there is any possibility of pregnancy (get consent!)

Anaesthesia

The emphasis is on rapid recovery to allow early ambulation with minimal postoperative pain, nausea, and vomiting.

- Local anaesthetic, nerve blocks and adequate doses of analgesics including NSAIDs may prevent significant postoperative pain.
- Severe pain may require treatment with opioid analgesics.
- Nausea and vomiting (📖 p. 252) may also occur, most commonly in gynaecological patients: around 1% of day surgery patients require admission to deal with these or surgical complications.

Discharge

- Discharge when vital signs are stable, the patient is fully ambulant, can tolerate oral fluids and has passed urine. The patient should be orientated and their pain adequately controlled. Check the operative site prior to discharge.
- Check arrangements for the patient's wound care, final briefing to carer before the patient leaves.
- Driving or working with machinery is not allowed for 24h after general anaesthetic.
- Make follow-up appointment in clinic.
- Give TTOs, usually just analgesia, with clear instructions.

The surgical drug chart

Antibiotics (📖 p. 88), analgesia (📖 p. 78), antiemetics (📖 p. 253), heparin (📖 p. 61), fluids (📖 p. 64).

How to write a postoperative drug chart

- Legibly, in capitals, in black pen! (📖 See Box 2.4 for abbreviations.)
- Generic (*not* trade) name, dose, route, frequency, date started, times for regular drugs, indication for prn drugs, sign (write your name if not clear from signature)—also good practice to add your pager number.
- *Regular drugs*: prescribe surgical meds first (easy to see):
  - Antibiotics, heparin, nebulizers, regular analgesia, laxatives, etc.
  - Patient's normal medication, change inhalers to nebulizers.
  - Omit warfarin, aspirin, clopidogrel, ACE-inhibitors, long acting hypoglycaemics (metformin) preop, and restart postop.
  - Consider supplementing oral steroids with IV hydrocortisone (📖 p. 281).
- *On request drugs (prn):* write up additional analgesia (📖 p. 78), two anti-emetics (📖 p. 253), laxatives (📖 p. 255), and sedatives.
- *Single dose drugs:* write up pre-medication (or check that anaesthetist has done so), bowel prep, single dose prophylactic antibiotics.
- *IV infusions:* write up postop fluids (📖 p. 64), insulin sliding scale (📖 p. 276), PCA (📖 p. 81) as required.
- *Changes to prescriptions:* don't alter the original—cross it out clearly, sign and date, and rewrite below.
- Routinely review charts for *duplicate prescriptions*.
- Review daily to see what can be safely discontinued.
- *Verbal orders:* repeat the prescription clearly to two nurses on phone.

Box 2.4 Abbreviations

Route and formulation

IV intravenous	IM intramusuclar	SC subcutaneous
PO by mouth	PR by rectum	PV vaginal
INH inhaled	NEB nebulized	top topical
disp dispersible	EC enteric coated	SR slow release
NGT by nasogastric tube		
PEG by percutaneous endoscopic gastrostomy tube		

Timing

od once a day	bd twice daily	tds three times day
qds four times day	prn as needed	STAT immediately
T one tablet	TT two tablets	TTT three tablets
1/7 1 day	3/52 3 weeks	4/12 4 months

Dose

g grams	mg milligrams	mcg micrograms
L litres	mL millilitres	mmol millimoles

Regular medication				Time	Date	
					8/7/09	9/7/09
Drug CEFUROXIME				(06:00)		𝒟𝒦
Route IV	Dose 750mg		Start 8/7/09	12:00		
Additional instructions 24 hours only				(16:00)		𝒟𝒦
Signature Miles	papger 2978	Pharmacy		(22:00)		𝒟𝒦
Drug ENOXAPARIN				(06:00)		
Route sc	Dose 40 mg		Start 8/7/09	12:00		
Additional instructions + TEDS until mobile				(18:00)		
Signature Miles	papger 2978	Pharmacy		22:00		
Drug SODIUM CHLORIDE 0.9%				(06:00)		
Route neb	Dose 5mL		Start 8/7/09	12:00		
Additional instructions				(16:00)		
Signature Miles	papger 2978	Pharmacy		(22:00)		
Drug PARACETAMOL				(06:00)		
Route PO/PR/IV	Dose 1g		Start 8/7/09	(12:00)		
Additional instructions				(16:00)		
Signature Miles	papger 2978	Pharmacy		(22:00)		
Drug ASPIRIN EC				(06:00)	𝒟𝒦	
Route po	Dose 75mg		Start 9/7/09	12:00		
Additional instructions				16:00		
Signature Miles	papger 2978	Pharmacy		22:00		

On request medication				Time	Date	
					8/7/09	9/7/09
Drug DICLOFENAC						
Route pr/po	Dose 75mg		Start 8/7/09			
Instructions For pain. Max 150mg in 24h						
Signature Miles	papger 2978	Pharmacy				

Fig 2.2 Sample surgical drug chart

Drugs and surgery

Key facts

- Even if patient is NBM they may still take oral medication.
- Withhold anticoagulants, antiplatelets, ACE-inhibitors, hypoglyacaemics.
- Continue all other medication up until surgery, and restart on day 1.
- Prophylactic antibiotics are used to prevent infection occurring due to surgical interventions and are usually very short course (1–3 doses).
- Heparin used to prevent VTE in surgical patients, until fully mobile.

Routine antibiotics

- Aim for high serum level of antibiotics at incision: *prescribe in advance so antibiotics are given at induction, giving at incision is too late.*
- Prophylaxis often 1 dose at the time of surgery (📖 see Table 2.4).
- Many clean wounds (e.g. skin lesion excision) don't require prophylaxis.
- High risk patients who may warrant extend ed or specific prophylaxis:
  - Neutropaenic, immunosuppressed, severely malnourished.
  - Prosthetic implants (e.g. heart valves).
  - 'Dirty' operation (open fracture, perforated viscus).

Table 2.4 Standard antibiotic prophylaxis (these change, so check local protocol)

Operation	Typical prophylaxis
'Clean' GI surgery e.g. acute non perforated appendicitis, elective colonic resection	Cefuroxime 1.5 g IV + metronidazole 500mg IV *or*
'Clean' hepatobiliary surgery 'Clean' gynaecological surgery	Gentamicin 120mg IV + metronidazole 500mg IV
ERCP, TURP	Gentamicin 120mg IV *or* ciprofloxacin 500mg po
Termination of pregnancy	Metronidazole 500mg PO
Elective orthopaedic surgery	Flucloxacillin 1g IV
'Clean' vascular surgery	Cefuroxime 1.5 g IV *or* ciprofloxacin 400mg IV

Single dose at induction if not stated otherwise

Bowel preparation (Table 2.5)

Table 2.5 Bowel preparation

Procedure	Bowel prep
OGD, ERCP, reversal ileostomy	None needed
Anal fissure, haemorroidectomy, EUA, flexi sigmodosopy	Phosphate enema on morning of operation
Colonoscopy, any colectomy, anterior or AP resection, Hartmann's reversal	Full prep: clear fluid only for 24h, then Picolax® or Klean-prep® 12:00 and 18:00 day before surgery, phosphate enema on morning. Consider admitting elderly preop for IV fluids to prevent dehydration

Heparin (Table 2.6)

- LMWH is usually given SC od as treatment or prophylaxis for AF/ DVT: *no need to monitor APTT.*
- Give unfractionated heparin IV to treat MI, known PE or DVT, patients with mechanical heart valves if off warfarin; monitor APTT every 4–6h until stabilized: *stop 6h before planned surgery.*
- Bleeding due to over-heparinisation should be treated with 1–2U of FFP (📖 p. 69) or usually 1 dose of protamine 25mg IV will suffice.

Table 2.6 Heparin prescribing

Indication	Dose
Routine DVT prophylaxis	Enoxaparin 20mg SC od 12h before surgery, then 20mg od for 7–10 days, TED stockings
	Double dose if BMI >30, reduce in renal failure
High-risk surgery (e.g. hip)	Enoxaparin 40mg 12h preop, then 40mg SC od for 7–10 days, TED stockings
Treatment of DVT, AF	Enoxaparin 1.5 mg/kg SC od
Treatment MI, PE, mechanical valve	IV heparin: 5000U IV bolus then 25,000U in 25mL NS, IV at 1 mL/h or 1000 IU/h, check APTT 4–6h after start or change in dose, and titrate dose to APTT 50–70s

Warfarin (📖 see also p. 398)

- Withhold preop to reduce risk of bleeding, haematoma, re-exploration.
- Stop 4 days before elective surgery and check INR the night before: *most surgery/procedures should be safe with INR<2.0.*
  - **High risk of VTE** (mechanical valve, recent PE): admit 2–3 days preop, start IV heparin as soon as INR <2.0; stop heparin 6h preop.
  - **Medium risk of VTE** (recent DVT, high risk AF 📖 p. 136): start routine prophylactic heparin/LMWH (Table 2.6) as soon as INR <2.0.
  - **Low risk of VTE** (low risk AF 📖 p. 136): no heparin needed, if surgery is delayed >24h start sc heparin prophylaxis.
- Restart warfarin after surgery, continue preop heparin until INR >2.0.
- *In emergency (bleeding or need for emergency surgery) reverse by:*
  - 2U of FFP over 30min, recheck INR in 1h; *or* 10mg vitamin K IM, and recheck INR in 6h.
  - Vitamin K slower, less predictable, may cause anaphylaxis; FFP faster but carries all the risks of transfusion (📖 p. 70)

Other drugs

- *Clopidogrel, aspirin*: should be stopped 5 days before major surgery, but if patient had recent coronary stent, this **must** be discussed with cardiology: stent occlusion may happen within days of stopping.
- *Steroids*: if on >10mg prednisolone, consider hydrocortisone (📖 p. 280).
- *ACE inhibitors*: withhold the night before major surgery.
- *Long-acting hypoglycaemics*: withhold night before surgery.
- *OCP*: stop combined OCP 4/52 before surgery, progesterone only ok.

Organizing the list

Key facts
- Ideally list order is decided by the consultant, typed and distributed by the secretary, by 3pm on the preceding day.
- Getting an accurate list out **early** helps your fellow surgeons, anaesthetists, theatre nurses, ward nurses, and blood bank prepare.
- Getting patient details wrong will result in cancellation at best, wrong surgery at worst: always check the list with someone senior.

Booking elective lists
- Fill in the form (may be kept at theatre reception), 📖 see Box 2.5.
- Any changes to the list:
  - Try to do this **before** the theatre deadline: within an hour multiple copies of your list will have been distributed to anaesthetists, wards, theatres, and blood bank, making changes much harder work
  - Write clearly on the top of the list "*NOTE CHANGE OF ORDER/ ADDITIONAL PATIENT", renumber clearly with the new order, contact theatre desk, wards, and anaesthetists if list already out.
- List order balances medical needs with logistics:
  - *Put short cases first:* they are less likely to be cancelled this way
  - *Patients needing HDU/ICU bed should go early:* lower risk of bed given away, periop problems can be managed more effectively during the day-time
  - *Diabetics, patients on heparin drips and children should go early.*
  - Try to put patients that have previously been cancelled early on the list to reduce the chance of them being cancelled again.
  - Avoid putting patients first who are on outlying/medical wards, or are coming in from home: they can delay the whole list.

Box 2.5 Mandatory details for booking theatre list

- Name of consultant surgeon and anaesthetist
- Theatre number
- Date and start time of list
- For every patient provide: Full name, hospital number, DOB, preop **and** postop location, operation including SIDE, SITE, approach, and number of units of blood crossmatched
- Other details: frozen section pathology / image intensifier / specimen collection for trials, etc.
- Leave your name (legibly) and bleep number.

Important extras to remember
- *Frozen section:* (histology for intraoperative staging of cancer which may change operative plan) phone up histopathology the day before.
- *Image intensifier:* (orthopaedics, long line insertion) phone radiology the day before to book.
- *Pacemakers:* book cardiac technician the day before to reset (📖 p. 144).

Booking emergencies

- *Always* check with a senior team member that surgery is definitely planned, what the urgency is, and what the approach is.
- Make patient NBM and find out *when they last ate*. Put this on the list together with all the details listed in Box 2.5.
- Usually you need to give the written details to theatre reception **and** *discuss with the on-call anaesthetist* who should be responsible for deciding patient priority. Factors which make your patient higher priority:
  - *Immediately* (ruptured AAA, chest trauma, splenic rupture, ectopic pregnancy) or potentially *life-threatening* (perforated viscus, septic shock, active bleeding), *limb threatening*.
  - Very elderly or young patient, particularly if NBM all day.
  - Asking politely displaying a clear understanding of context.
- You may also need to page the theatre co-ordinator.
- Check the patient has been consented; is blood available?

Organizing transfers

- **Never** accept a patient until you know that your consultant has accepted the transfer, **and** there is a bed available.
- Take patient name, DOB, problem, name of sending hospital, name and direct phone number of ward, name of responsible nurse, name and contact details of referring clinician.
- If the clinician phoning you hasn't already spoken to your bed-manager (in hours) or ward sister (out of hours) give them the contact details.
- Once transfer is agreed ask for an estimated time of arrival (ETA) and led the ward sister know.
- Always ask for a copy of the patient notes, a transfer letter, a copy of recent bloods **and all radiology** to be sent with the patient

Cancelling patients

- This miserable task is usually left to the most junior team member, as everyone else is conveniently scrubbed.
- Always double check before you tell the ward the patient can eat.
- Before you go to see the patient know your facts:
  - Why were they cancelled?
  - When is the new date for surgery?
  - How will delay affect things?
  - If patient is to be discharged, how will they get home?
  - How can they get something to eat and drink now?
- Being able to give the patient a clear plan, reassurance that this delay will not have a negative impact on their condition, and something to eat makes a difficult conversation a bit easier (see also p. 46).

Fluid management

📖 Fluid resuscitation p. 116.

Key facts

- The main aim of fluid management is to replace whatever fluid and electrolytes are lost, without overloading the patient.
- Success can make the difference between a short, uncomplicated post-operative course and the patient ending up on ITU.
- Most surgical patients are hypovolaemic with good hearts (but always look out for the overloaded patient in heart failure).

Maintenance crystalloid (Box 2.6)

Average daily loss of fluid and electrolytes is approximately:

- *Water loss 2500mL/day* (insensible loss from skin, respiratory and GI tract, and in urine,) MORE in sepsis, ventilation, diarrhoea, vomiting, high output fistulas, polyuric renal failure.
- Na^+ *100mmol/day* in urine, *more* in pyrexia, diarrhoea, vomiting, high output fistulas
- K^+ *80mmol/day* in urine, *more* in pyrexia, diarrhoea, vomiting, high output fistulas.

Box 2.6 Maintenance fluid regimens

Regime 1

- Suited to most adult patients with no significant comorbidity.
- Takes no account of age, size, cardiac function, or fluid loss.
- Gives 3L of fluid, 200mmol Na^+ and 80mmol KCl in 24h.
  - 1L normal saline (NS) with 40mmmol KCl over 8h.
  - 1L NS with 40mmol KCl over 8h.
  - 1L 5% glucose over 8h.
- If Na^+ >145mmol/L substitute 1L 5% glucose for 1L NS (⚠ in marked (>150 mmol/L) long-standing (>2 days) hypernatraemia, see also 📖 p.230)

Regime 2

- More suited to patients on HDU.
- This adjusts fluid given to fluid lost, but needs the nursing resources to run an hourly fluid balance chart, and infusion pumps.
  - 1mL/kg/h NS.
  - Gelofusine or 5% glucose fluid challenges to maintain CVP 8–12 or BP >120mmHg.
  - 10–40mmol KCL in 100mL 5% glucose via central line.

Regime 3—Alder Hey paediatric regimen

- Useful in all ages and all body weights except extreme starvation.
  - Fluid volume/24h = 100mL/kg 0–10kg of weight; 50mL/kg 10–20kg of weight; 20mL/kg weight >20kg.
  - Electrolytes Na^+ 2mmol/kg/24h, K^+ 1mmol/kg/24h.

Colloid

Colloids (especially blood) produce a more lasting expansion of intravascular volume than crystalloid, which rapidly enters the interstitial tissues.

- These are used as boluses (e.g. 250–500mL over 10–20min IV) to improve BP, or titrate to CVP: not as maintenance fluids!
- *Gelofusine* is based on bovine gelatin, which has a half-life of about 2h in plasma, and is associated with mildly ↑ bleeding times.
- *Dextran* is a glucose polymer mixture, which has a plasma half-life of about 2h, it has been associated with anaphylactic reaction.
- *HES preparations* are derived from hydroxyethyl starch: they have widely differing plasma half-lives and effects on plasma expansion.
- *Albumin* is a naturally occurring plasma protein, sterilized by ultrafiltration. 5% albumin is isotonic, 20% albumin is hypertonic. Specific indications for use of albumin as a volume expander are very limited.
- Blood, platelets, FFP, and cryoprecipitate (📖 p. 68)

Assessing volume status

This is usually straightforward, but in the HDU patient 24h post-complex surgery you need information from several sources: if patient is unstable ask nurses to start *hourly fluid balance chart.* (📖 See Table 2.7).

Table 2.7 Differences between dry and overfilled patients

	The dry patient	The overfilled patient
History and examination	Feels thirsty, dry mouth, may have been NBM several days or be dehydrated because of diarrhoea or vomiting. Low JVP, dry mucous membranes, reduced skin turgor.	May be SOB Raised JVP, normal skin turgor, may have dependent oedema or evidence of pulmonary oedema
Observations chart	Falling BP, rising pulse rate, low CVP unresponsive to fluid challenges, hourly urine output <1/2mL/kg/h, weight several kg below preop weight, net fluid balance (all input minus all output) may be hundreds of mL –ve each day	High CVP that rises/plateaus with fluid challenge, BP may fall with fluid challenge, not usually tachycardic. Weight several kg above preop weight, urine output unreliable indicator, but should have good response to furosemide (>5mL/kg/h), and calculated net fluid balance may be several litres +ve each day
Blood results	↑urea, may also have ↑Na$^+$ ↑K$^+$, ↑creatinine; urea usually raised more than creatinine (unless ARF)	May have ↓Na$^+$
CXR	No evidence of pulmonary oedema/effusions	May have both

Fluid balance troubleshooting

Fluid optimization

Patients who benefit most from fluid optimization

Optimization is essentially tailored preoperative fluid resuscitation aimed at reducing perioperative morbidity in high risk patients, particularly:

- Acute presentations with vomiting or diarrhoea, including intestinal obstruction, biliary colic, gastroenteritis.
- Acute presentations where the patient has been immobile or debilitated for a prolonged period e.g. pancreatitis, chest infections, acute on chronic vascular insufficiency, prolonged sepsis with pyrexia.
- Elderly patients:
  - Reduced renal reserve demands meticulous care with fluid balance.
  - Heart failure and fluid overload more common.
- Drugs which impair renal responses to fluid changes e.g. diuretics.
- Patients with low body weight with overall lower total body fluid volume in whom similar losses have a greater effect.

Basic principles of optimization

The key is estimating the fluid deficit (p. 64) and replacing this with suitable fluid over a period of hours: in sick patients admission to HDU for invasive monitoring will help. Other than exceptional circumstances, isotonic crystalloids are the fluid of choice to correct imbalances.

Table 2.8 Replacement fluids in surgical patients

Losses	Content (mmol/L)		Suitable replacement fluid
	Na$^+$	K$^+$	
Blood	140	4	Hartmann's, NS, colloid, blood products
Plasma	140	4	Hartmann's, NS, colloid
3rd space	140	4	Hartmann's, NS
NG losses	60	10	50:50 NS, 0.15% KCl and 5% dextrose
Upper GI	110	5–10	NS (check K$^+$ regularly)
Diarrhoea	120	25	NS, 0.15% KCl

Monitoring fluid optimization

- Skin turgor and mucosal hydration change slowly after optimization and are unreliable guides.
- Hourly urine output is a good guide to renal blood flow which indirectly relates to intravascular fluid volume and cardiac output: 0.5mL/kg/h is a commonly used minimum.
- Monitoring of serum urea is an approximate guide provided renal function is adequate and there is no acute GI bleeding or proteolysis.
- When patients require urgent surgery but require fluid optimization prior to anaesthesia, more rapid fluid infusions may be required and this should be monitored (HDU/ICU).

Box 2.7 Solutions to common fluid balance problems

Patient needing a LOT of fluid to maintain BP
- Exclude surgical bleeding (📖 p.98), early sepsis (📖 p.90), epidural-related hypotension (📖 p.85).
- If after major surgery, check the CVP and give 250mL fluid challenge.
- If CVP <14mmHg after major surgery and does not increase with fluid challenge, this may be due to capillary leak (see below).
- If no CVP, try to identify clinical signs of hypovolaemia (📖 p.116).
- Give 500mL colloid (📖 p.64), increase rate of crystalloid infusion to 200mL/h and re-evaluate hourly: may need inotrope.

My patient is hyponatraemic
- Unless the Na^+ was abnormal preop, hyponatraemia is due to a relative excess of water (excess 5% glucose, TURP syndrome: absorption of irrigation fluid at TURP, 10–30mL/h).
- Change IV fluids to NS, consider 1L/24h fluid restriction (📖 p.228)
- **Do not** use hypertonic saline, (too rapid correction leads to life-*threatening* pontine myelinolysis).

My patient is very oedematous but seems hypovolaemic
- Inability to keep fluid in vascular space (↓albumin, capillary leak syndrome in sepsis) requires IV fluid to maintain circulating volume.
- Look for an underlying problem. Sepsis or tissue necrosis is highly likely.
- Oedema difficult to improve as the fluid is often sequestered in the peripheries, and is only mobilized as the patient improves.
- Ensure good nutrition early on to increase albumin (📖 p.246).
- Give blood transfusion if anaemic and symptomatic.
- Concentrated albumin solution with loop diuretics does not improve outcome and should be avoided.
- Look for evidence of heart failure and treat.

What should I do in a patient with cardiac failure?
- Restrict fluid input, replacement fluids according to losses.
- Monitor urine output and CVP with major surgery.
- Although these patients are at risk of deteriorating with overenthusiastic IV fluid administration, they will do badly if underfilled.
- Consider involving HDU/ICU as invasive monitering may be required.

My patient is passing a lot of urine
- This is normal if it occurs 2–3 days after surgery when the patient is mobilizing fluids that have been sequestered in the tissues.
- If the creatinine and serum Na^+ normal, then this is the likely cause and no therapy is indicated: the polyuria settles in time.
- Other conditions may also present in this way (diabetes mellitus (📖 p.274), diabetes insipidus (📖 p.230), polyuric renal failure (📖 p.230), polydipsia.

Transfusion

📖 See Table 2.9.

G&S takes 5min, emergency XM takes 15min

Table 2.9 Suggested XM (check local protocols)

Category	Procedure	G&S/XM
General surgery	Oesophagectomy, oesophagogastrectomy, liver resection, pancreatic surgery, rectum AP/anterior resection	2U
	Gastrectomy, cholecystectomy, small bowel resection, colectomy, laparotomy, mastectomy, splenectomy, thyroidectomy,	G&S
Vascular surgery	Emergency aortic reconstruction	6U, FFP, plts
	Elective aortic reconstruction	2U
	Carotid endarterectomy, distal reconstruction, axillo-femoral bypass, amputation	G&S
Urology	Cystectomy	4U
	Nephrectomy	3U
	Open prostatectomy	2U
	TURP, reimplantation of ureter	G&S
Transplant	Renal	2U
	Liver	6U, FFP, plbs
Cardiothoracic	Reop CABG/valve	4U, FFP, plts
	Thoracotomy, CABG, MVR/AVR	2U
	Mediastinoscopy	G&S
Trauma	Major RTA	4U
ENT/plastic surgery	Major head/neck reconstruction	2U
	Free flaps	2U
	Breast reduction	2U
Orthopaedic surgery	Total hip replacement/revision	2U/4U
	Total knee replacement	G&S
	Total shoulder replacement	G&S
	Major spinal stabilisation	2–4U
Maxillofacial	Bimaxillary osteotomy	2U

Indications for blood products

- Young, fit patients tolerate haemodilution much better than elderly patients with cardiovascular and respiratory disease.
- *Blood*: transfuse to keep Hb above 7.0–9.0g/dL in older patients or those with cardiorespiratory disease, above 9.0–10g/dL.
- *FFP*: massive transfusion (📖 p. 71), or APTR>1.5 with active bleeding.
- *Platelets*: platelets $<50 \times 10^9$/L with active bleeding/recent clopidogrel/ before surgery. Even without bleeding, give platelets if $<5 \times 10^9$/L.
- *Cryoprecipitate*: massive transfusion, or fibrinogen <1g/L with bleeding.

Blood
- 1 unit of blood increases Hb by about 1g/dL in a 70kg adult.
- Blood is normally provided as packed red cells (1 unit ~350mL).
- XM blood can normally be provided within 20min.
- In dire emergencies O–ve blood (universal donor) can be given to recipients of any ABO/Rhesus group without incompatibility reaction.
- Autologous blood transfusion may be used: up to 2U of blood are withdrawn from patients preop, and stored for up to 5 weeks.
- Cell salvage reduces the need for allogeneic blood. Shed blood is collected intraoperatively, heparinized, spun with NS to remove all material including residual heparin, platelets, and clotting products, and repackaged as red blood cells suspended in saline for transfusion.
- Simple measures to reduce need for blood transfusion include:
  - Treating anaemia and coagulopathy preoperatively.
  - Stopping warfarin, heparin, aspirin and clopidogrel appropriately.
  - Good surgical technique
- Special methods to reduce homologous blood transfusion include:
  - Autologous blood transfusion.
  - Cell-salvage.
  - Antifibrinolytic drugs eg. tranexamic acid.
  - Erythropoietin (EPO) stimulates erythrocyte production, *do not use* without specialist input.

Platelets
- 1 unit of platelets increases platelet count by $5–10 \times 10^9$/L in 70kg adult.
- Platelets are provided as units (1U ~50mL), usually pooled, but single donor units available for platelet refractory patients.
- Platelets do not need to be XM but they should be ABO compatible (and Rhesus matched in women of childbearing age).

Fresh frozen plasma (FFP)
- 1 unit FFP contains all coagulation factors except platelets.
- 1 unit of FFP = 150–250mL, and 5–10mL/kg is normally given.
- FFP does not need to be XM but should be ABO compatible (and Rhesus matched in women of childbearing age).
- FFP must be stored at $< -18°C$: it must be thawed, usually over 20min, before giving, and discarded if not used within 2h.
- It is acellular and does not transmit CMV infection.

Cryoprecipitate
- 1 unit of cryoprecipitate contains 150–250mg fibrinogen, factors VII and VIII (80U), volume ~20mL, 5–10U are normally given.
- 10U contain same amount of fibrinogen as 5U of FFP.
- 10U of cryoprecipitate raise fibrinogen 0.6–0.7g/L in a 70kg adult.
- ABO and Rhesus compatibility is not relevant.

Special considerations
- CMV: use CMV –ve products in patients who are or may become BMT recipients or neutropaenic, and have unknown or documented CMV –ve status.
- HLA maternity: if repeated transfusions are likely to be required
- Iradiated products: any patient who had or may have BMT

Transfusion reactions

Acute haemolytic reaction

- Life-threatening medical emergency.
- Sudden onset of hypotension, tachycardia, pyrexia, breathlessness, tachypnoea and back pain on starting transfusion. Bilirubinaemia, anaemia, and haemoglobinuria as a result of haemolysis ensue.
  - Stop the transfusion immediately and give basic life support (📖 see inside cover).
  - Keep the bag and giving set for analysis, inform haematology.
  - Give crystalloid and furosemide to encourage diuresis.
  - Dialysis may be required.

ABO incompatibility (usually due to clerical, bedside, sampling or laboratory error) results in cytokine and chemokine release and sympathetic inflammatory response. Donor erythrocytes carrying either A and/or B erythrocyte antigens bind to the recipient's anti-A or anti-B antibodies, resulting in complement formation, membrane attack complex and immediate haemolysis. Other blood group determinants (Rh, Kelly, Duffy) can also trigger haemolytic reactions.

Anaphylaxis and allergic reactions

- Life-threatening anaphylaxis (📖 p.117) characterized by hypotension, bronchospasm, angioedema, loss of consciousness can occur after a few mL of blood (IgA deficient patients prone to IgA allergy).
  - Stop the transfusion immediately and disconnect connection tubing. Call for help
  - Give adrenaline 0.5mg 1M (0.5mL of 1:1000), chlorphenamine (10mg IV), and hydrocortisone 100mg IV.
  - Maintain IV access, give fluid.
- Mild allergic reactions are relatively common: characterised by erythematous papular rashes, wheals, pruritus and pyrexia.
  - Stop transfusion, give chlorphenamine (10mg IV), resume transfusion once symptoms have settled.

Non-haemolytic febrile reaction

- Mild pyrexia, typically over an hour after transfusion is started.
- Severe reactions feature high grade fever, rigors, nausea, and vomiting.
- Stop transfusion: antipyrogens such as paracetamol 1g po/pr limit pyrexia, but antihistamines are not helpful.
- Resume transfusion at slower rate once symptoms have settled.

Caused by recipient antibodies directed against donor HLA and leucocyte specific antigen on leucocytes and platelets. Severity of symptoms is proportional to the number of leucocytes in the transfused blood and the rate of transfusion. Leucocyte depleted blood helps prevent these reactions.

Delayed extravascular haemolytic reaction

- ↓Hb 5–7 days post transfusion, hyperbilirubinaemia and +ve Coombs' test due to accelerated destruction of transfused RBCs.
- As haemolysis is extravascular so haemoglobinuria is uncommon.
- May require further transfusion with careful matching.

Alloantigen reaction (commonly Rhesus E, Kelly, Duffy, Kidd). Recipient antibody levels too low to be detected at standard XM until anamnestic response on exposure to transfused antigen triggers production of large amounts of alloantibody binding donor erythrocytes.

Transfusion-related acute lung injury
- Non-cardiogenic pulmonary oedema within 6h of transfusion.
- Hypoxia and respiratory failure may need mechanical ventilation, but recovery without long-term consequences is the norm.

Mediated by donor antibodies against recipient HLA. Recipient leucocyte aggregates migrate to the lung releasing proteolytic enzymes causing capillary leak syndrome and pulmonary oedema.

Infection
Bacterial
- Recipient shows signs of sepsis: pyrexia >40°C, hypotensive, ± DIC. This may occur during the transfusion or hours after completion, and unlike febrile transfusion reactions, is not self–limiting.
  - Stop transfusion and disconnect tubing.
  - Fluid resuscitation (📖 p. 116).
  - Culture the patient and send bag and giving sets to microbiology.
  - Start empirical broad spectrum antibiotics (📖 p. 88).
- Serious bacterial contamination of stored blood may occur, although platelets, which are usually stored at room temperature, are at greater risk of this. Common organisms: *Staphylococcus*, *Escherichia*, *Yersinia*, *Pseudomonas*, *Actinobacter* sp. Contamination is difficult to detect.

Non-bacterial
- Pre-transfusion testing includes screening for hepatitis B (HbsAg, anti HBc), hepatitis C (anti HCV), HIV (anti HIV-1/2, HIV-1 p24 antigen), HTLV (anti TLC-1/2), and syphilis.
- HIV can be transmitted by an infective but seronegative donor for about 15 days after infection. The HCV window is 20 days.
- CMV is common in donor population (40–60%): CMV –ve recipients who are either immunocompromised or potential bone marrow transplant candidates ***must*** receive leukocyte depleted/CMV –ve blood.
- Malaria may be transmitted by blood transfusion as may nvCJD.

Fluid overload
- Characterized by high JVP/CVP, pulmonary oedema and low PaO_2.
  - Stop the transfusion.
  - Give high flow O_2 and loop diuretics (40mg furosemide IV).

Massive transfusion
Replacement of the patient's circulating volume within 24h.
- Stored RBC are ATP/2,3-DPG depleted, leak K^+, fluid contains citrate.
- Large volumes of RBC lead to a blood volume which has poor O_2 carrying capacity, ↑K^+, is hypothermic (if blood is not warmed), and does not clot well due to Ca^{2+} sequestration.
- Reduce the effect of massive transfusion by:
  - Use infusion warmers and a warming blanket.
  - Monitor central circulation and respiratory function closely.
  - Consider giving Ca^{2+} supplements (with care!).
  - Check platelets, APTT and fibrinogen: replace if needed.
  - Check K^+ regularly.

Critical care

Recognizing the critically ill surgical patient

It may be obvious that a patient needs a critical care bed: those needing ventilation, inotropes, or dialysis. But anticipating, and maybe avoiding this is more difficult. The first step is *recognizing compensated critical illness* (e.g. shock compensated by tachycardia and peripheral shut down, respiratory failure compensated by unsustainable respiratory effort). Also see Box 2.8.

Box 2.8 Signs that should ring alarm bells

History: 'I feel like I'm going to die.' *Timor mortis* (fear of dying) may accompany MI, hypovolaemic shock, respiratory failure. **Never** ignore the patient who thinks they are dying: they are often right.

Nurses: 'Mr Smith doesn't look right/looks sick.' Experienced nurses quickly recognize the patterns of critical illness, listen to them!

General: hypothermia/hyperpyrexia, cold and clammy sweating

Cardiovascular: ↓BP, ↑↓pulse, arrhythmias, peripheral shut-down

Respiratory: tachypnoea, difficulty getting full sentences out

Renal: oliguria <0.5 mL/kg/hr

Gastrointestinal: new anorexia, nausea and vomiting.

Neurological: confusion, agitation or drowsiness, fits.

Immediate management

First identify and treat potentially life-threatening conditions. *Then* quantify the problem: important for referring patients to other clinicians and for establishing a baseline by which to guide treatment and monitor progress. *Finally* start looking for the underlying problem. Some of these tasks overlap. *Keep* reassessing the patient and adjust your management.

- Quickly assess airway, breathing, and circulation: ALS algorithms are printed on the inside back cover of this book, management of shock is described on 📖 p. 116, and of haemorrhage on 📖 p. 98.
- Sit patient up and give high flow O_2.
- Secure IV access, take blood for FBC, U&E, amylase, glucose, LFTs, cardiac enzymes, clotting, G&S, blood cultures.
- Take ABG: good O_2 saturations do not rule out respiratory failure, and blood gases will also show acidosis and electrolyte abnormalities.
- Give 500mL gelofusine if patient not obviously fluid overloaded.
- Request a 12-lead ECG.
- Review drug, diabetic, and fluid balance charts.
- Perform a focused history and examination: ask about symptoms that have changed recently and focus your examination on that.
- Review recent bloods and XRs, and request appropriate radiology.
- If the patient needs HDU or ITU talk to your registrar or consultant.
- A patient may need to be discharged from HDU, or surgery postponed: think ahead.

High dependency unit

The HDU allows a level of care between ICU and the general ward. Invasive monitoring and inotropic support are routine but ventilation and dialysis are not supported. Nurse:patient ratio generally 1:2. Patients with single organ failure requiring basic respiratory support, including non-invasive support with CPAP (📖 p. 209), should be admitted to HDU. Also see Box 2.9.

Guidelines for admission to HDU

- Need for monitored bed.
- Need for invasive monitoring.
- Need for inotropes.
- Need for CPAP or other respiratory support.
- Epidural.
- Need for 1:2 nursing.

Box 2.9 Intensive care unit

The ICU offers advanced ventilatory and inotropic support, renal replacement therapy, full invasive monitoring, and 1:1 nursing care.

Patients suitable for ICU

- Needs mechanical ventilation, *or*
- Failure of two or more organ systems, *or*
- Need for advanced monitoring e.g. cardiac output monitoring or
- Need for escalating or multiple inotropes, *and*
- Primary pathology leading to admission should be reversible.

There are no ICU beds but patient needs ICU

- The ICU team may be able to discharge/swap a patient.
- Can the patient be managed on HDU, or CCU (for inotropic support), neuro ICU (ventilation), renal unit (dialysis)?

How do I know if my patient will need ICU or HDU?

- *The golden rule is 'If in doubt ask the advice of anaesthetist or Critical Care team—more patients can benefit than do'.*
- Elective patient in need of intensive infusional treatment prior to surgery (e.g. IV anticoagulation, IV clotting factors)? **HDU**
- Undergone major surgery with large transfusion requirements which might lead to haemodynamic and clotting abnormalities (e.g. elective extensive pelvic surgery, aortic surgery, extensive burns)? **HDU**
- Patient >80 years having major abdominal or thoracic surgery? **HDU**
- Known significant respiratory/neurological disease making prolonged mechanical ventilation likely? **ICU**
- Patient due for emergency surgery needing aggressive, closely monitored fluid resuscitation prior to anaesthesia? **HDU**
- Postop patient needing infusional inotropic support, renal replacement therapy, or invasive monitoring? **ICU / HDU**

Theatre

Theatre clothing
- In most theatre suites you need to wear *scrubs, theatre shoes, and a hat* which should cover all hair, to enter any part of the theatre area.
- If you don't have theatre shoes, disposable covers are available.
- To try to reduce infection, most hospitals either ban you wearing scrubs outside the theatre area (and white coats within theatre), or require you to wear a coverall over your scrubs outside theatre.
- Most theatres ban long sleeves under scrubs.
- Put a mask on before you enter any room where surgery is in progress.
- Most units ban all jewellery (except small ear studs), and nail varnish.

Theatre etiquette
- Ask before you scrub (Box 2.10).
- Introduce yourself to the scrub nurse, and the surgeon if you are scrubbing, or the circulating nurse and the anaesthetist if you aren't.
- If unscrubbed, *never* walk between two sterile fields, or between a scrubbed person and a sterile field.
- If in doubt, don't touch instruments, drapes or light handles.

Getting the most out of theatre
- If you are useful, people tend to teach you more in return.
- If you feel useful, you'll enjoy things more.
- Spending time with the anaesthetist will be useful to you: they are usually a font of medical knowledge and good teachers.
- Eat, drink, and micturate: you may faint or have to go to the toilet.

Before you scrub
- Know the patient: see them before surgery, know their age, history, clinical findings, and speak up if asked.
- Check the patient, operation, consent, and marking.
- Ask if patient needs a Foley catheter, and offer to do it.
- Fill in histology forms/TTOs.
- Find the relevant imaging, put it up on the light box, and reconcile the report with what you see and know.
- Find the surgeon, ask if you can scrub.

Once you're scrubbed
- When you are scrubbed, rest your hands gently on the patient.
- If you can't see, ask for a standing stool.
- Ask if you're not sure what's going on, unless there's a problem.
- If in doubt, ask before touching.
- Things that can be helpful:
  - Adjusting light (don't desterilize your arm on someone's head).
  - Holding a camera (takes a bit of getting used to).
  - Suctioning blood gently out of the field.
  - Cutting sutures (3–4mm) once they are tied.
  - Holding retractors exactly as they are given to you.
  - Touching the cautery onto forceps on request.
  - Help the scrub nurse do the dressings at the end of surgery.

- Things you may be able to do:
  - Skin sutures.
  - Ties if you have already practiced surgical knots.
  - Incision and basic dissection depending on your experience.
  - Improve your understanding of key conditions and treatment.

Once you unscrub
- Stay to remove the drapes and transfer the patient instead of disappearing off for a coffee.
- Check the histology samples are correctly labelled.
- Thank the scrub nurse/anaesthetist for keeping an eye on you, thank the surgeon for letting you scrub.

Box 2.10 Scrubbing up

- This is a crucial part of reducing infection risk.
- First time? Ask a theatre nurse to show you how.
- First remove all jewellery, tuck your hair into your hat, put on a mask and add protective eye wear if you are assisting.
- Open a gown onto the shelf in the scrub area in a sterile fashion, and drop a sterile pair of gloves on top.
  - If you're not sure of your glove size ♀ are usually 6 to 6 1/2, ♂ are usually 7 1/2 to 8.
  - Latex-free gloves are available.

Scrubbing
- Put the taps on, adjust temperature, open a scrubbing brush, and spend 1min cleaning under your nails.
- Then using either chlorhexidine or povidone-iodide spend 3–4min cleaning your hands and forearms, taking care not to miss out the backs of your nails or between your fingers.
- Rinse off holding your hands up so water runs from hands to elbows, not the other way around.
- Turn the tap off (elbow, knee, or foot control).

Putting on gown and gloves (if scrub nurse does not help)
- Dry your hands thoroughly on the sterile paper towel that comes with the gown—damp hands are difficult to glove.
- Only touch the inside of the gown from start to end.
- Pick it up, stand back from non-sterile surfaces, and let it unravel so that you can put your arms in the sleeves, but don't put your hands out of the openings at the end.
- It is easier if someone ties the gown at your back now.
- With your right hand inside its sleeve, pick up the left glove and pull it over your left hand also still inside its sleeve, then pull on the left sleeve to slide the glove onto your left hand.
- Repeat for the right glove: the white cuff of the gown should be completely inside the glove when you're done.
- Give the cardboard piece at the front of your gown to someone, turn round to your right, pulling the belt out of the card as you do so, and tie it.

Postoperative management

Routine tests

Protocols vary widely according to the complexity of surgery and the age of the patient: this is a rough guide to management of the older patient following major abdominal, cardiac surgery, or reconstructive surgery.

Blood tests
- FBC, clotting, U&E on day 1, day 2, day 3, day 5, and day 7. Look for:
  - Anaemia: consider surgical bleeding, dilutional, peptic ulceration.
  - Raised WCC: look for other signs of sepsis (📖 p. 90).
- Monitor INR daily if the patient is being warfarinized, and clotting before insertion of drains, or central lines.
- Check Na^+ and K^+ to guide choice of crystalloid (📖 p. 66).
- Monitor urea and creatinine especially in preop renal dysfunction, cardiac and aortic surgery, nephrotoxic drugs (e.g. NSAIDs, ACE-inhibitors, vancomycin/gentamicin, fluid restriction).

ECG
Important in cardiac and vascular surgery patients, and any patient with symptomatic IHD or valvular heart disease. Look for:
- Rhythm disturbances, e.g. atrial fibrillation/flutter.
- Evidence of new ischaemia.

CXR
Request daily if chest drains are present on suction, after drain removal and to check position of newly placed central lines. Look for:
- Position of indwelling lines.
- Consolidation, pneumothorax (on side of central line), pulmonary oedema, pleural effusion.

Ward rounds

See patients twice a day. In the evening review the blood results and other investigations from that day. For formal ward rounds:
- Make sure you have a nurse with you.
- Make sure someone writes a summary in the patient's notes.
- Ask the patient if they are experiencing any problems: establish whether they are mobilizing appropriately, eating and drinking, adequate pain control, passing urine, and opening bowels.
- Check the observation chart for: temperature, BP trends, O_2 saturations, weight, fluid balance/drainage if these are still being monitored.
- Feel pulse, look at JVP and ankles.
- Look at wounds, check evidence of infection, seroma, dehiscence.
- Listen to chest in all patients, and check most recent CXR.
- Check diabetic charts for blood sugar control.
- Review drug chart: restart regular oral medication as soon as possible, convert IV to oral where appropriate, look actively for drugs that can be discontinued to minimize polypharmacy.
- Review the previous day's blood results, and note any trends.
- Review the nutritional status and feeding rate of the patient
- Make a clear problem list, make a clear plan for each problem.

Special cases

Surgery for carcinoma
- Review histology as soon as it is available. Liaise with specialist nurses.
- It may be unit practice to explain the results of surgery in outpatients, if not, breaking bad news is discussed on 📖 p. 338.
- Refer patient to oncology as soon as diagnosis known and the patient has been informed. If further treatment is planned time is usually tight.

Plastic and reconstructive surgery
- Check perfusion of flaps at least daily.
- Check take of split-skin grafts on day 5.
- Book postop medical illustration for photos prior to discharge.

Orthopaedic surgery
Check XRs of prosthesis to assess position, fraction reduction.

Vascular surgery
- Check distal pulses/capillary refill after reconstructive surgery.
- Perform neurological examination to evaluate patients post-carotid endarterectomy
- Arrange prosthesis fitting for amputees

Cardiac surgery
- Check sternal stability daily—ask the patient to cough while you feel for abnormal sternal movement.
- Request transthoracic echo for day 4–5 postop in valve repair patients and auscultate daily.

Discharge
- Plan discharge from day of admission—use hospital discharge team and identify patients requiring special facilities, e.g. rehabilitation early.
- Make sure the patient understands what operation they have had.
- Tell them how to look out for common problems like wound infections, what is normal, and who to contact if they are worried.
- Make sure patient understands timeframe for return to normal activities and work.
- Tell them when they will be seen in clinic.
- Write informative but concise discharge summary for the GP

Rehabilitation
- The average time for patients to be fit to go back to work are:
  - 2–3 weeks after minor abdominal or thoracic surgery.
  - 6 weeks after major abdominal, cardiac or reconstructive surgery, as long as work does not involve heavy lifting.
  - Weight bearing takes up to 2 months after lower limb arthroplasty, and 3 months after lower limb fracture.
- Patients can usually drive once they are fully mobile as long as they have not experienced blackouts or fits.
- There are detailed rules for HGV drivers and pilots.

Pain management

Key facts
- Good pain relief reduces postoperative complications such as chest infections, nausea/vomiting, DVT, ileus.
- Acute pain is often badly managed: this need not be so. Pain control can often be improved by a simple strategy:
  - Assess the pain (site, source, severity, reversible causes).
  - Treat with drugs and techniques with which you are familiar.
  - Reassess the pain after treatment and be prepared to adjust the treatment accordingly.
- Follow the 'Ten Rules' religiously (Box 2.11) until you have developed a good feel for the more subtle points of pain management (often only by the time you are on the specialist training track).

Box 2.11 Ten golden rules of pain management

1. Severe pain after surgery is always preventable.
2. Prevention is much more effective than treatment, for management of both pain and side effects of pain.
3. Always look for treatable causes of pain.
4. Never withhold analgesia for fear of hiding surgical signs.
5. The maximum benefit with fewest unwanted effects is often obtained by a combination of different drugs given by different routes (e.g. opioid with NSAID, and local anaesthetic infiltrated into the wound before closure).
6. Know a few drugs well.
7. Opioids given for acute pain do not cause drug addiction.
8. The correct dose of an opioid analgesic is 'enough'.
9. The same surgical operation may produce widely differing analgesia requirements in different patients, and the same level of pain may be expressed in widely differing ways by different patients.
10. Patients who say that they are in pain almost invariably are: listen to your patients and believe them, as there are no physiological or behavioural patterns that can be used to prove that someone is fabricating pain. Give enough analgesia for the patient in front of you!

The pain team
- A pain team exists in many hospitals. *It is an invaluable source of help and information.* An anaesthetist usually heads the team, with a specialist nurse running the day-to-day service.
- Contact them early in patients with problematic pain management; they also help with epidural and PCA troubleshooting.

General principles of pain management

- Can the patient take *oral analgesics?*
- Do they need *IV administration* for speed of onset?
- Can *local anaesthesia* better treat the pain, or be used in combination with systemic analgesics?
- Can *other methods* be used to help ease the pain, such as splinting of fractures, dressing of burns, reassurance?
- Also see Box 2.12.

Box 2.12 The WHO analgesic ladder

- If one drug fails to control the pain, move up the ladder: do not try other drugs at the same level, they will not work.
- In severe pain, omit rungs 1 and 2.
- This approach is inexpensive and 80–90% effective.

Rung 3	Strong opioid: morphine, diamorphine, oxycodone, fentanyl
Rung 2	Weak opioid: codeine, dihydrocodeine, tramadol
Rung 1	Non-opioid: aspirin, paracetamol, NSAID (e.g. ibuprofen, diclofenac)

Always prescribe stat, regular, and prn analgesia for patients in pain.

Always consider adjuvant drugs e.g. anxiolytics, laxatives, antiemetics.

Give by the clock not PRN

Assessment of pain, analgesia, and sedation

- Scoring systems are used to assess pain and to measure the effectiveness of treatment.
- A *visual analogue scale* (VAS): a line whose end-points are 0 (no pain) and 10 (the worst imaginable pain). The patient puts a mark on the line to represent their pain severity. This may be difficult to apply if the patient is in severe pain. It is useful for charting pain over time.
- A *verbal rating scale* (VRS) is simpler. The patient is asked if they have no pain, mild, moderate, or severe pain and is scored 0 for no pain, 1 for mild pain, 2 for moderate pain, and 3 for severe pain.
- Assess pain both at rest and on movement. Patients whose pain is severe on movement will not mobilise.
- The patient should be assessed after gentle arousal. Sedation should be scored at the same time: 0 if awake, 1 if dozing intermittently, 2 if mostly sleeping, 3 if difficult to waken.
- Know a limited number of drugs well, and get help if they do not work (you will be able to deal with most painful episodes satisfactorily).

Opioids

Key facts

- *Weak opioids* (codeine, dihydrocodeine) have limited use on their own. They are best used in combination with paracetamol or NSAIDs. Weak opioids cause nausea and constipation as often as strong opioids but without the benefit of potent analgesia.
- *Strong opioids* (morphine, diamorphine, pethidine, methadone, fentanyl) are all pure agonists, acting on similar receptors. All have similar unwanted effects including nausea, vomiting, sedation, itching, reduced gut motility, constipation, and respiratory depression. Also see Box 2.13.

Box 2.13 Opioid overdose

- Drowsiness and respiratory rate <8/min in patient receiving opioids indicate overdose. Pinpoint pupils likely to be present.
  - Pinpoint pupils in alert patient do not indicate overdose.
  - A slow respiratory rate without over-sedation is acceptable, but requires extra vigilance: risk of aspiration, respiratory failure, respiratory arrest.
- Give naloxone 0.2mg IV and repeat every 2–3min until over-sedation is reversed (this will also result in reversal of analgesia).
- As long as patient breathing, you can afford to titrate slowly so as not to completely block the analgesic effect.
- Naloxone is shorter acting than the opioid, so observe carefully for several hours and repeat naloxone if needed

---

Morphine

- Morphine is the drug of choice for postoperative analgesia (Table 2.10)
- Rarely, morphine causes anaphylactoid reactions and bronchospasm. Avoid if actively wheezy or allergic, use *pethidine* or *fentanyl*. Urticaria along the vein is common, but does not indicate 'allergy'.
- Reduce frequency and dose in severe renal or hepatic impairment as repeated doses accumulate leading to excessive sedation and respiratory depression (and potentially inadequate analgesia).

Oral morphine

- Use oral morphine if absorption guaranteed, at 3 × parenteral dose.
- Prescribe oral morphine every 4h, with the same dose available for prn between each dose. Remember antiemetics/laxatives.
- If inadequate analgesia, increase dose by 50%.
- Once on stable dose of oral morphine, if this is required for more than a few days, convert to slow release.
  - Take daily total short-acting dose (regular *plus* all prn), divide by 2. This is the dose for slow-release preparations (MST, MXL) given bd.
  - Continue prn dose at 1/6 the total dose of slow-release morphine.

Sympathetic drive from pain dilates, opioids constrict pupils. Normally, with good analgesia, pupils will be normal to small. A patient with pinpoint pupils is receiving the maximum tolerated dose: if persistent pain, another form of analgesia is required (beware sudden analgesic effect of adjuncts leading to decreased sympathetic drive and subsequent sedation and respiratory depression).

Table 2.10 Options for giving opioid analgesia

Drug	Dose	Notes	Relative strength*
Oral			
Morphine-oral solution, tablets or modified release preparations	5–10mg/4h with equal dose for breakthrough pain 15–30mg bd po with morphine oral solution prescribed for break through (give 1/6 of total daily dose)	If delayed gastric emptying, overdose may occur when normal emptying resumes. Do not combine morphine by different routes.	1/3
Oxycodone	15–30mg po 8h		1
Tramadol	50–100mg po qds	Caution with SSRI	1/10
Codeine	30–60mg po qds		1/10
Parenteral			
IV gives fastest onset of action and repeat doses can be titrated; IM is much slower onset, longer acting and most effective if given regularly.			
Morphine	Severe pain: 5–10 mg IV 2–3min (1mg bolus for elderly/frail) or 7.5mg (40–65kg); 10mg (>60kg) IM 2–3-hourly	Diamorphine is 2 × more potent, no real benefits over morphine in surgical use.	1
Pethidine	Severe pain: 25–50mg slowly IV or 25–100mg IM (repeat after 4 hours if needed)	Use with caution: no better than morphine, Overdose: twitching/fits	1/10
PCA			
Very effective, lock-out period avoids overdose, generally anaesthetist sets this up			
Morphine	e.g. 50mg in 50mL NS, 1mg in 100 mL, 1mL bolus with 5min lockout 1mL bolus with 5min lock out.	Always use dedicated IV to avoid inadvertent bolus when flushed	1
Fentanyl			100
Transdermal			
Fentanyl	25/50/75/100mcg/h patch/72h	Slow, stable pain only	100
Suppository			
Oxycodone	30mg/8h	Opioid	1/2
Epidural			
Extremely effective: diamorphine/alfentanyl/fentanyl used with local anaesthetic. Smaller dose, less nausea/vomiting, respiratory depression. Set up by anaesthetist (📖 p.85)			

* mg for mg relative to parenteral morphine

NSAIDs and paracetamol

Key facts

- Have moderate analgesic potency, NSAIDs also are anti-inflammatory.
- Particularly effective after dental surgery and minor orthopaedic surgery, and reduce the requirement for opioids after major surgery.
- NSAIDs all work in a similar way, never prescribe two different NSAIDs at the same time. See Box 2.14 for contraindications.
- Increase the bleeding time, and may increase blood loss.
- Can be given by many routes: oral, IM, IV, rectal, topical. The oral route is preferred if available. IM diclofenac should be avoided as it is painful and may lead to sterile abscess formation.
- Paracetamol *CAN* be safely prescribed at the same time as a NSAID e.g. ibuprofen and the combination is very effective.

Box 2.14 Contraindications to NSAIDs

Avoid use if possible:

- History of peptic ulceration.
- Renal impairment or oliguria.
- Hyperkalaemia.
- Renal transplantation.
- Anticoagulation or other coagulopathy.
- Severe liver dysfunction.
- Dehydration or hypovolaemia.
- History of exacerbation of asthma with NSAIDs.

Use NSAIDs with caution in:

- Patients >65 years.
- Diabetics with nephropathy and/or renal vascular disease.
- Patients with widespread vascular disease, or hepatobiliary disease including current jaundice.
- Patients on ACE inhibitors, potassium-sparing diuretics, β-blockers, ciclosporin, or methotrexate, loop diuretic therapy, aminoglycosides e.g. vancomycin and gentamicin.

Avoiding renal dysfunction and peptic ulceration

- Electrolytes and creatinine must be measured regularly and any deterioration in renal function or symptoms of gastric upset is an indication for stopping NSAIDs.
- Prolonged courses of NSAIDs are more likely to cause unwanted effects than short perioperative courses, although a single dose of NSAID is enough to cause a significant deterioration in creatinine clearance, or gastric ulceration.
- H_2 blockers (e.g. ranitidine 150 mg po 12h) or proton pump inhibitors (e.g. lansoprazole 30mg od) given with NSAIDs help to protect against GI side effects.
- Give NSAIDS pr/IV in patients at risk of peptic ulceration, although they also have a systemic effect.

Table 2.11 Options for giving non-opiate analgesia

Drug	Dose	Notes
Oral		
Diclofenac	50–75mg 8h po up to 150mg/24h	Risk of peptic ulceration highest with oral administration, so avoid this route in high risk patients or prescribe lansoprazole 30 mg od
Ketorolac	10mg 6h po up to 40mg/24h	
Ibuprofen	200–400mg 6h po up to 1600mg/24h	
Paracetamol	500–1000mg 6h po up to 4g/24h	
Parenteral		
Avoid IM route if possible: it is painful, slower, can cause sterile abscess formation		
Paracetamol	500–1000mg 6h IV up to 4g/24h	Quick onset with IV injection, paracetamol has best efficacy via this route
Ketorolac	10–30mg 6h IM/IV up to 90mg/24h	
Diclofenac	50–75mg 8h IV up to 150mg/24h	requires slow infusion
Transdermal		
Ibuprofen	Topically every 8h	
Suppository		
Diclofenac	100mg pr 12–18h	Slower onset.
Paracetamol	1000mg 6h pr up to 4g/24h	Paracetamol has less efficacy by this route

---

Box 2.15 Patient is in pain despite maximum everything!

- Get patient to describe pain and show you exactly where it is:
  - Look for important causes of severe pain: pressure sores (📖 p.96), limb ischemia (📖 p.158), wound infection (📖 p.96), acute abdomen (📖 p.250), chest pain (📖 p.120)
  - Drain sites are often very painful–either take tension off sutures holding the drains by supporting with adhesive dressing, or consider injecting 1–2mL 0.5% bupivacaine around drain and suture site. Can the drain be removed?
- Review chart: patient may not be *getting* 'maximum everything'.
- Remember WHO pain ladder (📖 p.79):
  - Ensure patient has *regular and prn* analgesia (think maximum dose, contraindications, route/absorption).
  - Move up ladder, or increase dose of strong opioids.
  - Consider adjuncts (anxiolytics, laxatives).
- Contact pain team or duty anaesthetist if pain still uncontrolled.

Local anaesthesia

Key facts

- Provides additional analgesia for all types of surgery.
- Can provide excellent analgesia with no effect on consciousness: a simple technique such as local infiltration into the wound edges at the end of a procedure will provide short-term analgesia.
- Nerve, plexus, or regional blocks can be made to last many hours or days if catheter techniques are used.
- See Box 2.16 for complications.

Box 2.16 Complications of LA

- Systemic toxicity can occur from excessive dosage or accidental IV administration of LAs:
  - Mild: tingling round mouth, metallic taste, tinnitus.
  - Moderate: visual changes, confusion, seizures.
  - Severe: coma, cardiac arrhythmias, and cardiac arrest.
- Treatment: **stop** injection, check ABC, ALS protocols on inside cover. Give O_2, midazolam 2mg may prevent seizures.
- The commonest complications are related to technique.
- Accidental administration of wrong drug, or correct drug via the wrong route, or the incorrect dose is disastrous.

Reducing the risk of LA toxicity

- Calculate total dose of drug that is allowed according to Table 2.12.
- Use lower doses in frail patients or at the extremes of ages.
- Always inject the drug slowly and aspirate regularly looking for blood to indicate an accidental IV injection.
- Add adrenaline (epinephrine) to reduce the speed of absorption. This reduces the maximum blood concentration by about 50%. Use premixed local anaesthetic with adrenaline. *Adrenaline makes no difference to the toxicity of the local anaesthetic if inadvertently injected IV.*
- For the same total dose of LA you will get a better block with a larger volume of 1% than a smaller volume of 2%.

Table 2.12 Doses of LA*

Local anaesthetic	Duration	Suggested dose	Upper dose limit
Bupivacaine	40mins	10mL 0.25%	2mg/kg
Lidocaine	10–20mins	10mL 1%	3mg/kg
Lidocaine + adrenaline	20–40mins	10mL 1% 5mL 2%	7mg/kg

*See BNF and product literature for further information

Box 2.17 Trouble-shooting spinal anaesthesia and epidurals

- Spinal: LA (bupivacaine) injected in CSF at lumbar level for any surgery below the umbilicus.
- Epidural: LA delivered by small catheter into epidural space, continuing postop for pain relief up to 3–4 days.
- Both produce sympathetic block (less pronounced with epidural) the level of block is assessed by asking patient when sensation of cold touch disappears as you go down the chest wall's dermatomes right and left (📖 see p.422).

Hypotension

- Not due to epidural if infusion is opioid only (unless recent bolus of LA given)—look for other causes (📖 p.116).
- Give IV fluid bolus 250mL, and increase rate of maintenance fluid.
- If patient sitting out ask nurse to put them back into bed.
- Check level of block: if spinal block above T10 or thoracic epidural aboveT4, then ask nurse to halve rate of infusion and call anaesthetist.

Bradycardia

- Unresponsive? 📖 see ALS protocol on inside cover.
- If pulse <40bpm give 300mcg of atropine IV, repeat if no response, and give 500mL crystalloid IV fluid bolus.
- Check level of block: high thoracic epidural >T3 may be the cause.
- If in any doubt switch off epidural and call anaesthetist.
- If no evidence of opioid toxicity (📖 p.80) give 2.5mg morphine IM.

Respiratory depression

- Unresponsive? 📖 see ALS protocol on inside cover.
- Give 6L O_2 by tight fitting face mask.
- Suspect opioid toxicity: give naloxone 200mcg IV and repeat (📖 p.80).
- High epidural block? Switch off epidural and call anaesthetist.

Urinary retention

Common: insert Foley catheter.

Dural puncture headache

- Severe occipital pain worse on movement or sitting up, usually resolves in a few days but may be debilitating.
- Bedrest, paracetamol 1g po/IV 6h, keep patient well-hydrated contact anaesthetist.
- Caffeine may help (tablets, cola, or coffee).
- Blood patch (sterile injection of 30mL patients blood into epidural space).

Epidural abscess

- Local cellulitis ± pus around epidural site, ± meningism.
- Contact anaesthetist and medical microbiologist urgently.
- Take pus swab blood cultures, start broad spectrum IV antibiotics.

Surgical sepsis

Table 2.13 Expected wound infection rates after surgical procedures

Types of surgery	Rate of postop infection
Clean (no viscus opened) e.g. hernia repair	<2%
Clean contaminated (viscus opened minimal spillage) e.g. cholecystectomy	<10%
Contaminated (open viscus with spillage or inflammatory disease) e.g. simple appendicectomy	15–20%
Dirty (pus or perforation or incision through abscess) e.g. perforated appendicectomy	>40%

Universal precautions

Treat all patients as potentially infected/infectious.

- Double glove when scrubbed to reduce the risk of skin exposure.
- Wear eye protection (goggles, masks).
- Wear re-enforced gloves when high risk of sharps injury e.g. fracture.
- Wear plastic aprons in procedures with expected soiling.
- Handle all sharps using a transfer container—never pass them hand to hand, and *always* dispose in appropriate sharps bucket.
- Don't allow unnecessary blood or fluid spillage.

Commonest causes of surgical infections

Staphylococci

- Normal flora of skin, oropharynx, and nasopharynx
- *S. aureus*: important pathogen in surgical infections, only species that can coagulate plasma (coagulase +ve).
- 'Coagulase –ve': non *S. aureus* species (e.g. *S. epidermidis*), increasingly common in line/prosthesis infections, munocompromised patients.
- *Antibiotic sensitivities*: flucloxacillin, cefuroxime, gentamicin, vancomycin, teicoplanin (💻 see MRSA, p. 87).
- *Antiseptic sensitivities*: chlorhexidine, povidone-iodine.

Streptococci

- Normal flora of skin, oropharynx and nasopharynx.
- 'α-haemolytic' streptococci haemolyse blood agar e.g. *S. pyogenes*.
- 'β-haemolytic' streptococci also haemolyse RBCs e.g. *S. viridans*.
- *Antibiotic sensitivities*: penicillin, erythromycin, cephalosporins, clindamycin, fusidic acid.
- *Antiseptic sensitivities*: chlorhexidine, povidone-iodine.

Enterococci

- Normal flora of large intestine.
- Increasingly important in: wound, intra-abdominal, UTI, intravascular line infections, dialysis-related infections.
- *Antibiotic sensitivities*: highly resistant (e.g. to all cephalosporins) treat with combination, e.g. ampicillin/gentamicin (💻 for VRE see p. 87).

'The Gram –ve rods'
- Normal flora of large intestine.
- Gram –ve bacilli (rods, also known as **coliforms**) include *E. coli*, *Salmonella*, *Klebsiella*, *Enterobacter*, and *Proteus* spp.
- *Pseudomonas* and *Actinobacter* are non-coliform Gram –ve bacteria.
- *Antibiotic sensitivities:* most are intrinsically resistant to penicillin, and there is increasing resistance to amoxicillin and ampicillin: *cephalosporins are the commonest first line treatment for non-resistant forms or 'extended range' penicillins (e.g. piperacillin/tazobactam); aminoglycosides e.g. gentamicin, streptomycin, amikacin, tobramycin alone or in combination with cephalosporins offer good bacteriocidal action.*

Anaerobes
- Normal flora of skin, oropharynx, colon, terminal ileum, GU tract.
- Include *Bacteroides* and *Clostridia* spp. (bowel).
- *C. difficile* causes pseudomembranous colitis (📖 p.254).
- Cause anaerobic infections including cellulitis, gas gangrene, empyema, and colonize diabetic foot ulcers.
- Act usually with aerobes to produce 'synergistic' necrotizing infections of skin, fascia and muscle spontaneously or after trauma, or surgery.
- *Antibiotic sensitivities:* metronidazole is only active against anaerobes and resistance is rare; most anaerobes are also sensitive to penicillins, cephalosporins, clindamycin, erythromycin, co-trimoxazole.

Methicillin-resistant Staphylococcus aureus (MRSA)
- Resistant to flucloxacillin/methicillin, and all β-lactams, cephalosporins, and carbapenems that work by the same mechanism.
- Glycopeptides (vancomycin and teicoplanin) usually still cover MRSA, as does fusidic acid which has good bone penetration.
- Usually screening swabs to check for MRSA on admission, together with CSUs, tracheostomy swabs etc. whenever it is suspected. Increasingly, decolonization with a combination of topical disinfectants, nasal mupirocin, antiseptic gargles, etc. is attempted.
- Patients are usually barrier nursed in isolation where possible, until three consecutive –ve sets of swabs can be taken as clear.

Vancomycin-resistant enterococci (VRE)
- Low-grade pathogens resistant to aminoglycosides and cephalosporins and often ampicillin, trimethoprim, rifampicin, and imipenem.
- Increasing in incidence, usually only cause actual infection in transplant or immunocompromised patients.
- VRE can survive high pH and temperatures, thus living in the environment (e.g. mattresses etc.) for long periods.
- VRE infection control: barrier nursing in a side room, good handwashing. Discuss with microbiology, especially if septic.

Specific infections

See Tables 2.14–16.

Table 2.14 Antibiotics for common infections

Site	Organisms	First choice	Penicillin allergy
Skin or wound	Staphylococci Streptococci	Flucloxacillin **and** benzylpenicillin	Clindamycin **or** vancomycin
Urine—no catheter	Gram –ve	Trimethoprim **or** co-amoxiclav	Trimethoprim **or** ciprofloxacin
Catheter-associated	Gram –ve Pseudomonas	Gentamicin **and** cefotaxime	Gentamicin (1 dose) **and** ciprofloxacin
Gut (faecal peritonitis)	Coliforms Pseudomonas Anaerobes	Cefuroxime **and** metronidazole; **or** imipenem **and** metronidazole	Gentamicin **and** ciprofloxacin **and** metronidazole
Chest infection	S. pneumoniae H. influenzae	Amoxycillin **or** co-amoxiclav **or** cefaclor	Clarithromycin **or** levofloxacin
	Gram –ve	Cefotaxime **or** imipenem	Ciprofloxacin **and** gentamicin
Ulcers Amputations	Anaerobes	Co-amoxiclav **or** penicillin **and** flucox **and** metronidazole	Metronidazole ± clindamycin

Table 2.15 Coverage of commonly used antibiotics

	Gram +ve cocci		Enterobacteria (mostly Gram –ve)			
	Streptococci	Staphylococci	Coliforms	Pseudomonas	Enterococci	Anaerobes
Ampicillin						
Piperacillin						
Flucloxacillin						
Co-amoxiclav						
Cefuroxime						
Cefotaxime						
Carbopenems						
Aminglycosides						
Quinolones						
Glycopeptides						
Metronidazole						

Table 2.16 Management of the septicaemic patient

Signs	Possible organism	Treatment
Skin generally red ± confluent or peeling rash ± diarrhoea ± confused	S. aureus Group A Streptococci	Flucloxacillin 1–2g qds IV **or** clindamycin 450–1200mg qds IV *Drain and culture all collections*
Catheter *in situ* or recently catheterized	Coliforms Pseudomonas	Gentamicin 5mg/kg daily IV + cefotaxime 2g tds IV
Rampant cellulitis, blistering and dusky purple patches (necrotizing fasciitis)	Group A Streptococci	Imipenem 500mg qds IV + clindamycin 450–1200mg qds IV *Emergency debridement is mandatory*
Black blisters, foul smelling 'gas gangrene'	C. perfringens	Imipenem 500mg qds IV + clindamycin 1.2g qds IV + metronidazole 500mg tds IV
TPN/CVP line infection	Staphylococci If TPN line, consider fungal infection	Vancomycin 1g bd IV add fluconazole 400mg IV od if fungus likely or proven. *Line should be replaced at new site*
Community-acquired pneumonia	S. pneumoniae	Ampicillin 1g qds IV **or** cefotaxime 2g tds
Hospital-acquired pneumonia ± recent anaesthetic	Gram –ve	Gentamicin 5mg/kg daily IV + cefotaxime 2g tds IV **or** imipenem 500mg qds IV **or** ceftazidime 1–2g tds IV
No obvious focus	Anything!	Gentamicin 5mg/kg daily IV + cefotaxime 2g tds IV + metronidazole 500mg tds IV

Contact medical microbiology. Early referral to plastic surgery for cutaneous and deep fascial infections

See also:
- Chest infection p. 192.
- Diarrhoea p. 254.
- Wound infection p. 96.
- Septic shock p. 90.

The septic patient

Key facts

- Septic shock is a medical emergency. It kills.
- Worrying signs in a septic patient include cold, clammy skin, hypotension, WCC<2.0, ↑creatinine, oliguria, confusion, drowsiness.
- Always try to take cultures before starting antibiotics.
- Postop day 1–2: pyrexia usually due to non-infectious causes, e.g. atelectasis, systemic inflammatory response after major surgery.
- Postop day 3–5: pyrexia commonly due to chest, urinary, wound infections, but consider anastomotic leak and prosthesis infection.
- Postop day 7: peripheral/central lines are at highest risk of infection.

Clinical features

Systemic response to infection manifested by two or more of:
- Tachycardia >90 beats/min.
- Tachypnoea >20 breaths/min.
- Pyrexia >38°C (or hypothermia <36°C). (Box 2.18)
- WCC > 12×10^9/L (or <4×10^9/L).
- Look for localizing signs:
  - *Chest* (📖 p. 192): cough, pain, sputum, ↓air entry, bronchial BS, consolidation on CXR—smokers and COPD patients are highest risk but may not show infection on CXR.
  - *Urinary* (📖 p. 88): frequency, dysuria, nocturia, +ve nitrites/WCC on dipstick, +ve organisms on MC&S.
  - *C. difficile diarrhoea*: diarrhoea in patient on antibiotics, send stool for *C difficile* toxin, give *oral* metronidazole **or** oral vancomycin.
  - *Wound* (📖 p. 96): ↑ tenderness, cellulitis, pus, +ve swabs.
  - *Anastomotic leak* (📖 p. 262): abdominal tenderness/peritonism.
  - *Prosthesis infection*: inability to weight bear, pain on movement, XR: migration of prosthesis/surrounding lytic change.
  - *Line sites*: look for cellulitis around peripheral and central line, and drain sites, +ve cultures from lines.
  - *Epidural* (📖 p. 85): examine site for cellulitis.

Emergency management

1–5 minutes

- Address patient: if unresponsive start ALS protocol (📖 inside back cover).
- Sit the patient up and give 2–6L O_2 by face mask.
- Attach pulse oximetry, BP cuff, telemetry for continuous monitoring.
- Get IV access, send blood for blood cultures FBC, U&Es, LFTs, amylase, clotting, G&S, , blood glucose, and βHCG in ♀.
- If abnormal clotting: request D-dimers FDP, blood film to check for DIC.
- Start IV fluids: bolus 500mL over 10min if BP<120mmHg systolic, or pulse rate >100bpm, or clinical signs of shock: reassess BP immediately after fluid bolus to determine further resuscitation (📖 p. 120).
- Give cefuroxime 1.5g IV/metronidazole 500mg IV if not on antibiotics (or be guided by the clinical picture and Table 2.16).

5–10 minutes
- Proceed with focused history and exam concentrating on localizing symptoms and signs of sepsis as already described.
- Assess response to fluid bolus: repeat if necessary (📖 p. 116).
- 12–lead ECG in hypotensive, elderly patients.
- Call senior cover to discuss management early.

Establish a diagnosis
- Place urethral catheter (📖 p. 360), send CSU for MC&S, ABGs (📖 p. 174), consider CVP line (📖 p. 352).
- Request cultures of stool, sputum, any wound exudate.
- CXR, AXR.
- Consider chest, abdomen, and pelvic CT:
  - With IV contrast if renal function satisfactory.
  - With oral/enteral constrast if you suspect anastomotic leak.
- If blood cultures are persistently +ve despite appropriate antibiotic therapy:
  - Consider TTE or TOE to confirm bacterial endocarditis.
  - Surgical re-exploration if possible graft or prosthesis infection.

Box 2.18 Patient with pyrexia but no signs of infection

- POD 1–2? Likely just atelectasis, request saline nebs and physio.
- History and exam focusing on infection sources (📖 p.88): at a minimum ask about chills/rigors, cough, sputum, dysuria, wound pain, line pain, and look at all wounds, lines, and drain sites.
- Take blood cultures whenever temperature >38.0°C, and send urine, stool, sputum, any wound exudate.
- Request FBC, CRP (measure serially to monitor trend), CXR.
- If patient unwell/WCC >15.0 discuss choice of antibiotics with medical microbiologist.
- If patient well, and WCC <15.0 do not start antibiotics, consider DVT (📖 p.168), transfusion reaction (📖 p.70), SIRS (📖 see below), repeat cultures.

Systemic inflammatory response syndrome (SIRS)

- Any two or more of the four following signs:
  - Tachycardia >90 beats/min.
  - Tachypnoea >20 breaths/min.
  - Pyrexia >38°C (or hypothermia <36°C).
  - White blood count >12 ×10⁹/L (or <4 × 10⁹/L).
- **Without** identifiable bacteraemia or infectious source and in the setting of a known cause of endothelial inflammation such as:
  - Pancreatitis.
  - Ischaemia.
  - Multiple trauma and tissue injury.
  - Haemorrhagic shock.
  - Immune mediated organ injury.

Blood-borne viruses and surgery

Viral hepatitis

Hepatitis A
- Self-limiting hepatitis, common in children, young adults, after travel, diagnosed by finding anti-HAV antibody in blood.
- Spread by faecal–oral route, the incubation period is 2–6 weeks.
- Active or passive immunization recommended for travel to 3rd world.

Hepatitis B
- DNA virus causing acute hepatitis (UK: 4500 new cases in 2000), 5–10% fail to clear virus after infection. 6% of people worldwide are carriers.
- Transmission: blood, needle stick, IVDU, sexual intercourse, birth.
- After exposure, surface (HBsAg)/e antigen (HBeAg) appear in blood at 8–12 weeks, both imply infectivity (core antigen HBcAg intracellular).
- Antibodies in blood after 10 weeks (anti-HBe) to 24 weeks (anti-HBs)
  - **HBsAg / HBeAg +ve at >6 months**: carrier status, infectious.
  - **HBsAb +ve:** marker of immunization or infection.
  - **HBcAb +ve:** past infection (not immunization), check HBsAg.
- Chronic infection is infectious, and can lead to cirrhosis and hepatoma.
- Hospital staff are routinely offered vaccination against Hep B:
  - Infectious carriers may not perform exposure-prone procedures.
  - Vaccination voluntary, alternatives: frequent tests/limited practice.
  - The NHS Injury Benefits Scheme provides some benefits.
- *Treatment* for chronic infection: interferon and nucleoside analogues.

Hepatitis C
- RNA virus causing mild hepatitis (or asymptomatic), transmitted by blood, IVDU, sexual intercourse, acupuncture. There is no vaccination.
- Diagnosis by detecting Hep C RNA and anti-HCV in blood.
- In 85%, chronic infection occurs (UK prevalence 0.5%), 20–30% develop cirrhosis over ~20 years, ↑risk of hepatoma in these.
- *Treatment*: pegylated interferon/ribavirin, ↓chronic infection by 50%, durable virological response in chronic disease 50–80%.
- Surgeons are tested for Hep C, and may not operate if Hep C +ve.

Human immunodeficiency virus (HIV)
- RNA retrovirus, transmission: intercourse, IVDU, sharps, blood, birth.
- Prevalence in S. Africa adults is 15–30%, sub-Saharan Africa is 5–15%, in homosexual ♂ at London GU clinics is 10%, in UK IVDUs is 1%
- HIV infection results in widespread immunological dysfunction, a fall in CD4+ve T-cells, monocytes, antige presenting cells (APCs), and risk of opportunistic infections.
- Incubation period (3 months) may be followed by seroconversion illness (flu-like symptoms) after which ELISA test for HIV antibodies is +ve (patient infectious *before* antibodies detectable), leading to generalized lymphadenopathy (>1cm, >2 extra-inguinal sites)
- Untreated, AIDS-related complex (ARC) and acquired immunodeficiency syndrome (AIDS) develop over 5–10 years.
- Median survival with untreated AIDS is 2 years, treated is >15 years.
- Treatment: highly active anti-retroviral therapy (HAART), rotation of different drugs to avoid resistance.

High-risk procedures

The UK General Medical Council obliges surgeons, if required, to operate on patients regardless of patients' serological or infective status. High-risk procedures include:

- Any invasive procedure in HIV +ve patients.
- Invasive procedures in high-risk populations.
- Biopsies for the diagnosis of opportunistic infection or suspected HIV, or AIDS-defining malignancies, e.g. Kaposi's sarcoma, B cell lymphoma. Sharps injuries are avoidable but still occur regularly so you should know what to do if you or a colleague are injured (see Box 2.19).

Box 2.19 Help! I got a sharps injury, what should I do?

Treat all patients as potential infection risk. Avoiding infection depends on speed of treatment.

0–5 minutes
- Stop what you're doing immediately, get someone else to continue.
- Immediate basic treatment reduces infection risk:
  - Needlestick: squeeze wound to express blood, wash with soap and water, do not press on wound directly.
  - Splash onto eyes, mouth, nose: rinse well with water (NS if eyes).
  - Is patient known HIV/Hep B/C +ve (notes, nurses, high-risk).
  - Phone *occupational health* or *A&E* (*duty nursing manager* or *medical microbiologist* if out of hours and no A&E) to arrange blood sample/any treatment: *all* hospitals have clear protocols.
- Document exposure in patient notes and incident form.

5–30 minutes
- Assess risk posed by patient/nature of injury, document your vaccinations, take **your** blood for viral serology (voluntary baseline).
- If high risk, *first dose post-exposure prophylaxis (PEP) within 1 hour of injury for HIV, or 24 hours for Hep B.* Arrange follow-up with Occupational Health (or HIV clinic).
- Delegate colleague to talk to patient to identify high risk activity, request consent to take blood for HIV and hepatitis testing (voluntary).

Next few weeks
- Patient's blood results should be available in <24h.
- You should have a repeat blood test at 3/12 and 6/12 (voluntary).
- Safe sex, no blood donation but usually OK to operate (check!).
- PEP course is 4–6 weeks—nausea, vomiting, diarrhoea common.

	Hep B	Hep C	HIV
UK prevalence	<0.5%	0.5%	<0.1%
Transmission in needlestick	1 in 3	1 in 50	1 in 300
PEP	Ig/booster	None	Triple therapy

Wound care, drains, and stomas

Wounds

📖 Also see Wound infections and dehiscence (📖 p. 96), bleeding (p. 98), vacuum dressings (📖 p. 342).

- Surgeons should write instructions for removal of non-absorbable sutures in their operation notes, so check. Usually remove:
  - Abdominal and trunk sutures 7–10 days postop.
  - Face sutures 5 days postop.
  - Drain sutures 3–5 days post drain removal.
- Patients can shower or bath within 3–4 days of surgery, but should avoid letting the wound get soggy.

Drains

- Drains are used to remove or prevent abnormal collections of fluid including blood, exudate, pus, or air—complications include:
  - Damage to surrounding structures.
  - Potential route of introduction of infection.
  - Blockage or may move, allowing fluid to accumulate.
- Just like sutures, the operation note should outline when drains may be removed: if in doubt always check with the surgeon—generally:
  - Abdominal drains are removed when there are no concerns of intra-abdominal sepsis, and 24h drainage<50mL at 3–5 days postop.
  - Chest drains may be removed when there is no airleak (bubbles in underwater seal when patient coughs), 24h drainage <100mL, and no pneumothorax on CXR when drain is off suction >24h.
  - Wound flap drains may be removed at 5–10 days when 24h drainage <20mL
- Sudden increase in drainage should be reported to surgeon, as should a failure for self-vaccing drains to maintain their seal as this may reflect an important problem.
- Never clamp a chest drain, and always check the water seal is at the appropriate level.
- Most drains are removed by simple, gentle traction, *except chest drain:*
  - Patient must not inhale as drain is removed (risk of pneumothorax).
  - Ask patient to fully exhale and hold breath while you remove drain, get an assistant to tie drain hole closed.

Stoma

A stoma is created by joining any organ with a lumen to the skin:
- *Tracheostomy:* creating hole in trachea and passing ET tube through overlying skin into trachea, to help long-term ventilated patients.
- *Ileostomy/colostomy:* formed from ileum/large bowel respectively.
  - May be loop (often to 'rest' the distal bowel) or end (usually as a result of surgical removal of distal bowel).
  - Colostomies are usually flush, have flat mucosal folds, tend to be light pink in colour, they are usually on the left side of abdomen.
  - Ileostomies are usually spouted, have prominent mucosal folds, tend to be dark pink/red in colour, and right sided.

- *Urostomy:* formed from a short length of disconnected ileum into which one or both ureters are diverted (usually after radical lower urinary tract surgery).
- *Gastrostomy/jejunostomy:* either a surgically or endoscopically (PEG/PEJ) formed connection between anterior stomach and anterior abdominal wall (for gastric drainage or direct feeding).
  - Usually narrow calibre, flush with little visible mucosa, and are most common in the left upper quadrant of the abdomen.
  - They are usually fitted with indwelling tubes or access devices, with inflatable balloons to secure them (like Foley): removal when feeding no longer required by deflating balloon and gentle traction.
  - Once out they cannot easily be replaced.
  - Treat blockages by attempting to flush with cola or sodium bicarbonate, or *very carefully* passing down a flexible wire.

Box 2.20 What care do new stoma patients need?

Preoperative issues
- Consent for any bowel resection should include a discussion about the possibility of a stoma, or 'bag'. A stoma is unlikely in most elective resections, except the following where it is an integral part of the procedure: *AP resection, anterior resection, Hartman's stage 1, any 'defunctioning' surgery.*
- Most colorectal units have a stoma nurse, who should see all these patients preoperatively for counselling.
- The stoma site should be marked by the surgeon preoperatively.

Postoperative care
- Any patient with a new stoma should be seen by the stoma nurse for counselling and teaching stoma care.
- Find out from the surgeon if there is any option for reversal.
- There is a range of stoma bags with hypoallergenic adhesive skin barriers (like Duoderm®) to protect the surrounding skin from effluent, bags which in the case of ileostomies can be drained instead of changed, filters (including gas filters for pressure equalization during air travel), wipes and lotions.
- Patients should be taught diet modifications: increase fluid intake, avoiding certain foods (eggs/fish: odour; carbonated drinks: gas) to reduce problems with stoma output.
- Problems that need surgical input include *prolapse, para-stomal herniation, ischaemia, narrowing, involution.*

Wound problems

Pressure sores

Key facts

- Damage to skin from prolonged pressure: usually over bony areas especially sacrum, heels, ischium, scalp, elbows, scapula. Four stages:
  - I: persistent redness but skin not broken, may itch or hurt.
  - II: epidermis broken, may look like blister.
  - III: obvious ulcer, dermis and subcutaneous fat exposed.
  - IV: large wound, damage to muscle, bone, tendons or joints.
- Pressure sores decrease quality of life and life expectancy.
- Risk factors: age, immobility, sensory neuropathy, faecal and urinary incontinence, malnutrition, low BMI, smoking, vascular disease, diabetes mellitus.

Prevention and treatment

- Meticulous nursing care: frequent turning of immobile patients, attention to patient hygiene, avoid soiling, use of special mattresses and supports, extra attention to nutrition (📖 p. 244) and physiotherapy.
- Liaise with tissue viability nurse for stage II: involve plastic surgery for stage III and IV which may need debridement/vacuum dressing.

Wound infection

Key facts

- Most wound infections are acquired from the patient's own flora.
- The majority are skin organisms (e.g. *S. aureus*, *S. epidermidis*)
- The second commonest cause is contamination from opened viscera at surgery (e.g. *E. coli* from the GI tract, *Pseudomonas* from biliary tree).
- *Symptoms*: pain, discharge, malaise, anorexia and fever.
- *Signs*: fever, tachycardia; red, swollen, tender wound (may be discharging pus or fluctuant due to contained pus).
- *Complications*: bacteraemia is common but rarely significant, septicaemia reflects drug resistance or immunocompromised patient.

Emergency management (📖 see also p. 90)

- Get IV access—give crystalloid IV up to 1000mL if ↓BP/↑HR.
- Send any discharging pus for MC&S , and blood for FBC and cultures.

Early treatment

- IV antibiotics if there are systemic features. If no pre-existing infection, cover *Staphylococcus*: flucloxacillin 1g stat, then 500mg qds.
- If the patient is immunocompromised or very unwell, add broad spectrum cover to include anaerobes: metronidazole 500mg IV tds, cefuroxime 1.5g IV stat + 750mg IV tds.
- If MRSA infection possible, consult microbiology, consider adding vancomycin 1000mg IV bd.
- Open or aspirate the wound if there is contained pus.
- Consider a vacuum dressing particularly if there is prosthetic material in the wound that is at risk of infection.

Dehiscence

Key facts
- Wound dehiscence may be superficial (including skin and subcutaneous tissue) or full thickness (involving fascial closures or bony closures).
- Full thickness dehiscence will expose deep structures.
- In the abdomen this may include the viscera which may protrude through the wound (evisceration).

Causes
- Most wound dehiscences are 2° to wound infection.
- Contributory factors include immunosuppression, malnutrition, steroid use, poor surgical technique, previous surgery or procedures.
- Occasionally dehiscence is due to intracavity pathology (e.g. anastomotic leak causing enteric fistulation, outgrowth of residual tumour).

Symptoms and signs
- Usually painless
- Open wound, visible fat and fascia if superficial; visible viscera if full.
- Occasionally associated organ dysfunction if involved by the accompanying wound infection (e.g. pericarditis/anterior mediastinitis in sternal dehiscence)

Emergency management
- Ensure IV access, fluid resuscitation if low BP (📖 p. 116).
- Calm the patient, particularly if there is any degree of evisceration.

Early treatment
- If viscera exposed, cover these with saline soaked dressings.
- Give IV antibiotics if wound infection (📖 see Wound infection, p. 96).
- If dehiscence is superficial, ensure wound is open and any pus is fully drained. Lightly pack wound with absorbent dressing (e.g. Sorbsan®)

Definitive management

Superficial
- Continue regular wound lavage and dressings, treat infection.
- For large defects consider vacuum assisted closure.

Full thickness
- Resuturing/closure of the defect in theatre may be appropriate.
- Some clinical factors (presence of infection or intestinal contents, fistulae, severe immunocompromise, physiologically unstable patient, intracavity pathology causing the dehiscence) make it preferable for a chronic wound to form with closure by 2° intention, assisted by vacuum closure devices.

Postoperative haemorrhage

Key facts

- Postoperative haemorrhage may be arterial or venous.
- *Arterial haemorrhage* is rare and occurs from vascular anastomoses, or loose vessel ties: it is rapid, bright red in colour, and often pulsatile.
- *Venous bleeding* is commoner, usually due to the opening up of unsecured venous channels or from damage to the liver/spleen at surgery: it is non pulsatile, low pressure, and dark in colour but can be very large volume and just as life threatening as arterial bleeding.
- Most postoperative bleeding is contained within body cavities.
- Drains, even correctly placed, are an unreliable sign of bleeding: rely on your clinical instincts even if the drains are empty.

Clinical features

- *1° haemorrhage*: occurs immediately after surgery or as a continuation of intraoperative bleeding. Usually due to unsecured blood vessels (e.g. liver bleeding following trauma).
- *Reactionary haemorrhage*: occurs within the first 24h. Usually due to venous bleeding and is commonly thought to be due to improved postoperative circulation and fluid volume exposing unsecured vessels which bleed (e.g. delayed splenic bleeding following minor trauma at laparotomy).
- *2° haemorrhage*: occurs up to 10 days postoperatively. Usually due to infection of operative wounds or raw surfaces causing clot disintegration and bleeding from exposed tissue.

Symptoms

- Confusion/agitation from cerebral hypoperfusion 2° to hypotension.
- May be painful if blood volume within confined space.
- Drop in Hb may be early sign (also due to haemodilution from IV fluid).

Signs

- Overt signs of bleeding are rare—soaked dressings, blood in drains.
- Pallor, sweating, tachypnoea, tachycardia, hypotension (a late and ominous sign in children and young adults).

Emergency management

Resuscitation

- Establish large calibre peripheral IV access—give crystalloid up to 1000mL bolus if tachycardic or hypotensive, stop anticoagulants.
- **Only use O Rh –ve blood for resuscitation if patient in extremis.**
- Take blood for FBC, clotting, and XM 2–4U.
- Don't waste time inserting central venous catheter. They are unreliable measures of CVP at the bedside, and too long/fine calibre to be useful for rapid volume resuscitation.
- Attempt to control superficial bleeding with direct compression. Do not use tourniquets on limb wounds.
- Get senior help immediately if significant blood loss. Consider alerting theatres and/or ITU.
- Catheterize and place on a fluid balance chart if hypotensive but stable.

Establish a diagnosis
- Investigation of coagulopathy is described in Table 12.5 p. 401.
- The cause may be obvious from the bleeding or the operation.
- Read the operation note—is there any potential cause mentioned?
- If the bleeding is severe, the only way to establish a diagnosis may be at re-operation.
- If the patient is stable and re-operation is undesirable consider imaging:
  - CT scanning may reveal intra-abdominal or intrathoracic blood.
  - Angiography may reveal active bleeding sites and may be therapeutic (coil embolization).

Definitive management

Most postoperative bleeding does not require re-operation but if it does it should always be by a senior surgeon.
- If the surgeon who performed the original surgery is not available, try to contact them in case they can give useful information about the original procedure (it is also polite to inform them of complications).
- If re-operation is highly undesirable (e.g. rebleeding after solid organ trauma) then definitive conservative management might include:
  - Radiologically-guided embolization.
  - Fresh frozen plasma infusions.
  - Controlled, permissive, hypotension.
  - Monitoring on ITU.

Wound haematoma

This is a localized collection of blood beneath the wound, usually characterized by swelling and discoloration.
- If this occurs after *vascular surgery, flap surgery, or procedures on the limbs or neck* get senior help as urgent surgical exploration and evacuation may be indicated to avoid *ischaemia, compartment syndromes, airway obstruction, flap failure,* or *ongoing haemorrhage.*
- Apply firm pressure followed by a pressure dressing.
- Check clotting and FBC and treat appropriately (☐ p. 101).
- Withhold heparin and warfarin.
- Surgical management is the same as for haemorrhage (☐ p. 98).

Haematological complications

📖 See also Excessive anticoagulation, Tables 12.2, 12.4 and 12.5.

Anaemia

Key facts

- Defined as low Hb concentration (Table 2.17), due to ↓red cell mass or haemodilution (e.g. pregnancy, over-enthusiastic fluid resuscitation).
- In acute blood loss, blood volume drops, but Hb may not fall for several hours: do not rely on Hb to guide resuscitation.
- A drop of 1g/dL reflects roughly 1 unit of blood lost.
- Preoperative causes:
  - **Microcytic** (MCV <76fL): Fe deficiency from blood loss (GI bleed, menstruation) or low intake, chronic disease rarely sickle cell anaemia, thalassaemia.
  - **Normocytic** (76–96fL): chronic disease (cancer, renal or bone marrow failure), pregnancy, blood loss.
  - **Macrocytic** (MCV >96fl):, EtOH abuse, liver disease, ↓vitamin B12/ folate (Crohn's, gastrectomy, ↓intake), haemolysis, hypothyroidism.
- Commonest causes postoperatively: blood loss (intraoperative/ongoing from wounds), dilutional (excess fluid IV/retention), persistent preoperative cause.

Diagnosis

- Check Hb, MCV, reticulocyte count, blood film.
- Think about features of potential causes to direct further tests and management (📖 Box 2.21).

Treatment

- None if patient asymptomatic (young patients tolerate anaemia well).
- Treat fluid overload (📖 p. 65).
- Blood transfusion if compromised (📖 p. 69), oral B12, folate, FeSO₄.

Heparin induced thrombocytopaenia (HIT)

Key facts

- HIT occurs in up to 5% of patients receiving heparin (10 × more common with unfractionated heparin).
- Results from formation of complement-mediated heparin-dependent IgG platelet antibody, resulting in fall in platelet count to <100, 5–10 days after initiation of heparin, or after the first dose of heparin in patients with previous exposure to heparin within the last 3 months.
- Bleeding complications are uncommon given the level of platelets.
- HITT develops with major thrombotic episodes (e.g. CVA, in 25%).

Diagnosis

Fall in platelets to $<100 \times 10^9$/L, or by >50% **and** +ve for PF4 antibodies.

Treatment

- Discontinue all heparin therapy, including heparinized saline flushes.
- If anticoagulation is required then danaparoid, lepirudin, and fondaparinux are alternatives.
- They cannot be reversed, and require specialized assays.
- Start warfarin postop only once platelets have recovered.

Table 2.17 Normal values for blood

Hb	♀: 11.5–16.0 g/dL ♂: 13.5–18.0g/dL	MCV	76–96fL
WCC	4–11 × 10⁹/L	PT	10–14sec
Platelets	150–400 × 10⁹/L	APTT	35–45sec

Box 2.21 My patient's Hb has dropped to 7.2g/dL postop

- Think about: acute bleed (melaena, may be delayed after bowel surgery, haematemesis, epistaxis), intraop blood loss/continued loss from wound, NSAID/stress peptic ulcer, preop anaemia.
- Ask about: bleeding/swelling at wound, postural hypotension, dyspnoea, chest pain on exertion, weight gain >5kg from preop.
- Look for: ↑pulse, ↓BP, clammy, confusion, peripheral oedema.
- A sudden drop in Hb is more worrying than a steady decline.
- *Shock:* (📖 p.116) means active bleed: ABC, large bore IV access, 500mL NS bolus over 10min, XM 4U RBC, give 2U over 2h, correct clotting abnormalities.
- *Symptomatic:* SOB on exertion, tachycardia, postural hypotension: give 2U RBC over 6–8h. FeSO₄, folate and B12, stop NSAIDs, start omeprazole 20mg po/IV od.
- *Asymptomatic:* young patient start FeSO₄, B12, omeprazole, daily FBC. Furosemide 10mg IV/po if >5kg above preop weight.

Disseminated intravascular coagulation (DIC)

Key facts
- DIC may occur postop as a complication of sepsis, transfusion reaction, drug reaction, transplant rejection, aortic aneurysm repair, cancer.
- It is characterized by widespread activation of coagulation, resulting in the formation of intravascular fibrin, (which can shear red cells as they pass) fibrin degradation products, consumption of platelets and clotting factors, and thrombosis.
- Patients may present with bleeding from indwelling venous lines, wounds, and minor abrasions.

Diagnosis
There is no single diagnostic test. The following findings suggest DIC:
- Sudden fall in platelet count to <100 × 10⁹/L.
- Bleeding and/or thrombotic complications.
- ↑APTT, PT, INR.
- ↑fibrin degradation products and ↑ D-dimeers.
- ↓fibrinogen correlates with severity.
- Red cell fragments on blood film.

Management
The key is to treat the underlying disorder. Bleeding patients should receive FFP, platelets, blood and cryoprecipitate as indicated by coagulation screens. Patients with thrombosis should be heparinized. This condition may be fatal; involve your seniors and a haematologist without delay.

Alcohol-related problems

Delirium due to mild alcohol withdrawal

- The commonest alcohol-related problem in general surgery.
- Patient gives history of regularly drinking >2–3U/day, but often still within socially acceptable norms, γGT often elevated.
- 2–3 days postop they may be uncooperative, agitated, confused, paranoid. Tremor and seizures in severe withdrawal (📖 p. 306).
- Prevent withdrawal with *chlordiazepoxide (5–10 mg 6h po reducing dose over 7–10 days*, speed depends on severity of withdrawal)
- Treat delirium with *5–10mg diazepam po/IV 4h prn* to sedate, as haloperidol lowers seizure threshold in this context.
- Quiet side-room with regular observations if possible
- Rarely, it may be appropriate to give 1 unit spirits/beer/sherry.

Box 2.22 Avoiding alcohol-related problems

Identify problems before they happen

- Quantify drinking (how many glasses, of what, home measure >> pub measure) 4/4 CAGE questionnaire is very sensitive: (Do you think you should **C**ut down? Ever get **A**ngry if people criticise your drinking? Do you feel **G**uilty? Ever had **E**ye-opener? (early morning drink?)
- Ask about weight loss and history of GI bleeding, recurrent accidents, infections, drink-related convictions.
- Look for spider naevi, ascites, jaundice, bruising, malnutrition, fetor, neglect, tremor, peripheral neuropathy, psychosis, encephalopathy, hypertension, cardiac failure, arrhythmias.
- Investigations: ↑MCV, ↓Fe, marrow depression, coagulopathy, ↓glucose, ↓K^+, ↑triglycerides, ↑γ-GT/AST/ALT, ↓albumin.
- Blood alcohol 80mg/dL is legal driving limit in the UK: 200mg/dL causes severe intoxication; and >500mg/dL may be fatal.
- ECG: conduction defects, bifid T-wave, ST changes (similar to digoxin changes), arrhythmias (commonly AF).
- TTE if suspect alcohol dilated cardiomyopathy.

Prevent problems if possible

- Avoid elective surgery in the presence of acute alcohol toxicity.
- If emergency, ensure rehydration and avoid ↓K^+, ↓glucose.
- Correct any coagulopathy with FFP and/or platelets (📖 p.68)
- Treat anaemia (📖 p.100).
- Assume patient has a full stomach: may need NGT.
- *Prescribe Pabrinex® 2 pairs IV 8h or thiamine 200mg po od*, serious allergic reactions can occur, have resuscitation trolley ready.
- Multivitamins, chlordiazepoxide and diazepam.
- Patients with liver failure need ICU postop.
- Patients with GI bleeding and cirrhosis may develop hepatic failure and may need an NGT to stop digestion of blood.
- Anticipate alcohol withdrawal symptoms.
- Look for unusual infections in immunocompromised patients.

Other alchohol-related problems
Liver disease, upper GI bleeds, pancreatitis
- Three progressive phases of liver disease are described:
  - Fatty liver is reversible with abstinence and rarely causes illness.
  - Alcoholic hepatitis causes abdominal pain, weight loss, jaundice, fever. Can lead to acute liver failure and cirrhosis in severe cases, reversible if mild. Mortality (~40% at 1 year) improved by steroids.
  - Alcoholic cirrhosis is characterized by jaundice, ascites, portal hypertension, hepatic failure. Cirrhosis is irreversible and associated with ↑ bleeding risk (📖 p. 264) and 1° liver cancer.
- Gastritis, erosive gastric ulcers, Mallory–Weiss tears, oesophageal varices if severe disease with portal hypertension in chronic abuse.
- Both chronic and acute pancreatitis can be caused by alcohol misuse. The mortality rate in acute pancreatitis is 10–40%.

Cardiovascular disease
- *Cardiac arrhythmias:* AF complicates both binge drinking and chronic alcohol misuse. Ventricular arrhythmias are also reported.
- Hypertension: 7–11% of in ♂ (1% in ♀) due to alcohol ingestion >2U/day. Intracerebral and SAH are commoner in alcoholics.
- *IHD:* incidence increases if alcohol intake exceeds 2U/day.
- *Alcoholic cardiomyopathy* is caused by a direct toxic effect of alcohol (not by thiamine deficiency). Commonest in ♂ aged 30–60 years. Patients have CCF, and oedema worsened by low albumin.

Metabolic effects and malnutrition
- Hypoglycaemia: direct alcohol effect, liver and pancreatic disease.
- Ketoacidosis may present after binge drinking in association with vomiting and fasting. Blood alcohol concentrations may not be elevated.
- Metabolic alkalosis may be seen after prolonged vomiting.
- Many features of chronic alcohol misuse are due to substituting normal food with alcohol calories with no other nutritional value:
  - *Macrocytic anaemia:* from toxic effect of alcohol, megaloblastic change, folate deficiency, Fe deficiency, poor diet, GI blood loss.
  - *Marrow toxicity:* neutropenia: folate deficiency; thrombocytopenia can complicate clotting deficiencies.
  - *Cerebellar degeneration* due to toxicity and thiamine deficiency.
  - *Wernicke's encephalopathy* and *Korsakoff's psychosis:* ↓thiamine. *NB Wernicke's is reversible, Korsakoff's is not! Give thiamine!*
  - *Peripheral neuropathy:* B vitamin deficiency.
  - *Immunodeficiency* with ↑respiratory infections (including TB) due to malnutrition, neutropaenia, poor social conditions, and self neglect.
  - *Skin diseases:* psoriasis, eczema, rosacea, fungal infections, acne.

Intoxication, trauma, and coma
- Alcoholic coma has a mortality of up to 5%. Treat conservatively: prevent airway obstruction and aspiration of vomit. May require ICU.
- Blood alcohol concentration >400mg/100mL puts patients at risk of respiratory arrest. Seek other causes for coma (e.g. head injury, other drugs, methanol, metabolic causes, infection, hypoglycaemia).

Challenging patients

Pregnant patients

- Check *BNF* Appendix 4 when prescribing, use smallest effective dose.
- Acceptable drugs (avoid all drugs in first trimester): penicillins, cephalosporins, heparin, ranitidine, paracetamol, *avoid* NSAIDS, warfarin, ACE-I, thiazide diuretics, tetracycline, antiemetics. Use opioids cautiously.
- Avoid XRs and CT scans (consider MRI or U/S where possible).
- Cardiac arrest: call O&G + paeds in addition to arrest team.

Young children

- Always have chaperone: either nurse or parent.
- History: presenting problem, PMHx: pregnancy problems, weeks' gestation (37–42/40 is normal), type of delivery, special care, developmental milestones (are they doing everything their friends are?) immunization history, previous admissions, social history, family history.
- Examination: all systems as you would do for adult, additionally in young children check ears and throat, and position on growth chart.
- Check *BNF* or ask paediatric team before prescribing fluids or drugs.
- Obtaining consent is discussed on 📖 p. 51.
- More likely to need GA for minor procedures.
- Put EMLA® cream on cannula sites and cover with Tegaderm® 30min before cannulating young children, use butterfly needle for phlebotomy, and always ask nurse or parent to hold child.
- Avoid XRs and CTs (consider MRI—may need GA; or US).

IVDU

- Try to get accurate history of nature of drugs, most recent use.
- IV cannulation often difficult: consider femoral vein for phlebotomy, and central venous line for infusions, and *use universal precautions*.
- High risk for HIV and Hep B and C: sharps injury advice (📖 p. 93).
- Give analgesia po/pr if fears about drug seeking behaviour, do not undertreat pain. Remember that opiate users may need large doses to treat pain due to opioid tolerance.

Factitious

- Very, very rarely patients feign illness: e.g. Münchausen's disease (want medical attention even undergoing surgery for invented problems) or to obtain prescription drugs, or a warm bed for the night.
- Always err on the side of believing the patient, try to obtain old hospital records and speak to GP or carers for full background.
- Give medication pr/po if concerned about drug seeking behaviour.
- Involve psychiatrist at early stage if history of factitious illness.

Immunocompromised

- Splenectomy: require pneumococcal, *haemophilus* B, meningitis A+C vaccine before splenectomy, flu vaccine yearly, penicillin V 2 years post splenectomy, amoxicillin for any sepsis, in addition to standard prophylaxis.
- HIV: avoid elective surgery if CD4 <100, ensure patient on triple therapy and involve ID specialist in care: *universal precautions vital*.

Elderly patients

Key facts

- Surgical mortality increases with age due to chronic medical disorders, delays in seeking surgical opinion, and ↓physiological reserve.
- Medical causes of postop mortality outnumber surgical ones by 3 to 1.
- Common causes of death include pneumonia, MI, and CVA.

Prevention and management of postoperative complications

- *Infection:* immune responses are blunted, ↓WCC response to infection, central temperature regulation compromised so infection may be present without fever. Give standard antibiotic prophylaxis, look for other signs of sepsis (📖 p. 90), maintain meticulous wound care.
- *DVT and PE:* impaired mobility means PE common cause of death in elderly. LMWH should be routine, and started on admission in elderly patients whether or not surgery is planned (📖 p. 61).
- *Malnutrition:* due to ↑gut transit time but ↓food absorption associated with ↑surgical morbidity and mortality. ↓metabolic rate, ↓muscle mass; ↓turgor and elasticity of skin makes it poor sign of hydration/nutrition. Start oral supplements early e.g. Ensure® with NGT feed for those with major malnutrition (📖 p. 244).
- *Urinary retention, incontinence, infection:* common postop in the elderly. Place catheter for urine output monitoring, particularly in patients with cardiac and renal disease, immobile patients after orthopaedic/abdominal surgery. Minimize retention by catheter removal within 24h, in the evening if practical (📖 p. 216).
- *Delirium:* hearing, sight, cognition diminish. 2/3rds of elderly patients develop postop delirium causing ↑length of stay, complications, mortality, and subsequent institutional care. Take extra care to avoid metabolic disturbance, dehydration, infection, hypoxia, alcohol withdrawal, urinary retention, change in environment, opioids (📖 p. 80).
- *Falls:* from poor balance, sensory impairment: visual and hearing loss. ↓bone density and mass predispose to fractures. Avoid and treat delirium (📖 p. 294), help with incontinence to reduce unsupervized mobilizing, always X-ray hips and pelvis after falls and consider head CT.
- *Iatrogenic:* rationalize drug chart carefully to reduce polypharmacy, and always take care when rewriting not to omit key drugs.
- *Chest infection:* TLC↓ by 25% during ageing, ↓muscular strength, lung elasticity, gas exchange, and PaO_2. Kyphosis also reduces lung capacity. Always prescribe nebulizers, chest PT, and ensure analgesia adequate.
- *MI, CCF and AF* ↓ LV function/stress response, ↑arterial wall stiffness and ↑↑silent IHD. AF common. Always check patient on correct cardiac drugs, review cardiovascular system thoroughly and look at ECG!
- *Renal dysfunction:* poor autoregulation of renal blood flow, ↓GFR, ↓in renal concentrating ability, ↓response to fluid/dehydration. Ensure optimal hydration, maintain BP (📖 p. 116). If any concern, start hourly fluid balance chart (📖 p. 65), use NS instead of 5% glucose IV.

↓↓muscle bulk means lower creatinine: small elevation of the serum creatinine may conceal major renal impairment. Use Cockroft–Gault formula to estimate GFR = {(140−age[years]) × weight[kg] × constant/creatinine)}, where constant is 1.23 for ♂ and 1.04 for ♀ if creatinine in μmol/L. Normal range 55–140mL/min. If in doubt get EDTA GFR measurement from nuclear medicine.

Transplant patients

Key facts

- Transplant patients are usually admitted under a specialist team, but occasionally they require non-transplant surgery for complications related to chronic immunosuppression (neoplastic or infective disease), or unrelated conditions (most commonly old heart and kidney transplant patients).
- In patients experiencing rejection, supportive management follows the principles of organ failure (📖 see heart p. 124, kidney p. 212 or p. 220, liver p. 264).
- All transplant patients are on long-term immunosuppression to inhibit the immune response to alloantigen, but which may fail resulting in rejection, or predispose patients to infection (📖 p. 90) and neoplastic change. See Box 2.23.
- Never alter immunosuppressive therapy without expert advice.

Acute rejection

- Clinical features include low grade fever, malaise.
- Specific signs of transplant organ failure:
  - Cardiac: reduced exercise tolerance, pericardial rub, supraventricular arrhythmias, low cardiac output, and signs of congestive cardiac failure.
  - Renal: fluid retention, oliguria, rising creatinine and urea.
  - Liver: ascites, jaundice, deranged coagulation, elevated LFTs.
- Blood tests reveal a lymphocytosis.
- As all patients are on immunosuppresion, symptoms may be minimal until rejection is quite advanced, so routine surveillance is undertaken.
- Biopsies reveal lymphocyte infiltration and cellular necrosis which is used to grade the severity of cellular rejection.

Other long-term complications

Cardiac

- Early coronary artery disease as a result of chronic rejection (treat as for ischaemic heart disease 📖 p. 118) which may be silent as a result of dennervation, and may be underestimated by coronary angiography as the morphology is diffuse, smooth, intimal proliferation.
- Ventricular arrhythmias, congestive cardiac failure, and sudden death. There is no effective treatment apart from retransplantation.
- Renal failure: combination of associated polyarteriopathy, and nephrotoxic immunosuppression.

Box 2.23 Immunosupressive agents

Corticosteroids

Corticosteroids inhibit the immune response at many levels. They decrease production of γ-interferon and interleukins which would normally cause upregulation of the lymphocyte response; and reduce macrophage function.

Ciclosporin (CYA)

Ciclosporin is a calcineurin inhibitor: it inhibits the production of IL-2 by T-helper cells, selectively reducing the cytotoxic T cell response. May cause renal dysfunction. Monitor levels.

Tacrolimus (FK506)

Tacrolimus is also a calcineurin inhibitor with a similar profile. Monitor levels.

Mycophenolate mofetil (MMF)

MMF inhibits purine synthesis in lymphocytes, reducing clonal expansion, and lymphocyte counts.

Azathioprine (AZA)

Azathrioprine causes dose related bone marrow suppression by suppression of purine synthesis, May cause liver dyusfunction.

Sirolimus (rapamycin)

Sirolimus stops IL-2 triggering clonal expansion of T lymphocytes.

Daclizumub, basiliximab

IL-2 receptor blockers which prevent clonal expansion of T cells.

OKT3

OKT3 (Muromonab) is a monoclonal antibody produced in mice that binds the CD3 receptor site on cytotoxic T cells, preventing antigen recognition and clonal expansion.

Polyclonal antibody (e.g. antithymocyte globulin)

These are produced by animals after immunization with HLA: they attach to most circulating lymphocytes effecting a reduction in cell counts to less than 10% of normal.

Simvastatin

Simvastatin has a moderate protective effect against chronic rejection: it suppresses T cell function. May alter liver enzymes or cause rhabdomyolysis.

Death

Confirming death

There is no legal definition of death in the UK. It is generally regarded as the cessation of circulation and respiration. Clinically, there is:

- No respiratory effort, denoted by the absence of breath sounds on auscultation over 1min.
- Absence of a palpable pulse and heart sounds over 1min.
- No response to painful stimuli, e.g. sternal or supraorbital rub.
- Fixed dilated pupils (beware drugs such as atropine), absent ocular reflexes.
- If there is doubt, perform an ECG (check gain).
- Hypothermia (core temp <34°C) must have been corrected.
- Also ☐ see Box 2.24.

Brainstem death

The concept of *brainstem death* has arisen from the advances in ICU care and the ability to maintain cardiac and respiratory function artificially in patients who have sustained severe irreversible brain damage. Brainstem death is defined as the *irreversible cessation of all functions of the entire brain, including the brainstem*. This, alongside the traditional definition, is taken to equate to death in the UK, USA, Australia, and many other countries. Strict criteria must be met:

- An identifiable cause for the brain death must be established, e.g. severe head injury/intracerebral bleed, *and*
- Other causes, including CNS depressants, hypothermia, metabolic and endocrine disturbance, need to be excluded, *and*
- The patient is in a coma, on a ventilator, and does not make any respiratory effort even in the presence of CO_2 drive (i.e. $PaCO_2$ >6.7kPa), *and*
- A number of brainstem reflex tests, performed by the consultant in charge (or deputy of 5 years' registration) and another suitably experienced doctor, have been failed on two separate occasions, usually some hours apart.

Coroners

Discuss with senior if you need to contact Coroner's officer. Inaccurate information may mean death certificates being delayed or Coroner involved unnecessarily. *Deaths must be discussed with coroner's officer if:*

- Death has occurred during an operation.
- Death occurred before recovery from anaesthetic.
- More than 14 days has elapsed since the patient last saw a doctor.
- Death is thought to be suspicious (caused by overdoses of prescribed substances or alcohol, medical error, suicide, neglect, violence).
- There is doubt about the cause of death.

Box 2.24 How do I certify death?

- Examine patient to confirm death (📖 see p.108)
- Write your findings in the patient's notes.

12/09/09 3.50pm	Asked to certify death
	No response to verbal or painful stimuli
	No respiratory effort or breath sounds
	No pulse, heart sounds absent
	Pupils fixed and dilated, ocular reflexes absent
	Time of death 3.50pm
	Death Certificate I Pneumonia Ib stroke II
	Aortic Abdominal Aneurysm (operated on)
	Coroner not contacted. No pacemaker
	GP informed, family aware
	Dr A Khan, Pager 4568

The death certificate

This can be issued by anyone with full medical qualifications who looked after the patient during their last illness, or where referral to the coroner has been made and permission to issue the certificate has been granted.

- Write legibly: the record is retained by the relatives, and illegible or incomplete certificates may be rejected by the funeral director.
- *Part I*: the cause of death: events leading to Ia are listed in Ib and Ic.
- *Part II*: conditions that *contributed* but did not directly cause death.
- General terms like heart failure and sepsis may not be accepted.

Cremation forms

These forms vary slightly between regions, but certain rules always apply.

- There are two parts: the first is filled in by a doctor who attended the patient during the illness leading up to death, the second by an independent clinician who has been fully registered for at least 5 years.
- They should not be issued if the cause of death is not established or the case has been referred to the coroner.
- It is the responsibility of the issuing doctor to ensure that they have seen and identified the person after death and that there are no radioactive implants or pacemakers present.

Post-mortems

- A *coroner's post-mortem* is required for suspicious deaths but is most commonly performed where the Coroner's Office has 'taken' a case where cause of death is uncertain or may be related to surgery or interventions. The consent of relatives is not necessary to proceed.
- A *hospital post-mortem* may be carried out with the consent of relatives to investigate other deaths. In 60% of post-mortems a new diagnosis that would have changed management is found.

End of life issues

Do not resuscitate (DNR) orders

A DNR order should be considered when the frailty, comorbidity (e.g. inoperable disseminated malignancy, multiple organ failure), maximal medical treatment, or advanced age of a patient means that any attempt at cardiopulmonary resuscitation in the event of a cardiac or respiratory arrest would be futile. DNR decisions should be reached on a case by case basis: a blanket 'do not resuscitate' policy based on a specific patient group, such as elderly patients, is unacceptable. An 84-year-old patient that was an appropriate candidate for cardiac surgery is an appropriate candidate for CPR postoperatively, whereas a 72-year-old patient undergoing palliative care for end-stage hepato-renal failure is probably not.

- Never make a DNR decision without discussing it with a consultant.
- Patients, and where appropriate their relatives, must be involved.
- Document the clinical reasons for the DNR order and state explicitly whether 'full active medical management' is to be continued: DNR orders do **not** always include withdrawing treatment. In the case of many terminal diseases this is just what happens: treat to the best of your ability until death, but without recourse to ITU/HDU/CPR.
- Discuss each case with the nurses involved.
- Complete the appropriate documentation and review process which varies from hospital to hospital, and make sure nursing staff are fully aware so that they do not call the arrest team when the patient dies.

Euthanasia

Euthanasia is the painless termination of life at the request of the patient concerned. In the UK *it is illegal to administer any drug to accelerate death*, irrespective of how compassionate the motive may be. Withdrawing futile treatment is not euthanasia. UK law states that the intention to kill is malicious, and such action would be classified as murder. Terminally ill people, and the parents of terminally ill or severely disabled children, may have several reasons for requesting euthanasia. Effective palliative care, counselling and multi-disciplinary support should be able to address most or all of them.

- Pain.
- Loss of dignity.
- Disability.
- Disfigurement.
- Depression.
- Fear of being a burden, being unable to cope.

Palliative care

Palliative care (see p. 334 for a more detailed account) is surgical, medical, and nursing care aimed specifically at relieving the problems associated with terminal conditions, when the possibility of cure has been abandoned. Palliative care physicians specialize in:

- Control of symptoms including pain, anorexia, nausea/vomiting, confusion, dysphagia, dyspnoea, incontinence.
- Psychological aspects of terminal illness.
- Bereavement.

Suicide

The suicide rate in the UK is currently 12.5 per 100,000.

Patients at risk

- The recently bereaved.
- Cancer patients have a 5 × increased risk.
- ♂ >55 years with oral cancer and a history of alcohol abuse.
- ♀ of any age often suffering from gynaecological or breast cancer. (In both these latter groups the treatment of the disease involves disfigurement and a change of body image.)

Action

Patients about to undergo disfiguring surgery for any reason should be counselled carefully in the period after confirmation of the diagnosis and before surgery. Doctors should discuss all treatment options and implications clearly. The support of a 'mastectomy counsellor' or 'stomatherapist' is invaluable. Postoperatively:

- Look for symptoms of depression including low mood, tearfulness, anorexia, early morning waking, and suicidal thoughts, especially in long-term patients.
- Do not discontinue antidepressant medication.
- Ensure that arrangements for discharge include community nursing support and that the GP is aware of the patient's state of mind.

Organ donation

- When brainstem death is established, organ donation should be considered for all patients who were under 75 years of age with no history of malignant disease or major untreated sepsis.
- All donors should be tested for HIV, hepatitis B and C, HSV, and CMV.
- Organ donation is usually co-ordinated by regional transplant teams.
- The body should be identified and the next of kin contacted.
- If despite reasonable attempts, the identity of the corpse or next of kin remains unknown, the body becomes the property of the health authority.
- If a donor card is present, it is reasonable to assume that the deceased wished to donate their organs, and the transplant team can proceed.
- If relatives are identified, and do not wish organ donation to proceed, even though there is a donor card, their wishes should be respected.
- Relatives should be asked to act as agents in expressing what they believe to be the wishes of the patient. Ideally, the person seeking permission should be someone whom they already know. This may be the consultant in charge, but on occasion a senior staff nurse, chaplain (or other religious figure), or the family GP may be more appropriate.
- In the case of accidental deaths, the coroner's permission should be sought before proceeding.
- Speed is of the essence, as 'organ quality' rapidly declines after brainstem death.

Cardiovascular

Investigations

ECG

Indications
Non-invasive, easy to carry out: if in doubt, do one.
- Preoperative:
  - All patients >60 years.
  - Any patient with CVS PMH, risk factors, symptoms or signs.
  - Patients with respiratory or renal disease undergoing major surgery.
  - *Not* necessary in the asymptomatic patient <40 years.
- Postoperative:
  - Chest pain, palpitations, hypotension, dyspnoea.
- NB normal values: PR = 120–200ms, QRS <120ms, Q <40ms and <2mm deep, QT_c = 380–420ms, and $QT_c = QT/\sqrt{(RR)}$ in seconds, ST isoelectric (<1mm elevation and <0.5mm depression), T upright.

Look for
- Current ischaemia (p. 118).
- Old infarction (deep Q waves, poor R wave progression V_1-V_6).
- Conduction disturbances and arrythmias (p. 135).

Stress testing
- Exercise treadmill ECG may be used to assess perioperative cardiovascular risk.
- The best indicator of significant myocardial ischaemia during an exercise ECG is ST segment depression.
- Chest pain, a fall in systolic BP, the development of ventricular arrhythmias, and a poor effort capacity may also be due to myocardial ischaemia.
- The predictive value of a +ve exercise test is poor, but a normal exercise test correlates very strongly with freedom from perioperative cardiac complications.
- Echo and radioisotope scans can be carried out with physical (exercise bike) or pharmacological stress (e.g. dobutamine) to further evaluate changes in myocardial contractility and perfusion (see opposite).

Transthoracic echo

Indications
- Most commonly to investigate new cardiac murmur.
- Evaluate LV function in patients with CVS history undergoing major surgery (see Nuclear cardiology, p. 115).
- Diagnose bacterial endocarditis in patient with persistent +ve blood cultures (TOE is much more accurate).

Look for
- Valvular heart disease (p. 146).
- LV function: regional wall motion abnormalities suggest ischaemia or infarction.
- If you ask, may give you information about filling status which may be useful in the postoperative hypotensive patient.
- Pericardial effusions/tamponade.

Nuclear cardiology

(Myoview/MUGA/thallium/technetium/sestamibi scan.) Radioisotopes bound to molecules target specific tissues. Decay of radioisotopes produces γ rays detected by γ camera. Technetium (99mTc) is used to label sestamibi taken up by red blood cells. Thallium (201Tl) mimics K$^+$. There are two types of nuclear cardiac imaging: 1) myocardial perfusion which compares regional cardiac blood flow in stress and at rest to identify areas of ischaemia and infarction, and 2) ventriculography.

Indications
Discuss with cardiologist: evaluation of angina prior to major surgery (e.g elective AAA), especially in the patient with known coronary artery disease.

Look for
- LV ejection fraction (<30% is poor).
- Reversible defects suggest (potentially treatable) ischaemia.
- Fixed defects suggest previous infarction.

Cardiac catheterization

Indications
Must be discussed with cardiology. Not a part of routine non-cardiac pre-operative assessment, but patients may have undergone angiography for evaluation of ischaemic heart disease.

Look for
- Left main stem disease: untreated this is very high risk for MI.
- Multiple vessel disease: moderate risk of MI if untreated.
- Previous coronary stents: high risk of thrombosis and MI with certain stents if antiplatelet medication is stopped perioperatively.
- If left ventriculography has been performed: Gradient across aortic valve, Mitral regurgitation, LV function.

How to make a cardiology referral

> **Box 3.1 How to make a cardiology referral**
>
> - Introduce yourself; check you're talking to the right person.
> - State if you'd like advice or a review (be clear how urgent it is).
> - Name, age of patient, timing of surgery and nature of operation.
> - Clear description of symptoms, and haemodynamic status.
> - Know the relevant PMHx:
>   • Preop exercise tolerance.
>   • Previous MI/angina/PCI/cardiac surgery/pacemaker.
>   • Cardiac risk factors (📖 p. 118).
> - Know the results of relevant investigations:
>   • Troponin, CKMB.
>   • U&Es, particularly for arrhythmias.
>   • ECG changes.
>   • Echo/myocardial perfusion scans/coronary angiography.
> - Know preop cardiac medication:
>   • Antianginals, Antihypertensives, Anti-arrhythmics.
>   Antiplatelet, ACE inhibitors, Diuretics.

Hypotension and shock

Key facts
- *Hypotension* is low BP which may cause symptoms.
- Shock is inadequate, end-organ perfusion leading to ↓ tissue oxygenation and compensatory responses.

Hypotension
- Systolic BP <100mmHg, u/o<30mL/h, transient postural dizziness.
- Most hypotensive post-op patients need fluid, but *always* think about other causes of hypotension, especially in elderly patients.
- Hypotension does not always lead to shock, but shock is almost always associated with hypotension (📖 see Box 3.2).

> ### Box 3.2 Recognizing shock
> - ↓BP, ↑pulse and *usually* cold, clammy, pale, sweating.
> - ↓urine output <<30mL/h.
> - Confused—may be agitated *or* drowsy.
> - Young patients will compensate with the only signs being ↓pulse pressure, tachycardia and ↓urine output.

Emergency management
- Assess airway and breathing: if patent and breathing spontaneously give 15L/min O_2 by facemask with reservoir bag.
- Check carotid/femoral pulse: 📖 see ALS guidelines—inside cover.
- Secure IV access and start giving 500mL crystalloid over 5min.
- Recheck BP—if low and falling fast call crash team.
- Take a focused history and examine patient to differentiate between hypovolaemia, septic shock, cardiogenic shock, and anaphylactic shock.

Hypovolaemia
- *Causes:* post-op haemorrhage, persistent diarrhoea/vomiting, trauma, ruptured AAA, ruptured ectopic pregnancy, major GI bleed, burns, pancreatitis, excess diuretic use.
- *Clinical features:* as described above with history of trauma/ surgery/ illness
- *Treatment:*
  - Lie patient flat, high flowO_2, put bed in Trendelenberg position (head down) to auto-transfuse if no IV access.
  - Repeat fluid infusion 500mL IV rapidly: you should see rise in BP.
  - Take blood and send for FBC, U&E, clotting, and cross match.
  - Take ABG: estimates Hb, K^+, as well as blood gases.
  - Treat any abnormalities found in investigations.
  - If no rapid improvement in BP look for other causes.
- Definitive management of haemorrhage (📖 p. 98).

Septic shock
- *Causes:* overwhelming sepsis (📖 p. 90)
- *Clinical features:* may be the same as hypovolaemic shock, or if established with circulatory collapse. Patient may look 'septic'—pyrexial, flushed, bounding pulses. Septic shock kills so time is short.

- *Treatment:*
  - As for hypovolaemic shock but with two extra imperatives: *culture*, and *give antibiotics*.
  - Take blood cultures immediately then give IV cefuroxime 750mg tds.
  - Send samples for sepsis screen (urine, sputum, stool, wound swab, others as indicated).
  - Get and follow microbiology advice on antibiotic management.
  - Surgery may also be needed e.g. draining pus, debriding dead/ infected tissue.

Cardiogenic shock

📖 See also pulmonary oedema p. 182.
- *Rapidly reversible causes:* cardiac tamponade (trauma, post cardiac surgery), arrythmias, tension pneumothorax.
- *Other causes:* fluid overload and CCF, MI, PE, SBE, aortic dissection, decompensated valvular heart disease.
- *Clinical features:* history of recent surgery/trauma, chest pain, dyspnoea, palpitations.
- *Treatment:*
  - Give high flow O2.
  - Give 2.5mg morphine IV (anxiolytic, venodilator, analgesic, anti-arrhythmic).
  - Put patient on cardiac and sats monitors, request 12-lead ECG.
  - Treat arrhythmias (📖 see ALS algorithm, inside cover).
  - Treat myocardial ischaemia with 0.1mg GTN, 300mg aspirin PO.
  - Ascultate heart sounds and lung fields: treat tension pneumothorax (📖 p. 203), cardiac tamponade (📖 p. 128).
  - Discuss with ITU.
  - Consider central venous and peripheral arterial monitoring.
  - Send blood for ABGs, FBC, U&E, clotting, troponin.
  - Catheterize the patient.
  - Request CXR—look for pulmonary oedema.
  - Treat fluid overload (📖 p. 65) with diuretics: furosemide 40mg IV.
  - Consider TTE to exclude pericardial effusion and valvular lesions, and to assess LV function.

Anaphylactic shock

- ***Death can occurs within minutes of first symptoms!***
- *Causes:* drug or blood product reaction, allergy: latex, nuts, fish.
- *Clinical features:* history of rapid onset after exposure. Stridor or bronchospasm, tachypnoea, hypotension, tachycardia, angioedema, urticaria, pruritus, rash.
- Sit patient up, give high flow O_2, call anaesthetist if stridor.
- Give:
  - 0.5mL of 1:1,000 adrenaline IM.
  - 10mg chlorpheniramine IV, then 5mL NS flush.
  - 200mg hydrocortisone bolus IV.
- Repeat again in 5–10min if no improvement.
- If wheezy, 5mg nebulized salbutamol (and treat as asthma (📖 p. 186). Alternatively, 1mg nebulized adrenaline will also act as a bronchodilator.

Ischaemic heart disease

Tables 3.1 and 3.2.

Key facts

- MI within 6 weeks greatly increases risk of operative mortality, the risk slowly declines for 3–6 months then plateaus: ***delay elective surgery for 3–6 months after ACS***. 📖 See Tables 3.1 and 3.2.
- ⚠ Stopping warfarin and clopidogrel preop decreases risk of bleeding but increases risk of major adverse cardiac events (MACE).

Table 3.1 Increase risk and IHD

Cardiac problem	Major risk	Intermediate risk	Minor risk
IHD	Recent (< 1 month) MI Unstable angina Drug eluting stent	Past history of MI Stable angina	Abnormal ECG (LVH/LBBB, ST/T-wave abnormalities)
Heart failure	Decompensated failure (i.e. LV dysfunction with pulmonary and/or peripheral oedema)	Compensated failure (i.e. LV dysfunction optimally treated)	Limited exercise capacity
Arrhythmia	Malignant ventricular arrhythmia SVT with rapid ventricular rate Profound bradycardia	New AF Complete heart block	Abnormal cardiac rhythm (e.g. AF)
Other	Severe valvular disease particularly AS Recent CVA	Diabetes. Prosthetic valve, warfarin	Past CVA Uncontrolled hypertension

Table 3.2 Surgery-specific risk in patients with IHD

Risk level	Type of surgery
High	Major emergency surgery, elderly patients, aortic or major vascular surgery, prolonged procedures with major fluid shifts or blood loss
Intermediate	Carotid endarterectomy, head and neck/orthopaedic/prostate surgery, intraperitoneal or intrathoracic procedures
Low	Superficial/cataract/endoscopic/breast surgery

Risks

- Any patient with coronary artery disease is at risk of ACS.
- Risk correlates poorly with severity of coronary stenoses: patients with trivial stenoses may still develop plaque rupture, thrombosis, and AMI.
- Risk ↑ with age, diabetes, HT, renal disease, ♂ sex, smoking.
- 60% of patients with peripheral vascular surgery have coexistent IHD although they may be asymptomatic. 20% have triple-vessel IHD.

Clinical features of IHD
- 📖 for *acute coronary syndrome (ACS)*—including NSTEMI, STEMI, and unstable angina see p. 122.
- 📖 for *chest pain* see p. 120.

Symptoms
History is the most important determinant of cardiovascular risk: the main focus should be on the patient's functional capacity. Patients with an exercise capacity ≥4 metabolic equivalents (METs) (i.e. can climb a flight of stairs in one go or walk up hills) have a low risk (see Table 3.3). Ask about:
- Angina, especially recent change in frequency or severity, cardiac drugs.
- Pain at rest—a worrying feature.
- Previous MI, PCI, or CABG.
- Heart failure—dyspnoea and oedema.
- Symptomatic arrhythmias—palpitations and syncope.
- Risk factors: smoking, hypertension, ↑ cholesterol, diabetes, related disease: PVD, renal.

Physical examination
- Pallor, cyanosis, breathlessness on minimal exertion, obesity or poor nutritional status, scars from vascular or cardiac surgery.
- Measure the BP yourself.
- Assess the arterial pulse (rate, rhythm, volume, and character), the JVP, and precordial pulsations.
- Check the peripheral pulses and listen for carotid bruits.
- Heart sounds: a 3rd heart sound at the apex implies a diseased LV, but its absence is not a reliable indicator of good ventricular function.
- Abdominal examination should include assessment of liver size and palpation of the aorta to identify aneurysmal dilatation.
- Look for peripheral and sacral oedema

Special investigations
- Troponin and cardiac enzymes (📖 p. 122).
- Electrocardiography (📖 p. 114).
- Echocardiography (📖 p. 114).
- Stress testing—discuss with cardiology.
- Coronary angiography—discuss with cardiology.

Table 3.3 Patients to discuss with cardiology preoperatively

Cardiac risk	Major	Intermediate		Minor	
Exercise tolerance	Any	poor	good	poor	good
Surgery risk					
High	Refer	Refer	Refer	Refer	Operate
Intermediate	Refer	Refer	Operate	Operate	Operate
Low	Refer	Operate	Operate	Operate	Operate

Chest pain

Emergency management: patient in shock

Resuscitation

- Sit the patient up, give 4–6L/min O_2 via face mask: aim for SaO_2>98%.
- Continuous ECG monitoring.
- Establish good venous access.
- Pain relief: 2.5–5mg morphine IM/IV initially (with antiemetic).
- Give 500mL fluid challenge if ↓BP or ↑pulse and no evidence of CCF.

Establish a diagnosis

- Ask for a 12-lead ECG and look for:
  - New ST segment changes-ACS. Occasionally, ↓ ST segments indicating angina may resolve with correction of precipitating factor e.g. BP, hypoxia, tachycardia, anxiety.
  - Change in rhythm: AF is common (🕮 p. 136) and predisposes to PE.
- Send bloods for U&Es, troponin, amylase, FBC, G&S, clotting; look for:
  - ↑troponin confirms ACS.
  - ↓Hb may be haemodilution BUT actively look for haemorrhage (upper and lower GI tract, wound, haemothorax, haemolysis).
  - ↑WCC suggests sepsis: look for source.
  - ↑amylase suggests pancreatitis/perforated peptic ulcer.
- Request a CXR and look for:
  - *Pneumothorax*—especially if COPD/asthmatic/central line recently sited/lung biopsy/renal biopsy/liver biopsy.
  - *Lobar collapse.*
  - *Haemothorax/pleural effusion.*
  - *Air under diaphragm* if you suspect perforated peptic ulcer.
  - *Widened mediastinum* if you suspect aortic dissection.
  - *CXR usually clear in acute PE.*
- If SaO_2 <90 despite >6L O_2 do ABGs.
- TTE to detect tamponade or CCF.

Early treatment

- ACS (🕮 p. 122), aortic dissection.
- Pneumothorax (🕮 p. 202), PE (🕮 p. 194), chest infection (🕮 p. 192).
- Peptic ulcer (🕮 p. 258), perforated oesophagus.
- Musculoskeletal pain is *not* the diagnosis: patients do not get shock from musculoskeletal pain.

If the patient is stable your two immediate aims are to a) decide if this is likely to be cardiac pain or not, and b) continue supportive management.

Think about: causes

Cardiac/aortic/upper GI/pleuritic/musculoskeletal (Box 3.3)

Cardiac chest pain is usually:

- Central, dull, constricting (commonly described as 'tight', 'like a band around my chest', or 'crushing').
- Radiates to left or both shoulders and arms, neck, and jaw.
- Brought on by exertion, emotion and relieved *by rest or GTN.*
- It is *not* usually:
  - Well localized. 'Can you point to it with a finger?' Answer no.
  - Stabbing, shooting, or lasting <30sec.
  - Reproducible by pressing over the ribs or sternum.
  - Relieved by Gaviscon®.

Box 3.3 Common patterns of chest pain

- *Dull, central ache or 'tightness'*—myocardial (usually brought on by exertion), gastric distension.
- *Central pain radiating through to back*—thoracic aortic dissection, peptic ulcer, oesophagitis, pancreatitis.
- *Pain on movement, well localized*—musculoskeletal pain/chest drains.
- *Pleuritic pain*—pneumonia, pneumothorax, PE, collection (pus/blood), chest drain.

Ask about: symptoms

A history will get you most of the way to the right diagnosis so take one!

- Think SOCRATES: Site, Onset, Character, Radiation, Associated symptoms, Timing, Exacerbating and relieving factors, Signs.
- Ask about breathlessness, cough, nausea, dyspepsia, calf pain.
- Ask about surgery, recent invasive investigations/lines:
  - OGD/TOE—think oesophageal perforation.
  - Central lines—think pneumothorax/haemothorax.
- Ask about PMH: angina, peptic ulcer disease, malignancy (↑risk PE).

Look for: signs

- **Sweaty, pale, hypotensive, tachycardic: get senior help.**
- Take BP in both arms: different BP may be only sign of aortic dissection.
- Hypotension with ↑JVP suggests tamponade, CCF, or PE:
  - If patient also has unilateral ↓breath sounds and/or ↓SaO2 think of tension pneumothorax (📖 p. 203): decompress and get senior help.
- ↓unilateral breath sounds suggests pneumothorax.
- Bronchial breath sounds suggests LRTI.
- A tender epigastrium suggests peptic ulcer disease.
- Look for warm, swollen leg: ?DVT with embolization to lung (i.e. PE).
- Chest pain reproduced by pressing on chest is *usually* musculoskeletal, but again in the hypotensive, tachycardiac patient, it is inot the sole cause.

Acute coronary syndrome

Diagnosis of ACS (Fig. 3.1)

Symptoms
- Central crushing chest pain (often radiating to left arm/jaw) at rest:
  - >20min = STEMI/NSTEMI.
  - <20min probably unstable angina.
- Dyspnoea, nausea, sweating, palpitations, anxiety.

Signs
- Tachycardia, cold and sweaty (clammy), pallor.
- Worrying signs: ↓BP, pulmonary oedema, new heart murmurs.

Investigations
- ECG: always interpret changes in light of clinical history.
  - STEMI: peaked T waves, ↑ST, new LBBB, later Q waves, T inversion.
  - NSTEMI: ↓ST, may have Q waves later and T-wave inversion.
  - Unstable angina: ↓ST.
- Cardiac markers:
  - STEMI: ↑troponin I and T, CKMB.
  - NSTEMI: ↑troponin I and T, CKMB.
  - Unstable angina: troponin I and T may be raised *but* CKMB should be less than twice normal upper limit.
- Markers rise 3–4h after pain, peak 10–24h, CKMB remains elevated 24–36h, troponins for 7–14 days.
- NB In the acute setting, (<4h) cardiac markers are not helpful, and diagnosis relies on history and ECG.

Coronary blood flow mostly occurs during diastole and is driven by the gradient between the (aortic) **diastolic pressure** and **the ventricular end-diastolic pressure**. Low diastolic BP may thus cause a critical reduction in flow through a stenosed coronary artery, leading to myocardial ischaemia. A downward spiral ensues and measures to 'improve coronary blood flow' by vasodilatation will be counterproductive if they simply further reduce the, coronary perfusion pressure.

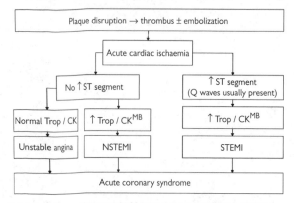

Fig 3.1 Definition and diagnosis of ACS (unstable angina, NSTEMI and STEMI)

Management of ACS

Think OAOAOA: O_2/Aspirin/On telemetry/Access/Opiate/Antiemetic.
- Sit the patient up, give 2–6L O_2 via face mask: aim for SaO_2 >98%.
- Give 300mg aspirin.
- Continuous ECG monitoring.
- Establish good venous access.
- Pain relief: start with diamorphine 2.5–5mg IM (or 1–2mg IV).
- Antiemetic: 50mg cyclizine *slow* IV/PO.
- GTN 2 puffs; consider IV GTN infusion (50mg GTN in 50mL at 4mL/h), increase by 2mL/h to max 10mL/h, titrate against pain and BP >90mmHg systolic).
- β-blocker, if no LVF or heart block, e.g. metoprolol 50mg qds PO or commence with 5mg IV.
- ACE-inhibitor if creatinine and BP allow: ramipril 2.5mg PO od.
- Manage on CCU.

NSTEMI
- Therapeutic dose LMWH e.g. enoxaparin 1mg/kg/12h SC.
- Clopidogrel or GIIb/IIIa glycoprotein IIb/IIIa inhibitors (tirofiban) may be part of local protocols involve cardiology early.

STEMI
Very important to make this diagnosis early—if in any doubt refer to cardiology. The definitive treatment is revascularization: thrombolysis (recent major surgery is an absolute contraindication) or PCI. Aim for pain-to-needle time <60min as outcomes much improved.

Complications
- Arrhythmias (📖 p. 132)—heart block, bradycardia, VF/VT.
- Mechanical: acute MR, ischaemic VSD, LV aneurysm—high mortality.
- Failure: pulmonary oedema, cardiogenic shock— high mortality.
- Pericarditis, mural thrombus and embolic complications e.g. stroke.

Secondary prevention
- Notify GP of perioperative MI.
- Refer to cardiology team while in-patient.
- Management of reversible risk factors: cholesterol, smoking, hypertension, sedentary lifestyle, diabetic control, dietician.
- All patients should be on: aspirin, statin, β-blocker, ACE inhibitor if BP and renal function sufficient.
- All diabetics should be switched to insulin for 3 months.
- Consider Ca^{2+} channel blocker/nitrate/K^+ channel activator for symptom control.

Heart failure

Key facts

'Heart failure' describes patients with a variety of symptoms and signs due to impaired ventricular function (Table 3.4). Several patterns including:

- Acute LVF with low cardiac output (cardiogenic shock) or pulmonary oedema.
- Chronic LVF with congestive heart failure (CCF), peripheral oedema and raised central venous pressure.
- LV/RV or biventricular failure.
- Heart failure may be primarily systolic or diastolic.

Table 3.4 Causes of heart failure

IHD	Chronic infarction, local aneurysm, 'stunned' myocardium
DCM	Idiopathic, alcohol, viral myocarditis, familial
Hypertension	'Essential', renal disease, endocrine disorders
Drugs	β-blockers, Ca^{2+} channel blockers, anti-arrhythmic
Others	End-stage valvular heart disease, septicaemia, HOCM, restrictive cardiomyopathy, thyrotoxicosis or hypothyroidism, chronic persistent tachycardia, heavy metal poisoning, haemochromatosis, amyloidosis

Common clinical presentations

Left ventricular failure

- Symptoms and signs of pulmonary oedema: tachycardia and often ↑BP.
- Treatment: reassure, keep sat up, high flow O_2, IV furosemide, IV opioids (small doses, titrated to effect), and IV GTN infusion (as long as BP >100mmHg).
- Notify HDU/ITU as CPAP may be indicated if medical therapy fails.

Chronic right ventricular failure and cor pulmonale

- Isolated RV failure with normal LV.
- Usually chronic lung disease: emphysema, chronic pulmonary thromboembolic disease, 1° pulmonary hypertension, right ventricular cardiomyopathy
- RV failure as a result of pulmonary hypertension is cor pulmonale.
- Perioperatively, any ↑pulmonary vascular resistance (hypoxia, hypercarbia, acidosis, atelectasis, pneumonia) will worsen RV failure and should be managed appropriately.

Acute right ventricular failure

- Acute RV failure may complicate inferior MI.
- Low BP, high systemic venous pressure (oedema), clear lung fields.
- Increasing circulating volume: cautious IV fluids to increase LV filling.
- Do not give diuretics in this situation.
- The diagnosis is made on enzyme rises and ECG changes and the condition may be confused with pulmonary thromboembolism.

Cardiomyopathy

Three forms of cardiomyopathy are identified: dilated, hypertrophic, and restrictive. Each form has a distinct pathophysiology, and treatment strategies are different.

Dilated cardiomyopathy

In the early stages there may be little or no increase in LV cavity size, simply impaired LV systolic function characterized by reduced amplitude of wall motion on echocardiography. At cardiac catheterization, there is impairment of LV function with normal coronary arteries. The prognosis is poor.

- Clinical features:
  - Signs and symptoms of LV failure.
  - ECG always abnormal with non-specific features of LV disease.
  - CXR: enlarged cardiac silhouette, pulmonary venous congestion, pleural effusions.
- Complications:
  - Heart failure.
  - Arrhythmia (particularly AF and VT, rarely bradycardia).
  - Thromboembolic disease from left atrial or LV thrombus.
- Treatment:
  - Diuretics, ACE inhibitors and, **in expert hands only**, β-blockers.
  - Vasodilators (nitrates, α-blockers) and inotropes (particularly digoxin) may prove helpful in advanced cases.
  - Many patients are given prophylactic warfarin.
  - Anti-arrhythmics only if evidence of arrhythmia.
  - Avoid alcohol, Ca^{2+} channel blockers, NSAID as they can be cardiotoxic.

HOCM

A genetic disorder characterized by excessive cardiac muscle mass which obstructs the outflow of blood from LV. Hypovolaemia and tachycardia worsen obstruction. Patients rarely present with classical 'heart failure'.

- Symptoms:
  - May have unrestricted exercise capacity, but severe cases suffer breathlessness, angina, fatigue, and dizziness.
  - Syncope is a sinister feature needing urgent investigation.
- Examination:
  - Pulse character: normal or sharp upstroke, apex beat heaving and/or double.
  - Often harsh systolic murmur.
- The diagnosis is made with echocardiography.
- Treatment is usually with β–blockade.

Restrictive cardiomyopathy

Rare disease caused by infiltrative diseases, e.g. amyloid. Echocardiography reveals normal or mildly impaired systolic function but profound diastolic dysfunction. Patients often refractory to conventional medication, but may be very sensitive to diuretics. The condition needs to be distinguished from constrictive pericarditis which may be 'cured' by pericardectomy. Treatment is similar to that of HOCM.

Management of heart failure

General principles

- Patients compromised by heart failure (unable to climb stairs without symptoms) are high risk, particularly in an emergency setting, with major surgery and where large fluid shifts occur.
- Patients with acute, untreated heart failure have very high perioperative mortality. Consider whether nonoperative treatment could be appropriate.
- Minor surgery is often best performed under local anaesthesia.
- Although it is possible to perform much major surgery under regional anaesthesia, this does not avoid major haemodynamic disturbances.
- Early discussion of all cases with anaesthetist and possibly cardiologist. For elective major surgery these patients are best reviewed by a cardiologist before admission for surgery. An echocardiogram will give an indication of LV reserve. Perioperative risks increase with the degree of ventricular impairment.
- HDU/ICU should be considered perioperatively if major surgery is planned. Some patients benefit from pre-operative fluid optimization on HDU or ITU (📖 p. 66).
- Patients with severe HOCM need special perioperative attention. The vasodilator action of some anaesthetic agents and hypovolaemia will increase the gradient across the outflow tract and may lead to circulatory collapse. Strict attention to fluid balance is necessary.

Table 3.5 Perioperative prescribing in heart failure

Dosing	Diuretics	Digoxin	β-blockers	Nitrates	ACE inhibitors
Continue therapy: IV if unable to absorb from gut	Yes	Yes, but requires monitored bed			No
Give normal preoperative dose; resume when stable postoperatively	Yes	Yes	Yes	Yes	Only for minor/ intermediate surgery
Omit preoperative dose if NBM; resume when stable postoperatively	No	No	No	No	Yes, if major surgery

Perioperative management

- Careful postoperative monitoring of BP, fluid intake, urine output, SpO_2. Remember surgical drains, NG tubes, and diarrhoea as other sources of fluid loss.
- Optimal medical therapy of heart failure involves balancing volume status, vasodilatation, and inotropic drugs and also ensuring that BP is not symptomatically low (Table 3.5). Perioperatively this balance may be upset by the following factors:
  - General anaesthesia may cause vasodilatation and hypotension;
  - Spinal anaesthesia may cause similar magnitude disturbance;
  - Perioperative dehydration may lower BP;
  - Excess postoperative fluids may provoke pulmonary oedema.
  - Increases in systemic vascular resistance (pain, hypertension) may result in acute heart failure.
  - Opioids can contribute to hypotension and bradycardia.
  - Patients with pulmonary hypertension and cor pulmonale may develop critical hypotension if volume depletion and vasodilatation are excessive.
- Perioperative hypotension may be difficult to diagnose and treat. It should be managed in the HDU/ICU. It may be caused by hypovolaemia, cardiac failure, vasodilated state or any of the problems described on 📖 p. 116. Ask the ICU team for assessment and help.
- Fluid balance is critical. A central line is usually required with major surgery. Selected patients may benefit from a Swan–Ganz catheter or other means of monitoring cardiac output; the anaesthetist will advise. Every patient is different and all need regular review postoperatively. Restricting fluids rather than prescribing diuretics is often the choice in the immediate postoperative period.
- Renal perfusion is frequently compromised and the risk of renal failure with major surgery is increased. Oliguria is a frequent problem (📖 for management see p. 215).

Pericardial disease

Pericarditis and pericardial effusion

Pericarditis is an acute or chronic inflammation of the pericardium. It may result in a pericardial effusion. Pericardial effusions also occur in cardiac failure, without pericarditis.

A large, chronic effusion may have much less impact haemodynamically than a smaller, acute effusion.

Causes
- Infectious: viral, bacterial, tuberculous, fungal.
- AMI, or post MI (Dressler syndrome).
- Uraemia, sarcoidosis, trauma.
- Malignancy.

A large, chronic effusion may have much less impact haemodynamically than a smaller, acute effusion.

Clinical features
- Pain common (in acute setting), retrosternal, constant, may be pleuritic, relieved by sitting forward, features of ↓cardiac output if tense effusion.
- Pericardial friction rub present in 85%.
- Faint heart sounds, absent apex beat.
- Effusions may tamponade (☐ see Cardiac tamponade, below).

Investigations
- ECG: widespread ↑ST, late T inversion, no Q waves, can be difficult to tell from AMI (patient often too well for ST changes to be AMI). Electrical alternans of P, QRS, T may be present if tamponade.
- Cardiac markers may show small rise (again not enough to be AMI).
- TTE diagnostic of effusions, can identify tamponade, volume of effusion.

Treatment
- Symptom relief e.g. NSAIDs for pain and inflammation.
- Treat underlying cause.
- Watch for tamponade.

Cardiac tamponade

Cardiac tamponade is an emergency, and requires prompt treatment. It restricts ventricular filling and ↓cardiac output.

Comon causes
- Penetrating chest injury (including elective surgery)
- Malignancy.
- Idiopathic pericarditis.
- Uraemia.

Clinical features
- ↑↑JVP, paradoxical pulse (>10mmHg systolic drop on inspiration).
- Hypotension.
- Soft or absent heart sounds.

Investigation and treatment
Urgent TTE is diagnostic and therapeutic: pericardiocentesis should be performed under US guidance whenever possible.

Constrictive pericarditis
Can follow acute pericarditis, especially if caused by trauma, irradiation, neoplasm. Perioperative management is similar to restrictive cardiomyopathy, and but needs to be distinguished long term as pericardectomy is an effective treatment.

Causes of dysrhythmias

Identify dysrhythmias preoperatively. It enables you to plan your later management and it's the only way you'll know whether that post-op AF is acute. A number of common factors contribute to perioperative arrhythmias; these need to be identified and specific treatment started. (📖 p. 134).

Preoperative causes

Age: postoperative arrhythmias are commoner in older patients.

Preoperative arrhythmias: Patients with pre-existing AF usually revert to AF even if their initial rhythm after anaesthesia is sinus rhythm.

Pre-existing heart disease
- Mitral valve disease leading to an *enlarged left atrium*.
- Patients with *dilated left ventricles* (ischaemic cardiomyopathy, decompensated valvular heart disease).
- *Hypertrophic left ventricles* (aortic stenosis (AS), HOCM) are more prone to ventricular dysrhythmias.

Intraoperative causes

Lung and cardiac surgery have higher risk of post-op arrhythmias.

Postoperative causes
- *Cardiovascular:*
  - Myocardial ischaemia should be excluded as a cause of dysrhythmias. *Get an ECG.*
  - Hyopvolaemia, pulmonary artery catheter, less commonly, central venous catheter insertion.
- *Respiratory:*
  - Hypoxia, hypercapnia, acidosis.
  - Endotracheal tube irritation, pneumothorax, atelectasis, pneumonia.
- *Electrolyte imbalance:* hyperkalaemia, hypokalaemia, hypomagnesemia, hypocalcaemia.
- *Drug related* (withdrawal/toxicity):
  - β-blockers, digoxin, Ca^{2+} channel blockers, bronchodilators, tricyclic antidepressants, adrenergic and dopaminergic infusions.
  - Alcohol.
- *Metabolic:* hyper- and hypothyroidism, hypoglycaemia.
- *Systemic:*
  - Fever, hypothermia, anxiety, and pain predispose to tachyarrythmias.
  - Bradycardias are common when the patient is asleep.
- *Vagal stimulation:* NGT insertion, gastric/bowel dilation, intubation, nausea and vomiting.
- *Mechanical:*
  - Pericardial effusion, tamponade, tension pneumothorax.
  - Cold fluids injected into right atrium via central line.
  - Chest contusion.

Lethal dysrhythmias

If you need to read this page in the peri-arrest situation, then you did not do enough bookwork—**know the ALS algorithm!**

Box 3.4 Management of cardiac arrest in the monitored patient

- The ALS algorithms on the inside cover.
- Defibrillate VF or VT.
- Open airway. Look for signs of life
- Call resuscitation team.
- Start external cardiac compressions at a rate of 100/min if defibrillation not indicated (EMD, asystole).
- Look for symmetrical expansion. Listen for bilateral breath sounds.
- Get IV access, check electrolytes, blood sugars, blood gases.
- Look for reversible causes: mechanical—cardiac tamponade, tension pneumothorax, massive PE; and metabolic—hypokalaemia, hyperkalaemia, acidosis, hypoxia, hypovolaemia and hypothermia.
  - Give 1mg (10mL 1:10,000) adrenaline IV.

Ventricular fibrillation

Features Irregular, fine, sinusoidal trace (Fig. 12.8(a)). No cardiac output.
Therapy Immediate defibrillation. Do **not** delay defibrillation for **any** other procedures e.g. intubation.

- Give 1 shock (150–360J biphasic or 360J monophasic). The next step is Immediately resume CPR 30:2 for 2 minutes.
- Give 1mg adrenaline IV (10mL of 1:10,000), repeat at 3-min intervals.
- Correct acidosis and electrolytes; consider 1mg/kg lidocaine.

Pulseless ventricular tachycardia

Features Wide complex tachycardia (Fig. 12.8(b)), no cardiac output.
Therapy Treat as VF.

- Sometimes runs of VT are short and self-limiting. These are best treated with lidocaine or amiodarone infusions, magnesium and correction of acid–base and electrolyte abnormalities.
- Sustained and non-sustained VT may degenerate into VF so do not ignore these dysrhythmias.

Asystole

Features Flat ECG trace/low amplitude fibrillation (Fig.12.8(c)), p-waves may be visible. No cardiac output.
Therapy Check leads and gain on machine, commence CPR immediately.

- Give atropine 3mg IV once, and adrenaline 1mg IV at 3-min intervals.
- Pace externally if possible.
- An absolutely straight line suggests lead disconnection.

Electromechanical dissociation (pulseless electrical activity)

Features No cardiac output despite ECG trace compatible with output.
Therapy Commence CPR immediately.
- Pace externally if possible.
- Look for a treatable underlying cause (4H, 4T).
  - Hypoxia.
  - Hypovolaemia.
  - Hypo/hyperkalaemia/metabolic.
  - Hypothermia.
  - Tension pneumothorax.
  - Tamponade, cardiac.
  - Toxins.
  - Thrombosis (coronary or pulmonary).

Complete heart block

Features Wide complex <35bpm with poor cardiac output. P-waves may
be visible but are not related to QRS complex (🕮 Fig 12.8 (d)).

Therapy

- If there is a cardiac output do not commence CPR which may convert
  heart block into VF. Treat pharmacologically (atropine, isoprenaline
  infusion).
- The risk is of asystole, but patients can be remarkably tolerant of low
  ventricular rate.
- Stop AV node blocking agents (β-blockers, digoxin, Ca^{2+} antagonists).
- If patient remains conscious, urgently plan intervention, but be sure that
  everything is in place: once patient is supported, intrinsic ventricular
  rhythm may no longer be sufficient to maintain adequate output.
- Transvenous pacing until permanent pacemaker can be implanted.
  Externally pacing is a stopgap only.
- If no cardiac output, commence CPR, give atropine 3mg IV once, and
  1mg IV (10mL of 1:10,000) adrenaline IV.

Dangerous dysrhythmias I

Ventricular tachycardia (pulse present) (Fig.12.10)

Features Wide complex, regular tachycardia, impaired cardiac output.

Therapy
- If at any stage the patient loses cardiac output start the ALS algorithm for VF/pulseless VT. Distinguish from SVT with conduction defect: also regular broad complex tachycardia with different management (📖 p. 137)
- Correct hypoxia (📖 p. 172).
- Correct hypokalaemia: give 20mmol KCl in 50mL 5% glucose via a central line over 30min, or 20mmol KCl in 500mL 5% glucose over 4h via peripheral IV, aim for serum K^+ of 4.5–5.0 mmol/L.
- If patient is haemodynamically compromised, sedate with anaesthetist present and give $1 \times 200J$ synchronized monophasic shock, and repeat up to 360J if not in sinus rhythm.
- Amiodarone 300mg in 50mL 5% glucose over 1h iv, followed by amiodarone 900mg in 250mL 5% glucose over 23h IV may achieve rate control and is first choice agent in most units.
- Alternatively, lidocaine 1mg/kg IV over 2min, followed by IV infusion of 4mg/min for 30min, 2 mg/min for 2h, then 1 mg/min.
- Look for and treat any evidence of myocardial ischaemia (📖 p. 120)

Torsades des pointes
- Polymorphic VT with point of QRS twisting from +ve to −ve and back that at first glance can look like VF.
- Long QT interval predisposes, look for and correct triggers: antiarrhythmic drugs (class Ia + III), $\downarrow Mg^{2+}$, $\downarrow K^+$, $\downarrow Ca^{2+}$, hypothyroidism, AV block, AMI, congenital syndromes, erythromycin, tricyclic antidepressants, ketoconazole.
- Treat with 8mmol (2g) of magnesium sulphate over 15min.

Ventricular ectopy (ventricular premature beats)

Although ventricular ectopics occurring <1 per screen are usually benign, particularly if present preoperatively, in a small number of patients they reflect myocardial ischaemia or structural heart disease and may herald lethal dysrhythmia.

Features Wide complex QRS that may occur occasionally or in couplets (ventricular bigeminy), may be uni- or multifocal, and is usually followed by compensatory pause.

Therapy
- Look for signs of myocardial ischaemia and treat accordingly (📖 p. 120).
- Correct hypoxia (📖 p. 172) and acidosis (📖 p. 174).
- Correct hypokalaemia (📖 p. 232).
- Do not use antiarrhythmic drugs to suppress isolated ventricular ectopic beats.

Second-degree heart block

Classification

- *Mobitz type I*: PR interval increasingly prolonged until QRS dropped. This is also known as the Wenkebach phenomenon.
- Mobitz type II: every n^{th} p-wave is not conducted (1:2, 1:3 etc. block).
- Bifascicular block: RBBB + block of either of the left fascicles.
- Trifascicular block: bifascicular block + 1st degree HB.

Features

- 2nd degree HB of Mobitz type I and II has abnormal PR interval and narrow QRS complex.
- Bi-fascicular block has normal PR interval, but broad QRS complex.
- Tri-fascicular block has prolonged PR interval and wide QRS complex.

Therapy

- Stop AV node blocking drugs (β-blockers, digoxin, Ca^{2+} antagonists).
- Refer to cardiologist, normally with a 24-h tape. A permanent pacemaker is indicated in:
  - 2nd degree HB associated with symptomatic bradycardia (also if caused by essential drug therapy), periods of asystole >3sec.
  - Asymptomatic tri-fascicular or Mobitz type II block.

Left bundle branch block (Fig. 12.7)

- Wide QRS complex (>120ms).
- The ST segment cannot be interpreted: elevation or depression is **not** well correlated with ischaemia in left bundle branch block.
- Therapy as for tri-fascicular block.
- New acute-onset LBBB may result from an acute coronary syndrome (□ p. 122)

Dangerous dysrhythmias II

These dysrhythmias are potentially dangerous in patients with borderline cardiac output. The tachyarrhythmias are particularly poorly tolerated in patients with stiff, non-compliant hypertrophic ventricles (AS, HOCM) where reduced filling times lead to ↓stroke volumes and low cardiac output. Loss of synchronized atrial contraction may further reduce stroke volume by up to 30%. Ventricular ectopy may herald the onset of lethal dysrhythmias.

AF and atrial flutter

Features Irregularly irregular usually narrow complex tachycardia. Atrial rate >380 in fibrillation, atrial rate <380 in flutter. (Fig. 12.2)

Box 3.6 Rationale for treating AF and atrial flutter

These are not benign arrhythmias. In addition to the haemodynamic compromise already described:

- 30% of patients without an embolic event can be shown to have intra-cardiac thrombus by TOE within 72h of onset of AF.
- TTE has a much lower sensitivity than TOE in the detection of left atrial thrombus.
- 5% of non-anticoagulated patients undergoing DC cardioversion for AF will have an embolic event compared to 1% of anticoagulated patients.
- The rate of stroke in patients with AF <65 years is approximately 1% per year, increasing to approximately 5% per year in patients >65 years.
- Although the natural history of AF following CABG is not well docu-mented, non-anticoagulated patients with a history of angina or MI have a 6–8% risk of stroke per annum.
- The risk of intracranial haemorrhage in anticoagulated patients is about 0.5% per year, increasing to about 1% in patients >80 years.

Therapy (depending on the clinical state of the patient):
- *Pharmacological cardioversion*: this is indicated in haemodynamically stable postoperative patients (📖 see p. 137).
- *Synchronized DC cardioversion*: 📖 this is dealt with in more detail on p. 140. It is indicated in two main groups of postoperative cardiac surgical patients:
  - Acute haemodynamic compromise.
  - The stable patient that is adequately anticoagulated (📖 p. 61), and who has not responded to appropriate antiarrhythmic and electro-lyte management.
- *Rate control*: usually the aim of treatment in chronic AF.

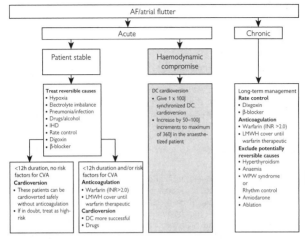

Fig 3.2 Algorithm for the management of AF. (Reproduced from Chikwe J, Beddow, E, Glenville, B (2006). *Cardiothoracic Surgery*, Oxford University Press, Oxford with permission.)

Specific management steps for atrial fibrillation or flutter (Fig. 3.2)

- Risk factors for CVA: previous CVA/TIA, mitral stenosis, HT, DM, age>75, LVF, LA diameter >5.0cm.
- β-blocker withdrawal common cause of post-op AF: check and restart.
- Digoxin 0.125mg in 50mL 5% glucose over 20min IV, repeat until good rate control, up to a maximum of 1.25mg in 24h. Digoxin is preferable to amiodarone for rate control in patients with poor LV.
- Amiodarone (📖 p. 134).
- Start regular LMWH e.g. enoxaparin 150U/kg od SC.
- Start warfarin on first postoperative evening for patients still in atrial fibrillation, with no bleeding problems. The target INR is 2.0–2.5.

Supraventricular tachycardia

Features Narrow complex, regular tachycardia, rate 150–250bpm. It is sometimes difficult to distinguish between an SVT and atrial flutter.

Therapy
- DC cardioversion as described for AF.
- Adenosine (3mg IV bolus ↑ by 3mg increments and repeated at 2-min intervals) produces a transient complete AV block sufficient to terminate most SVTs. Contraindicated in asthma.
- Calcium channel blockers (diltiazem 0.25mg/kg IV over 2min repeated 15min later if necessary) convert 90% of patients. Alternatively verapamil 5mg by slow IV injection, but do *not* use in patients taking β-blockers as prolonged complete heart block may result.
- Digoxin helps gain rate control in refractory SVT.
- Carotid sinus massage may slow ventricular response rate and can also reveal atrial rhythm. There is a risk of CVA from carotid plaque disruption in arteriopaths.

Benign dysrhythmias

'Benign' is a relative term. For some patients, *any* dysrhythmia is dangerous, so look at the patient as well as the ECG.

Sinus tachycardia

Although this is an essentially benign response to sympathetic overactivity, sinus tachycardia increases myocardial O_2 demand and decreases time in diastole. This interferes with coronary blood flow and ventricular filling. In borderline left ventricular function, or stiff, non-compliant ventricles (e.g. in preoperative AS), this can result in myocardial ischaemia. Sinus tachycardia may be a compensatory response to poor cardiac output, but can also exacerbate it.

Features Sinus rhythm with rate >100bpm. Rate >140bpm suggest SVT.

Therapy
- Look for and treat the common underlying causes: pain, anxiety, pyrexia, gastric dilatation, hypercapnia, hypovolaemia, and anaemia. Have the patient's usual β-blockers been accidentally omitted?
- Salbutamol nebulizers may be an unavoidable cause.
- If you are sure that the tachycardia is not compensating for poor cardiac output, **and** if the patient is not requiring inotropic support, **and** if the systolic BP is at least at preop values, **consider** restarting at a low dose β- or Ca^{2+}-channel blockers if these were discontinued preoperatively. Short acting drugs (metoprolol 25mg tds PO) are safest.
- Some inotropes (e.g. adrenaline, dobutamine, dopexamine, dopamine) cause tachycardia. It may be appropriate to wean or change the inotrope. Are the high doses of inotropes only necessary because the circulation is so hypovolaemic? Consider a fluid change.

Junctional tachycardia

Junctional tachycardia is caused when junctional tissue has a faster intrinsic rate than the sinus node. Drugs slowing the sinus node should be stopped. Although it is a benign dysrhythmia, loss of synchronized atrial contraction can reduce cardiac output by up to 30%.

Features Narrow complex tachycardia without P waves.

Therapy
- Stop digoxin and β-blockers.
- Consider atrial or dual-chamber pacing.
- Consider metoprolol (25–50mg PO tds) a short acting β-blocker, or diltiazem 60mg tds PO to slow the junctional focus, with atrial or dual-chamber pacing if the underlying sinus rate is slow.
- Overdrive pacing may help establish synchronized AV contraction.

Sinus or junctional bradycardia

Features Narrow complex, rate <60bpm. P-waves, if present, not related to QRS in junctional rhythm. At <40bpm, cardiac output will be very low. The aim of therapy is to alleviate symptoms, sinus bradycardia is not associated with ↑mortality.

Therapy
- Stop any drugs causing bradycardia, including amiodarone, β-blockers, and digoxin.
- Give a bolus of atropine (0.3mg IV) repeated in increments up to 1mg, in the acute setting in symptomatic patient.
- Refer for pacemaker implantation if persistent and symptomatic.

Atrial ectopics

Features P-waves with a different morphology, associated with altered PR interval to the following QRS complex.

Therapy Premature atrial ectopics are benign but sometimes herald the onset of AF or atrial flutter, and they are worth treating perioperatively.
- Correct hypokalaemia (📖 p. 232).
- Correct hypomagnesaemia: infuse 2–4g $MgSO_4$ in 50mL 5% glucose via the central line empirically if it has not already been given.
- Correct hypoxia (📖 p. 172) and acidosis (📖 p. 174).
- Give digoxin (125–250mcg IV over 1h, repeat up to a total of 1250mcg). Digoxin decreases the frequency of atrial ectopics and reduces the ventricular response rate if AF does develop.
- β-blockers decrease frequency of ectopics (e.g. metoprolol 25mg tds)

First-degree heart block

This is benign. In a patient that has undergone aortic valve surgery it suggests damage to the conduction pathways passing close to the aortic annulus. This often resolves over the weeks postoperatively as oedema and haematoma settle.

Features PR interval >200ms.

Therapy
The patient warrants follow-up by a cardiologist as occasionally insertion of a permanent pacemaker may be required, if first-degree heart block is accompanied by a new left bundle branch block or symptomatic bradyarrhythmias.

Further investigations warranted
- If history of (pre-) syncope, first-degree HB can indicate intermittent complete HB, 24h-ECG can help make diagnosis.
- In infective endocarditis, new first-degree HB can indicate aortic root abscess, refer for urgent echo.

Cardioversion

Synchronized DC cardioversion is the treatment of choice for AF and SVT compromising cardiac output, and for AF refractory to chemical cardioversion. See Box 3.7.

Box 3.7 Checklist for elective DC cardioversion

- Is it indicated?
  - Is the patient still in AF?
  - Is treatment of any new triggers (pneumonia, electrolyte disturbance) already underway?
- Is it safe? (📖 see p. 136)
  - **Either** AF has lasted <12h and no risk factors for CVA (📖 p. 141);
  - **Or** the patient must have had at least 6 weeks of formal anticoagulation;
  - **Or** a TOE excluding intracardiac thrombus.
- Is the patient ready?
  - The potassium should be 4.5–5.0.
  - The INR if anticoagulated should be >2.0.
  - The patient should have a valid consent form.
  - The patient should be starved for 6h.

DC cardioversion for AF and SVT

Patient should be anaesthetized, but some anaesthetists prefer not to intubate, using a bag and mask. You can use self-adhesive defibrillator pads (which remain on the patient until the procedure is completed), or hand held paddles and gel pads. Once the anaesthetist is happy:

- Self adhesive defibrillator pads can usually be used to monitor the ECG too. Otherwise place ECG electrodes on the patient and connect them to the defibrillator so that it displays the patients' ECG clearly.
- Self-adhesive defibrillator pads can usually be used to monitor the ECG too. Otherwise place ECG electrodes on the patient and connect them to the defibrillator so that it displays the patient's ECG clearly.
- Switch defibrillator on and turn dial to an appropriate power setting (100J, 200J, 360J).
- *Press the SYNC button, and ensure that each R wave is accented on ECG: failure to do this could deliver shock while myocardium is repolarizing resulting in VF. Check that the SYNC button is on before every shock for AF.*
- If you are using hand-held paddles press them firmly onto the gel pads.
- Perform a visual sweep to check that no-one (including you) is in contact with patient, at the same time say clearly, 'Charging. Stand clear'.
- Press the charge button.
- Press *and hold* the shock button when the machine is charged.
- If the shock has been delivered successfully the patient's muscles will contract violently: anyone in contact with the patient may experience a large electric shock.
- Check the rhythm.
- If still AF check with the anaesthetist then press the charge button (repeating the warning to 'stand clear') and repeat the sequence.

Complications of DC cardioversion

- Complications of general anaesthesia.
- Systemic embolization.
- Failure to cardiovert.
- Burns from incorrect application of gel pads.
- Muscle pain from involuntary contraction.
- Arrhythmias including VF and bradycardia.

Common pitfalls

Failure to deliver a shock

Check that the defibrillator is switched on and adequately charged. Ensure you press *and hold down* the shock button until the next R wave is detected. Check that the correct power setting has been selected. Change the machine.

Failure to cardiovert

Check the latest available serum potassium was 4.5–5.0. Check that the correct power setting has been selected. Replace gel pads with fresh ones. Reposition the patient on their side and the pads as shown and try two further shocks at 200J (Fig. 3.3). Don't start at too low a power setting: each shock leaves the myocardium less sensitive to further shocks. There is some evidence that 360J as the first power setting results in less myocardial damage and a better conversion rate than multiple shocks at lower power settings.

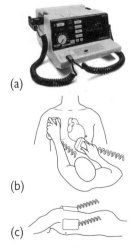

(a)

(b)

(c)

Fig 3.3 Using defibrillators. (a) Standard defibrillator console. (b) Correct positioning for defibrillation and cardioversion. (c) Alternative positioning for synchronized DC cardioversion. Parts (b) and (c) reproduced with permission from Chikwe J, Beddow E, and Glenville B (2006). *Cardiothoracic Surgery*, Oxford University Press, Oxford.

Defibrillation

Defibrillation is the treatment of choice for VF and pulseless VT.

Defibrillation for VF and pulseless VT

Do not delay defibrillation for manoeuvres such as intubation, chest compressions, or administration of drugs.

- Expose chest
- Place gel pads on chest in position shown in Fig 3.4: the aim is to direct as much of the current as possible through the heart.
- Switch defibrillator on and turn dial on to appropriate power setting (150–360J biphasic, or 360J monophasic)
- If you are using hand-held paddles instead of adhesive external defibrillator pads, place them firmly onto gel electrodes and hold.
- Perform a visual sweep to check that no-one is in contact with the patient. Press the charge button at the same time as saying clearly, 'Charging. Stand clear'.
- When the defibrillator has charged, press the shock button.
- If the shock has been delivered successfully the patient's muscles will contract violently: anyone in contact with the patient may experience a large electric shock.
- Check the rhythm.
- If still VF immediately resume chest compressions (30:2) for 2 minutes then check the rhythm.

Common pitfalls

- *Failure to deliver a shock:* check that the defibrillator is switched on and adequately charged. Check that the correct power setting has been selected. Check that the 'SYNC' button is **off** if you are trying to defibrillate VF. Change the machine and paddles.
- *Failure to defibrillate:* exclude reversible causes
  - Hypoxia
  - Hypovolaemia
  - Hypo/hyperkalaemia/metabolic
  - Hypothermia
  - Tension pneumothorax
  - Tamponade
  - Toxins
  - Thrombosis (coronary or pulmonary).

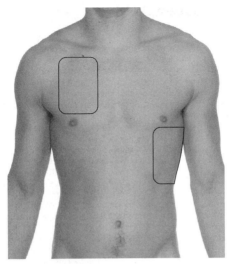

Fig 3.4 Correct positioning for defibrillation. Reproduced with permission from Thomas J and Monaghan T (2007). *Oxford Handbook of Clinical Examination and Practical Skills*, Oxford University Press, Oxford.

Cardiac pacemakers

Key facts

- Cardiac pacemakers are implantable electrical devices which generate a cardiac rhythm via electrodes in contact with cardiac muscle.
- They can stimulate atria, ventricles, or both, and be on demand (pace at a preset rate when detected heart rhythm is too slow) or asynchronous (pace irrespective of detected heart rhythm).
- In addition, modern pacemakers may have a built-in defibrillator capacity (implantable cardioverter defibrillator or ICD).
- Pacemakers and defibrillators need to be reprogrammed before and after surgery as electrical cautery can cause the defibrillator to fire potentially causing VF or VT, and inhibit pacing modes potentially revealing underlying asystole or profound bradycardia.
- These devices are absolute contraindications to MRI scans.

Basic principles

- Pacemakers are permanently implanted in the left or right subclavian area, with access to the heart via the left subclavian vein, easily palpable on examination, and clearly visible on CXR.
- The pacing modes are generally designated with a 4 or 5-letter code (Table 3.6); the most common single and dual chamber modes are VVIR (pacing and sensing the ventricle, inhibited by ventricular activity, and rate responds to detected demand) and DDDR (pacing and sensing both atria and ventricles, can be inhibited by activity in either chamber and responsive to detected demand), respectively.

Table 3.6 Cardiac pacemaker mode designation

1st	Paced chamber	**O** none	**A** atrium	**V** ventricle	**D** dual	**S** single
2nd	Sensed chamber	**O** none	**A** atrium	**V** ventricle	**D** dual	**S** single
3rd	Response to sensed event	**O** none	**I** inhibition	**T** triggered	**D** both	
4th	Rate responsiveness	**R** responsive				
5th	Antitachycardia function	**O** none	**P** pacing	**S** shock	**D** both	

(Letter)

Complications

Acute

- Infection, haematoma.
- Lead displacement (requires resiting).
- Pneumothorax (📖 p. 202).
- Phrenic nerve stimulation.
- Cardiac perforation with pericardial haematoma (📖 p. 128).

Chronic (often requiring replacement)
- Lead failure.
- Erosion.
- Infection.
- Inappropriate programming.
- Rotation of pacemaker in subclavian pocket.

Pacemaker syndrome
- Loss of co-ordinated AV activity leading to palpitations, fatigue, cough, exertional dyspnoea, neck pulsations, syncope.
- Signs of congestive heart failure (📖 p. 124), ↑JVP ± cannon waves.
- ECG: evidence of pacemaker activity, uncoordinated P and QRS.
- Reprogramming or exchanging pacemaker restores normal function and relieves symptoms: seek cardiology advice.

Patients with pacemakers/defibrillators
Day before surgery
- Establish why the device was inserted: sick sinus, complete heart block, heart failure with episodes of VT, VF.
- Try to find out what the make of device is e.g. Medtronic®; some patients carry a card, otherwise check hospital records.
- Contact pacing technician or cardiology the day before the list to plan reprogramming which should normally be done in the anaesthetic room immediately before surgery, and again in the operating room immediately after surgery
- Inform the anaesthetist that the patient has a device and what arrangements have been made to check reprogramme it.

On the day of surgery
- Patients should continue all antiarrhythmic medication as normal.
- If the patient has an implanted defibrillator place external defibrillator pads on the patient out of the way of the planned incision, before adjusting device function, and leave in place for the duration of surgery.
- A pacing technician should turn off the defibrillator function and change the pacemaker to an asynchronous pacing mode (one that will not be inhibited by the signal from electrocautery)—the machine they use to interrogate the pacemaker depends on the make, but if in doubt they will usually bring two or three kits.
- Bipolar cautery should ideally be used instead of monopolar if possible.
- Once surgery is completed the pacemaker should be re-interrogated and returned to its previous mode.
- If there is no facility to interrogate the pacemaker/defibrillator, holding a magnet against the device will reset most to default: asynchronous pacing at 60, defibrillator off.

Valve disease

Valve disease is found in around 5% of patients >65 years. The treatment of severe valve disease is usually surgical. Medical therapy often has little to offer. Surgical care of patients with valve disease entails delicate balancing of risks and precise anaesthetic care.

Principles of anaesthesia and surgery in valve disease

- The timing of valve surgery in relation to elective non-cardiac surgery is uncertain, but any patient who fulfils the accepted criteria for valve surgery should normally have this done beforehand.
- For emergency surgery, valve replacement is impractical.
- Volume depletion or vasodilatation may lead to drastically reduced cardiac output.
- Volume overload or vasoconstriction increases risk of pulmonary oedema.
- Perioperative monitoring of haemodynamics/fluid balance is essential.
- Antibiotic prophylaxis against infective endocarditis must be remembered in procedures likely to produce bacteraemia: check local guidelines, if not available, the *BNF* contains the latest recommendations.

Assessment of a new murmur

Any cardiac murmur may represent valve disease, but the intensity of a murmur is a poor guide to severity. Patients with severe AS may have no murmur at all, simply a low volume, slow-rising pulse. Even the detection of trivial valve lesions should be documented since these patients may be at risk of endocarditis should perioperative bacteraemia occur.

In general, any patient with a new murmur should be referred for echocardiography preoperatively, particularly if:
- The murmur is diastolic (benign flow murmurs are usually systolic).
- There are symptoms suggestive of heart disease.
- Major surgery is planned.

Clinical assessment
- Breathlessness is the single most important symptom of significant valve disease.
- Left ventricular disease frequently leads to heart failure with functional mitral regurgitation.
- Syncope and/or angina are features of severe AS.
- BP:
  - Systolic pressure is low in severe AS.
  - Diastolic pressure low in severe aortic regurgitation (AR).
- Investigations:
  - *ECG*: LV hypertrophy is typical in severe aortic valve disease.
  - *CXR*: cardiac enlargement, and possibly pulmonary congestion.
  - *Echocardiography* should be performed whenever clinical features and simple investigations raise the possibility of significant valvular disease.

Patient with a prosthetic valve

Key facts

- Prosthetic heart valves in any of the four positions may be:
  - Tissue (porcine, bovine, homograft—human donated).
  - Mechanical (mostly ceramic, some older valves are metal valves).
- Tissue valves more than a few years old may have structural degeneration resulting in stenosis or regurgitation: always take a careful history and examination (📖 p. 148 and p. 150)
- Management is focused on preventing the life-threatening complications of prosthetic valve endocarditis, thrombosis, and bleeding.
- All patients should be evaluated for need for prophylactic antibiotics to protect against endocarditis:
  - Regularly updated guidelines for best choice of antibiotic and which procedures should be covered are listed in the BNF; also check local guidelines.
  - Traditionally *any* instrumentation of the GI or GU tract has been preceded by antibiotic prophylaxis.
- If operating on an infected area, antimicrobial therapy will be targeted against that area obviously.
- Warfarin should be stopped before surgery.
  - Patients with tissue valves do not need to be heparinized unless they have a history of thromboembolic complications.
  - Patients with mechanical valves must be therapeutically heparinized once INR <2.0: in the setting of life-threatening haemorrhage it may be appropriate to tolerate a lower INR for 24–48h as the risk of valve thrombosis during this time frame is small, although not non-existent.

Aortic stenosis

Key facts

Untreated severe AS poses such a big risk of perioperative MI or death that elective surgery is usually cancelled until the AS has been treated.
- Up to 3% of elderly patients have clinically significant AS.
- The commonest cause is calcific degeneration.
- 1–2% of population born with bicuspid valve: these calcify earlier.
- Rheumatic disease eventually causes AS but this is less common.
- Critical AS is a valve area <1cm^2 or a valve gradient >50mmHg.
- The problems in AS result from:
  - Compensatory LVH and ↓coronary blood flow.
  - Resulting mismatch between myocardial O_2 supply and demand.
  - The stenosis fixes the cardiac output which therefore cannot rise to meet to ↑ demands. e.g. stress response to surgery

Clinical features

Symptoms

May be asymptomatic, but most aren't. Symptoms give a good guide to life expectancy—the average survival of the patient with untreated AS and dyspnoea is 2 years. In order of worsening prognosis symptoms are:
- Exertional syncope.
- Angina.
- Breathlessness (suggests CCF).
- Sudden death.

Signs

- Slow rising, low amplitude pulse.
- Sustained apex beat.
- Soft 1st heart sound.
- Single 2nd heart sound if valve calcified.
- Ejection systolic murmur loudest in aortic area radiating to carotids.
- Soft early diastolic murmur if AR also present.

Diagnosis and investigations

- TTE will both establish the diagnosis, and quantify the severity of the stenosis, as well as other valve lesions and LV function.
- Most patients with severe AS will go on to have coronary angiography.

Treatment

- Aortic valve replacement:
  - Operative risk of death from 2% for patient <65 years, upwards.
  - As this is much lower than the risk of dying if the lesion is untreated, most patients will be considered for surgery.

Perioperative management
Problems
- In severe or symptomatic AS, cardiac output cannot increase to compensate for hypovolaemia, sepsis, anaemia, hypoxia, or the inflammatory response to injury, resulting in *cardiogenic shock*.
- For the hypertrophied, stiff LV to fill, adequate time is needed in diastole, as is co-ordinated atrial systole (i.e. sinus rhythm). Tachycardia and AF cause *haemodynamic compromise* and *myocardial ischaemia* quickly ensues.
- Hypotension—from any cause—also has the potential to establish a vicious circle of myocardial ischaemia, and further hypotension, ending in death.
- Structurally abnormal heart valves are susceptible to endocarditis, so have a high index of suspicion.

Management
- ⚠ *Surgery should be deferred wherever possible.*
- Seek *cardiology advice*: the safest option is almost invariably elective aortic valve replacement followed by the non-cardiac surgery after an interval of at least 6 weeks.
- Operation under regional may be *worse* than general anaesthesia: spinals and epidurals result in hypotension, surgery causes hypovolaemia and both cause reflex tachycardia—a perilous combination.
- If surgery cannot be deferred, e.g. perforated ulcer, *speak to anaesthetist* early to decide if you need *HDU or ITU bed* post-op.
- A senior member of the team should discuss the options with the patient and obtain informed consent.
- Pre-op cardiology review to optimize antianginals and antiarrhythmics.
- Check local protocols or *BNF* for prophylactic antibiotics for endocarditis.
- Perioperatively maintain sinus rhythm at a rate of 60–80, and BP close to preoperative values by optimizing:
  - Oxygenation: aim for SaO_2 >98%.
  - Filling: usually hypertrophied ventricles need higher CVPs (14–16mmHg) than normal patients to maintain cardiac output.
  - Treat bleeding aggressively to minimize risk of hypovolaemia and anaemia and coagulopathy.
  - Electrolytes: keep K^+ 4.5–5.0mmol/L and Mg^{2+} 0.8–1.2mmol/L to minimize the risk of postoperative AF.
  - *Be vigilant: hypotension, low SaO_2, pulmonary oedema, ↓urine output, acidosis signal cardiogenic shock.*
  - Analgesia: reducing pain and anxiety reduces myocardial O_2 demand.
  - Treat sepsis aggressively: take cultures, including blood cultures, early and repeatedly, and involve a microbiologist early.
  - Have a low threshold for suspecting bacterial endocarditis if sepsis persists: TTE may not identify small vegetations, think about TOE.
- Ensure discharge is with cardiology f/u already in place and that all information is on discharge summary *and* letter to the GP.

Other valve diseases

Aortic regurgitation

Key facts

- Most cases due to rheumatic heart disease, bicuspid valve, AV prolapse. Rare causes: Marfan's, ankylosing spondylitis.
- Long latent period before onset of symptoms, even if AR severe.
- Patients progressively complain of sinus tachycardia on exertion and stress, exertional dyspnoea, orthopnoea, PND, angina-like pain.

Clinical features

Rapidly rising/collapsing pulse, wide pulse pressure, low diastolic BP, displaced apex, 3rd heart sound, early diastolic murmur.

Investigations

- *CXR*: look for cardiac enlargement and pulmonary congestion.
- *TTE*: gives a guide to LV function and the severity of AR.

Implications for surgery

- In contrast to AS, patients with AR tolerate vasodilatation well. This lowers arterial impedance and reduces the degree of regurgitation.
- Vasoconstriction will have a deleterious effect and should be avoided.
- LV function tends to recover after valve replacement, provided the period of LV dysfunction was <12 months. AV replacement should therefore come first only if patient symptomatic and LV dysfunction >12 months.

Mitral regurgitation

Key facts

Much commoner than MS. Many associations: ischaemic heart disease, dilated and hypertrophic cardiomyopathy, floppy mitral valve, rheumatic heart disease, extensive annular mitral calcification, and others. May reflect severe LV dysfunction and the risks and management of these patients are as for the underlying LV dysfunction.

Clinical features

Evidence of a volume overloaded LV (displaced apex, 3rd heart sound). Pansystolic murmur at the apex radiating to the axilla.

Investigations

- *ECG*: look for evidence of old MI or LV hypertrophy.
- *CXR*: look for cardiac enlargement and pulmonary congestion.
- *TTE*: gives a guide to LV function and the severity of MR.
- *Electrolytes and creatinine*: Many patients will be taking diuretics.

Implications for surgery

- Patients usually tolerate surgery well unless the leak is severe.
- Vasodilatation helps to encourage forward flow from the LV into the aorta and also reduces also the regurgitant volume.
- Vasoconstriction and fluid overload should be avoided.

Mitral stenosis

Key facts
- Incidence is declining in the northern hemisphere due to a decline in the incidence of rheumatic fever, which accounts for virtually all adult cases. More common in patients from developing countries.

Clinical features
- Insidious decline in exercise tolerance over many years.
- Complicated by AF and arterial thromboembolism e.g. CVA.
- Physical signs are an irregular pulse (if in established AF), a tapping apex beat (corresponding to a loud 1st heart sound), a right ventricular heave, a mid-to-late low pitched diastolic murmur, and an opening snap.

Investigations
- *ECG*: evidence of left atrial enlargement (p-mitrale) right ventricular hypertrophy, and/or right bundle branch block.
- *CXR*: left atrial enlargement (a straight left heart border, double right heart border, and splaying of the carina).
- *Echocardiography* to assess the severity of the stenosis by estimating the cross-sectional area of the valve orifice (>1.5cm^2 mild, 1–1.5cm^2 moderate, <1cm^2 severe).

Implications for surgery
- Patients with MS tolerate volume overload poorly and this may precipitate pulmonary oedema.
- An abrupt change from sinus rhythm to AF may have a similar effect due to sudden loss of atrial contraction. The ventricular rate in AF is critical. Rapid rates reduce the diastolic filling period; since rapid ventricular filling is impossible through a stenosed mitral valve this will lead to a fall in cardiac output (cardiogenic shock) and pulmonary oedema.
- Patients with MS and AF are at high risk of arterial thromboembolism and are normally anticoagulated with warfarin 📖 see p. 61 for perioperative care.
- Treatment of severe valve disease is by valvotomy or valve replacement. This should be undertaken before elective surgical procedures.

Tricuspid and pulmonary valve disease

Less commonly encountered as clinical problems. They are usually associated with other conditions that determine risks and prognosis.
- *Tricuspid regurgitation*: rarely due to structural valve disease, usually due to chronic LV or mitral valve disease. JVP very high with V-wave. Liver is enlarged and pulsatile. Pansystolic murmur at the left sternal border varies with respiration. Attempts to lower JVP by diuresis are futile and result in a low output state, and venous pressure will still be high. Surgical and anaesthetic risks are same as congestive heart failure.
- *Tricuspid or pulmonary stenosis*: usually due to rheumatic or congenital disease. Reduction in right-sided filling pressures due to venodilatation or hypovolaemia will lead to low cardiac output.
- *Pulmonary regurgitation*: usually occurs 2° to chronic pulmonary hypertension which gives rise to problems e.g. respiratory failure.

Hypertension

Key facts

- One in seven patients is hypertensive. Many are well-managed in primary care; many others do not know they have hypertension.
- There is no clear cut-off for hypertension, but there appears to be an increase of complications from 120/75mmHg upwards (📖 see Grades of hypertension, p. 153).
- Major complications of untreated hypertension are:
  - Ischaemic heart disease: angina, MI.
  - LV hypertrophy and failure.
  - Cerebrovascular disease: stroke, TIA.
  - Renal impairment.
- Implications for surgery and anaesthesia:
  - ⚠ You **must** try to get BP control preoperatively, consider delaying elective cases to allow appropriate investigation and management.
  - There is an ↑risk of perioperative MI, stroke, and renal impairment.
  - Hypertensive patients have a greatly ↑incidence of coronary artery disease.
  - Underlying causes may need investigation and treatment.
  - Both drugs and physiological stimuli which affect vascular tone result in much greater swings in BP in the hypertensive than in a normo-tensive patient. The more poorly controlled the hypertension, the bigger these swings will be.

Box 3.9 Autoregulation

- Organs (brain, heart, etc.) maintain nearly constant blood flow across a wide 'range' of systemic BPs, by varying the resistance of their own arterioles—a process known as autoregulation. However, if the BP falls below the lower limit of this range, blood flow to vital organs drops precipitously.
- In patients with severe and chronic hypertension, this entire 'range' has shifted upwards to compensate for the persistently raised BP. The concern, therefore, is that in these patients blood flow to their vital organs may actually be severely reduced at a BP which appears normal and healthy for the rest of the population.
- With antihypertensive treatment, the patient's BP comes down over a few days. 'Resetting' the body's autoregulation range—so the patient might now safely tolerate a degree of hypotension—takes several weeks, however. This is why elective surgery, especially if it requires prolonged hypotension in order to perform the operation at all, is deferred for longer than just a day or two.

Causes

- 95% are 'essential' hypertension, with no cause found.
- Alcohol consumption and obesity are important aggravating factors.
- Smoking adds to the underlying vascular disease.

- Identifiable causes include: renal disease, endocrine disease, drugs (legal, e.g. TCAs, MAOIs inhibitors, and otherwise, e.g. cocaine) and rarities such as coarctation of the aorta.
- Pre-eclampsia is a common cause of hypertension in pregnancy: any patient with pre-eclampsia needs specialist care.

Preoperative preparation

Patients frequently have ↑BP on admission to hospital (white coat hypertension). The BP should be re-measured several times to get an accurate assessment. Automatic BP monitors with a printout are an easy and accurate way of doing this.

- Cancellation of an uncontrolled hypertensive is reasonable (📖 see p. 63), **providing** a true estimation of BP has been obtained.
- Continue therapy. All patients on anti-hypertensive medication must remain on treatment during the perioperative period unless compromised by bleeding or sepsis. In such cases, stop the drug until cardiovascular stability is restored.

Grades of hypertension

- Patients with severe hypertension (diastolic 115mmHg or greater) should be started on medication or have existing treatment optimized. Elective surgery should be deferred if possible to allow the benefits of treatment to accrue (at least 4 weeks—📖 see Box 3.9).
- Moderately hypertensive patients (diastolic pressure 100–115mmHg) should have their operation deferred if possible and be treated, or their treatment optimized, especially if there is evidence of target-organ damage.
- Mild hypertensives (diastolic pressure <100mmHg) may benefit from the addition of a B-blocker with their premedication—the anaesthetist will decide on this. Clonidine may be considered if β-blockers are contraindicated.
- Even those with mild hypertension may need to be postponed for BP control if their surgery requires deliberate hypotensive techniques e.g. some ENT procedures. Check with a senior.

Postoperative care

- Careful monitoring is required. Try to minimize haemodynamic instability. Resume oral therapy as soon as the patient is stable.
- The treatment of uncontrolled hypertension in the postoperative period is similar to that outlined above.

Adult congenital heart disease

Key facts
- Congenital heart disease occurs in 8/1000 live births.
- Endocarditis prophylaxis: (check local policy as it is subject to change)
  - Traditionally required for all patients with congenital heart disease having dental or general surgery except:
    —isolated os secundum atrial septal defect repaired without a patch >6 months previously.
    —patent ductus arteriosus ligated and divided >6 months previously.
- Adults with congenital heart disease may have totally uncorrected, palliated, or corrected lesions.
- *Tell the anaesthetist early.*

Uncorrected disease
Such patients have developed physiological changes that have made surgical correction impossible (e.g. irreversible severe pulmonary hypertension associated with a large ventricular septal defect). They have a limited life expectancy and are likely to be severely incapacitated. Perioperative mortality is high even with minor surgical interventions. They are best cared for in specialist cardiac centres.

Palliated disease
- These patients have had a palliative operation that has not returned the anatomy to normal. Examples include the Senning or Mustard procedure for transposition of the great vessels or the Fontan procedure for various single ventricle anomalies (e.g. hypoplastic left heart syndrome, tricuspid valve, or pulmonary artery atresia). They usually have some limitation of functional capacity.
- Care of such patients requires a detailed understanding of the palliative procedure and its haemodynamic consequences. Even the most trivial of surgical procedures is best undertaken in a specialist cardiac centre, but if this is impractical, there should be discussion with the centre that undertook the initial cardiac surgery.

Corrected disease
These patients have a congenital defect that has either resolved spontaneously or has been completely corrected. If they have a normal functional capacity they can be treated normally. Remember that there may be associated non-cardiac abnormalities that might affect perioperative management.

Vascular surgery complications

Complications may occur in the perioperative, early or late postoperatively periods. In general vascular patients are older and have an ↑ cardiac, cerebral, pulmonary, and renal comorbidity. This is due to the associated risk factors of hypertension, diabetes mellitus, hypercholesterolaemia and smoking.

General

Cardiac (📖 p. 118)

- Atherosclerosis is a systemic disease with a predilection for the cerebral, coronary, peripheral arterial, and renal circulations.
- 40% of patients with PVD have at least 2 of the other circulations affected.
- 20% of patients undergoing non-cardiac vascular surgery have evidence of silent myocardial ischaemia.
- 70% of the mortality associated with aortic surgery is attributable to perioperative cardiac dysfunction.

Pulmonary (📖 p. 190)

- Worsened by pre-existing pulmonary disease, smoking, and obesity.
- Ensure adequate analgesia with PCA or epidural and good physiotherapy and early mobilization.

Haemorrhage (📖 p. 98)

- Perioperative: bleeding from uncontrolled blood vessels.
- Post-operative: usually due to breakdown of vascular anastomoses. Recognized by acute hypotension, shock, abdominal swelling, and pain. Return to the operating theatre.

Renal failure

- Many vascular patients have pre-existing renal impairment due to renovascular disease, drug treatments, or surgery.
- Acute perioperative risks include dehydration, use of IV contrast, use of NSAIDs and nephrotoxic antibiotics.

Specific

Post-declamp shock

- Due to reperfusion of ischaemic region, with sudden release into circulation of all its accumulated metabolites and toxins.
- Features of acute haemodynamic instability and release of toxins (↑ potassium, myoglobin).
- Prevented by controlled gradual reperfusion with fluid resuscitation and vasopressor treatment to maintain a good perfusion pressure to the coronary, cerebral, and renal circulations.

Trash foot

- Embolization of debris to the skin or feet after aorto-iliac surgery.
- Avoided by careful surgical technique and distal vessel clamping first.

Swollen limb

- Most are due to reperfusion injury of previously ischaemic limbs.
- Consider D-dimers and lower leg Doppler US if DVT a possiblity.

Lymphocoele
- Occurs mostly after groin surgery.
- Presents as a fluctuant, non-tender swelling.
- Most will settle spontaneously, although larger collections may be aspirated under **strict** aseptic conditions.
- Rarely require further surgery to oversew the lymphatics.

Gut ischaemia
- May follow aortic surgery (ischaemic colitis), 2.5% after ruptured AAA surgery, and < 1% of elective aortic aneurysm surgery due to loss of gut blood supply.
- May present as vague abdominal pain or blood stained diarrhoea.
- Sigmoidoscopy usually confirms the diagnosis.
- If there is no evidence of peritonitis then fluids to rehydrate and close observation are required.
- If there is evidence of peritonitis then an urgent laparotomy is needed with resection of the ischaemic bowel.

Impaired sexual function
Due to damage to the peri-aortic or hypogastric plexus and underlying vascular disease of the blood supply to the pelvis

Late complications
Graft occlusion
- Early failure <30 days—technical cause. Recognized by acute deterioration in symptoms or acute limb ischaemia.
- Late failure—usually due to intimal hyperplasia, continued smoking, or disease progression. Recognized by progressively worsening symptoms

False aneurysm
- Usually 2° to infection or occasionally fatigue of graft material (long term). Further surgery is usually required.

Graft infection
- Mostly gut bacteria or coagulase –ve staphylococci. MRSA an increasing problem.
- Can be minimized by prophylactic antibiotics, meticulous technique, and infection control policies on vascular wards.
- Once infected, the graft usually has to be removed and alternative extra-anatomic reconstruction required.
- Recognized by signs of low grade or chronic sepsis (↑CRP, ↓Hb, fever).

Acute limb ischaemia

Key facts

- An emergency: irreversible tissue damage can occur in <6h leading to loss of limb, and mortality up to 20%.
- 2/3^{rds} due to acute thrombosis in setting of chronic atherosclerotic narrowing, 1/3rd due to emboli (cardiac—think intramural thrombus from AF or MI, more proximal aneurysmal disease).
- May also be associated with displaced limb fractures.
- *Postoperatively, particularly after:*
  - AAA repair (intraoperative embolism of atherosclerotic debris).
  - Fem–pop/fem–distal bypass graft thrombosis.
  - Cannulation of femoral, radial, or brachial artery for any reason.
- Predisposing factors include dehydration, hypotension, malignancy, polycythaemia, or inherited prothrombotic states.
- Rarely inadvertent intra-arterial injection can cause acute ischaemia.

Clinical features of acute limb ischaemia

Six Ps: Pain, Pallor, Pulselessness, Paraesthesia, Perishing cold.

Emergency management

Resuscitation

- Give 100% O_2.
- Get IV access and consider crystalloid fluid up to 1000mL if dehydrated
- Take blood for FBC, troponin, clotting, glucose, G&S.
- Request CXR and ECG (look for dysrhythmias especially AF and evidence of previous MI).
- Give opiate analgesia (5–10mg morphine IM).
- Call for senior help.

Establish a diagnosis

- Type (embolism/thrombosis): thorough history and examination will help identify whether there was previous claudication (suggests thrombosis) or no evidence underlying vascular disease (suggests embolism), as well as any iatrogenic potential causes.
- Limb viability assessment—involve senior help early:
  - Irreversible—fixed mottling of skin, petechial haemorrhages in skin, woody hard muscles which are painful to touch.
  - Complete—white, cold, pulseless limb.
  - Incomplete—reduced pulses, severely reduced capillary refill.
- Underlying cause: echocardiography, 24h tape, angiogram.

Early treatment

- Consider giving heparin (5000IU unfractionated heparin IV bolus and start an infusion of 1000IU per hour) if there are no contra-indications (e.g. aortic dissection, multiple trauma, head injury).
  - Recheck activated partial thromboplastin time (APTT) in 4–6h.
  - Aim for a target time of 2–2.5 times the normal range.
- Patients are at ↑ risk of renal failure: monitor hourly fluid balance and ensure adequate systemic BP and hydration.

Definitive management

Depends on the severity of ischaemia:

- Irreversible (non-salvageable limb): amputation is inevitable and urgent to prevent the systemic complications of muscle necrosis (□ p. 212).
- Complete (acutely threatened limb): requires expert vascular input— thrombolysis, angioplasty, embolectomy or urgent arterial bypass.
- Incomplete (viable limb): needs heparinization to prevent propagation of thrombus, urgent imaging and definitive intervention (thrombolysis, angioplasty, arterial surgery).

Management of inadvertent intra-arterial injection

- This may result in loss of limb, depending on substance injected, amount injected and management.
- Early signs include pain, pallor, mottling, cyanosis due to arterial spasm.
- Very late signs included trophic skin changes, ulceration and oedema: gangrene or contractures are late features of severe cases.

Management

- If arterial cannula *in situ*, leave in place.
- Discuss with plastic or vascular surgeons *immediately*.
- Inject 1000IU heparin down cannula to reduce risk of thrombosis.
- Inject warm NS down cannula to dilute substance.
- Dexamethasone 8mg IV may reduce arterial oedema.
- Consider anticoagulation for 7–14 days.
- Give 2.5–5mg morphine IV.

Critical limb ischaemia

- Ischaemia which is likely to progress to limb loss or progressive tissue loss if it remains untreated, diagnosed by:
  - Rest pain for >2 weeks not relieved by simple analgesia, or
  - Doppler ankle pressure <50 mmHg (toe pressures <30mmHg if diabetic), or tissue necrosis (i.e. gangrene or ulceration).
- Rest pain typically worsens at night and during elevation of the limb; the pain is relieved by dangling the limb over the side of the bed.
- Arterial ulceration is typically painful, shallow, non-bleeding with few signs of healing.

Diagnosis and investigation

- Identify and treat risk factors: serum glucose, cholesterol, BP.
- Identify location and severity of all arterial stenoses involved: colour duplex Doppler ultrasound, angiography (usually Digital Subtraction Angiography (DSA)), magnetic resonance angiography (MRA).

Treatment

- Medical: analgesia—opiates (morophone oral solution, tablets or m/r preparations).
- Endovascular treatments: angioplasty ± stent proximal stenoses.
- Surgery: femorodistal bypass or amputation.

Aneurysms

Key facts

- An aneurysm is an abnormal localized dilatation of a blood vessel
- Affects 5% of ♂ over the age of 65, increasing with age, ♂:♀ = 9:1
- True aneurysms (all 3 layers of artery) usually due to atherosclerosis (associated with: hypertension, smoking, and family history).
- False aneurysms do not contain all 3 arterial wall layers: often traumatic e.g. femoral puncture, or infective.
- Common sites include thoracoabdominal, abdominal and peripheral (iliac, femoral, popliteal, visceral, carotid, or subclavian).

Clinical features

Thoracoabdominal

- Often asymptomatic, may present with acute chest pain (angina/MI), back pain, hoarseness, AR or cardiac failure due to complications.
- 50% diagnosed by widened mediastinum on CXR.
- Rupture has high mortality, rare without prior symptoms, risk is directly proportional to size.

Abdominal aortic

- Most are asymptomatic, 40% are detected incidentally (clinical examination, US, AXR, IVU).
- Increasingly there is a case for a national screening programme.
- 6-monthly scans for surveillance if size 4–5.4cm (1% per annum risk of rupture).
- 95% start below the origin of the renal arteries 'infrarenal'.
- 15% extend down to involve the origins of the common iliac arteries.
- Associated with other peripheral aneurysm (e.g. popliteal).
- 5–10% are 'inflammatory' (have gross connective tissue changes around the aortic wall in the retroperitoneum).

Peripheral aneurysms

- *Iliac:* 2% of patients >70 years. Mostly common iliac, often silent. Rarely palpable and rupture may be missed as acute abdomen or renal colic.
- *Femoral:* common site of false aneurysm, mostly asymptomatic pulsatile groin swelling or pain (25%). May present with lower limb ischaemia.
- *Popliteal:* many asymptomatic and over half are bilateral. May present with acute limb ischaemia and has a high limb loss in thrombosis.
- *Carotid:* rare and may be bilateral. May present with neurological or pressure symptoms. May present simply as a pulsatile neck swelling.
- *Visceral:* account for 1% of all aneurysms. Generally small and often asymptomatic until rupture. Splenic artery most common followed by hepatic and renal arteries.

Complications

Risk of rupture and mortality increase with increasing aneurysm diameter: 30–80% of those with ruptured abdominal aortic aneurysms will die even with surgery.

Preoperative management
- Discuss new findings of an aneurysm with vascular surgery: all except large or symptomatic aneurysms can generally be managed by monitoring size.
- Presence of a known asymptomatic aneurysm should not delay other surgery: contact vascular surgery for advice if the patient reports symptoms that could be due to the aneurysm (pain, nerve compression syndromes), or if the aneurysm has enlarged >0.5cm in last 6 months.
- Careful BP control: aim to maintain systolic BP <150mmHg.
- Look for other complications of atherosclerotic disease and treat appropriately: IHD (📖 p. 118), renal dysfunction (📖 p. 212), stroke (📖 p. 298).

Postoperative management
Continue careful BP control and preventative measures aimed at avoiding renal dysfunction (📖 p. 212), and myocardial ischaemia (📖 p. 120).

Carotid disease

Key facts

- Management of stroke is described on 📖 p. 298 and p. 300.
- A cerebrovascular accident (CVA) or 'stroke' is 'a sudden onset of irreversible neurological deficit': a transient ischaemic attack (TIA) is 'a sudden onset of neurological deficit which resolves within 24hrs'
- CVA has an incidence of 2 per 1000 population: roughly 15% of these are due to atherosclerotic disease of the carotid arteries.
- Atheromatous plaques form at the bifurcation of the common carotid artery and progress into the external and internal carotid vessels.

Clinical features

- Patients may give a history of previous stroke or TIAs: neurological *features* depend on the territory supplied by the vessel affected by the embolism, the degree of collateral circulation to that territory, and the size/resolution of the embolism.
  - *Amaurosis fugax:* transient monocular visual loss (described as a curtain coming down across the eye), lasting for a few seconds or minutes—*central retinal artery.*
  - *Internal capsular stroke:* dense hemiplegia usually including the face—striate branches of the middle cerebral artery.
  - *Hemianopia:* loss of vision in one half of the visual field.
- Carotid bruits are detectable in over 10% of patients >60 years of age and do not correlate well with the degree of stenosis or risk of CVA.
- Patients with a significant stenosis may have no audible bruit.
- 80% of TIAs are in the carotid territory and the risk of stroke following a TIA is around 18% in the first year, 20% of which may occur in the first month of the TIA. The overall risk is 7 × the risk of stroke for an age-matched population.

Diagnosis and investigation

- Carotid colour duplex scan—all patients who have had a TIA or stroke within the last 6 months. 95% accuracy for assessment of degree of stenosis.
- MRA is reserved for those patients when duplex is inconclusive or difficult due to calcified vessels.

Preoperative management

- Asymptomatic carotid stenosis is not normally a reason for delaying other surgery.
- Discuss any patient with symptomatic, significant (70–99%) carotid stenosis with vascular surgery, who will need to see the patient in clinic after surgery.
- In patients undergoing cardiac surgery, vascular and cardiac surgeons should liaise to perform staged cardiac and vascular intervention (stent or surgery) to reduce the risk of perioperative stroke.
- *Best medical therapy:* a antiplatelet agent (e.g. aspirin, dipiridamole), smoking cessation, optimization of BP and diabetes control, and a statin for cholesterol lowering.

Surgery

- Carotid endarterectomy: offered to patients with symptomatic >70% stenosis of the internal carotid artery: there is no significant benefit to symptomatic patients with <70% stenoses, and low benefit for asymptomatic >70% stenosis.
- Endovascular stent may be an option.
- Complications:
  - Death or major disabling stroke 1–2%.
  - Minor stroke with recovery 3–6%.
  - MI.
  - Wound haematoma.
  - Damage to hypoglossal nerve, ansa cervicalis, vagus nerve.

Foot ulcers

Key facts

- Foot ulceration commonly results from diabetic vascular complications, critical limb ischaemia, chronic venous insufficiency, neuropathic disease, as well as cutaneous malignancy.
- Established ulcers are very resistant to treatment: prevention is key.
- Evidence of sepsis may mean that elective surgery, particularly that involving prosthetic implants e.g. orthopaedic and cardiac valve surgery, may be postponed until adequate control of sepsis is obtained.

Causes and features

Table 3.7 Differentiating foot ulcers

Ulcer type	Clinical features
Diabetic (mixed ischaemia / neuropathic)	diabetes, infection, sensory neuropathy, failure to heal trivial injuries: look for evidence of peripheral arterial disease (🕮 p.156)
Ischaemia	vascular disease, painful ulcers over extremities – toe tips, ± gangrene, pain relived by dependency, ↓pulses, ↓ABPI
Neuropathic	diabetes/stroke/other neuropathy, painless ulcers over pressure areas (heel, Achilles tendon, metatarsal head), warm foot with good pulses, sensory loss
Venous (chronic venous insufficiency)	DVT, varicose veins, painful shallow ulcer over medial malleolus, varicose eczema, leg oedema, lipodermatosclerosis, pain relieved by elevation
Malignancy	Punched-out, irregular edged ulcer, dorsum foot

Investigation

- Calculate ABPI (Box 3.10).
- Venous Duplex to detect deep venous thrombosis or incompetence and to look for superficial venous disease.
- If clinical features suggest ischaemia component request US, contrast angiography, or MRA study of arterial tree.

Perioperative management

- Care of the diabetic surgical patients is described on 🕮 p. 274, Care of critical limb ischaemia is described on p. 159.
- Involve specialist tissue viability team with multidisciplinary input.
- Careful inspection for evidence of pressure/ulceration/infection.
- Treat local or systemic infection:
  - Broad spectrum antibiotics (local guidelines).
  - Debride obviously dead tissue.
  - Drain collections of pus.
  - Take plain XR for signs of underlying osteomyelitis.
- Refer to vascular surgery if re-vascularization or amputation is considered.

- If concern that malignancy is underlying pathology refer early to plastic surgery or dermatology: this should not delay important elective surgery (unless ulcerating melanoma).

Venous ulcers
- Elevation, bed rest, and elevation of foot of bed.
- Graduated compression hosiery (when ulcers healed) to prevent complications of oedema and varicose veins.
- Treat stasis ulcers with 4 layer compression bandaging (Charing Cross). 75% ulcer healing at 12 weeks as long as ABPI >0.7 or Doppler pressures >50mmHg.
- Skin grafts (split skin and pinch grafts).
- Ulcer bed clearance of slough/infection.
- Surgery for superficial venous disease only.

Box 3.10 How to do ankle-brachial pressure index (ABPI)

- Position patient flat in bed.
- Inflate syphgmanometry cuff in normal position on upper arm and record pressure at which ipsilateral brachial pulse disappears.
- Now re-position cuff over calf.
- Locate Doppler dorsalis pedis pulse, inflate cuff slowly, and note the pressure at which the Doppler pulse disappears.
- Repeat for posterior tibial pulse, and other leg.
- Divide ankle pressure by branchial pressure to obtain ABPI.
- 120mmHg/120mmHg = 1.0 (normal).
- Values <1.0 suggest arterial stenosis: ABPI 0.3 = critical limb ischemia.
- Values >>1.0 suggest calcification of leg vessels.

Amputations

Key facts
- 90% for arterial disease (20% of which are in diabetics), 10% for trauma, 1% for pure venous disease.
- Amputation may be a very beneficial treatment for pain, to restore mobility or occasionally to save a life in trauma or acute limb ischaemia.
- Amputation for arterial disease carries a significant mortality and a major morbidity.
- The surgical aim is to achieve a healthy stump for a suitable prosthesis and successful rehabilitation.
- Amputees are at the centre of a large team including surgeons, nurses, physiotherapists, prosthetists, occupational therapists, counsellors, and the family.

Causes and features
- 'Dangerous'—life saving:
  - Spreading gangrene e.g. necrotizing fasciitis, gas gangrene.
  - Extensive tissue necrosis following burns or trauma.
  - Uncontrolled sepsis (diabetic foot) with systemic infection.
  - Primary malignant limb tumours not suitable for local excision.
- 'Dead'—vascular events:
  - Critical limb ischaemia with unreconstructable disease.
  - Irreversible acute limb ischaemia.
- 'Damn nuisance'—neuropathic or deformed:
  - Failed, complicated orthopaedic surgery with severely impaired gait

Level
- The level is chosen according to:
  - Lowest level tissue is viable for healing.
  - Include as many working major joints as possible to improve function.
  - Ideally sited between large joints to allow prosthesis fitting.
- *Above knee:* most will heal and some achieve walking with a prosthesis.
- *Through knee:* fewer heal and some achieve walking.
- *Below knee:* about 2/3rds heal and many more achieve walking than with above knee amputations.

Types
- *Hip disarticulation:* rarely needed but indicated for trauma or tissue necrosis above high thigh.
- *Above knee (AKA):* bone transected at junction of upper 2/3rds and 1/3rd of femur (12–15cm above knee joint), common in end-stage vascular disease.
- *Gritti–Stokes (supracondylar above knee amputation):* increasingly popular for bilateral amputees as creates a long stump. Especially good for wheelchair-dependent patients.
- *Through knee (TKA):* produces a wide stump which is difficult for prosthesis fit.

- *Below knee (BKA):* weight bearing on patellar tendon with good prosthetic fit, good knee function essential:
  - Skew flap is best technique as it produces a better stump for prosthetic fitting.
  - Alternative is a posterior flap which is bulkier and leads to longer time to mobilization but better healing.
  - The tibia is transected 8–10cm distal to the tibial tuberosity and the fibula 2cm more proximally.
  - Postoperative mobilization is early and temporary limb aids can be used when the wound is sound.
- *Symes (ankle):* few indications for this in vascular patients and best avoided other than in trauma or diabetics. Prosthetic fitting is difficult and a good BKA is better for walking
- *Transmetatarsal:* useful in diabetics or when several toes are gangrenous.
- *Ray:* used when digital gangrene extends to forefoot, especially useful for diabetics when infection tracks up tendon sheath.
- *Digital:* usually only for diabetic disease or local trauma.

Treatment

Preoperative care
- Restore haemoglobin levels and correct fluid and electrolyte balance.
- Ensure good diabetes control.
- XM 2U of blood.
- Adequate pain relief.
- ECG and CXR.
- Optimize cardiac function.
- Prophylactic antibiotics with cephalosporin/metronidazole with additional gentamycin if MRSA +ve.
- Counselling if available.

Postoperative care
- Pain control with epidural ± PCA.
- Regular physiotherapy to prevent muscle atrophy or contractures as well as upper limb exercises.
- Early rehabilitation on temporary limb aid.
- Own wheelchair to aid early mobilization.

Complications
- Infection.
- Non-healing of stump.
- Progression of underlying disease and higher level amputation.
- Phantom limb pain: due to hypersensitivity in divided nerves, can be helped with gabapentin, amitriptyline, or carbamazepine.
- Failed mobilization: early regular analgesia and physiotherapy are important.
- Perioperative cardiovascular events in arteriopathic patient

Venous thromboembolism

Key facts

- DVT incidence is highest in patients over 40 years who undergo major surgery (Box 3.11).
- A postoperative increase in platelets coupled with venous endothelial trauma and stasis all contribute (Virchow's triad).
- Without prophylaxis, 30% of surgical patients develop DVT, 0.1–0.2% will die from pulmonary thromboembolism (PTE).

Box 3.11 Patients at high risk of DVT and PE

- Patients undergoing pelvic surgery.
- Patients undergoing hip replacement surgery.
- Patients with malignant disease, especially pelvic tumours.
- Patients on the contraceptive pill, or pregnant.
- Previous history of DVT or PTE.
- Older patients: increase in DVT is almost linear with age.
- Other factors: immobility, dehydration, obesity, diabetes mellitus, polycythaemia, varicose veins, cardiac and respiratory disease, SLE.

Clinical features of DVT

Symptoms

- Swollen, painful, warm, erythematous leg, usually unilateral.
- May present with symptoms of PE (📖 p. 194).

Signs

- Calf tenderness and ↑circumference >3cm on affected side.
- Mild pyrexia at 7–8 days postoperatively.
- Assess likelihood of alternative diagnosis (Baker's cyst, cellulitis).

Investigations

- Duplex Doppler: less sensitive for calf DVT than thigh DVT, but in conjunction with –ve D-dimer excludes significant DVT in pre-op patient (NB D-dimers increase in response to surgery).
- Ascending venography: more sensitive than duplex but invasive.

Preoperative management

- In newly diagnosed DVT, consider deferring surgery until patient anti-coagulated (INR 2–3) for 5–10 days, and clinical signs improved.
- Stop warfarin 4 days preoperatively in patients with known DVT (📖 p. 61 for managing pre-op anticoagulation).
- Ensure patients at high risk of DVT receive heparin prophylaxis (e.g. 20–40mg enoxaparin SC od), TED stockings and early mobilization.
- Consider stopping OCP 6 weeks pre-op.

Postoperative care

- All thrombi should be treated with heparin for 4–7 days (see BNF for dosing) (40 000U/24h), checked by APTT (5000–10 000U by bolus then 1000–1500U/h IV), or followed by anticoagulation for 6–12 weeks with warfarin (checked by INR) or LMWH (by U/weight).

- In bilateral ileofemoral DVT or recurrent embolism, IVC filter at the level below the renal vessels may prevent pulmonary embolism.
- Postphlebitic syndrome reduced with graded compression stockings.

Prevention

Mechanical devices (only if foot pulses present)
- Thrombo-embolic deterrent stockings (TEDS)—reduce stasis in infra-popliteal veins by continuous direct compression.
- Intermittent pneumatic compression (IPC) 'boots'—reduce stasis in infrapopliteal veins by intermittent compression of lower leg veins, improving venous blood flow.

Drugs acting on the clotting cascade
- Heparin activates anti-thrombin III.
  - Prophylaxis: 5000IU SC bd.
  - Treatment: 75IU/kg loading dose IV, 18IU/kg/h IV maintenance (1000IU per mL NS), check APTT 4–6h after starting and every dose change, titrate to APTT 50–70. Daily APTT once stable.
- LMWH inhibits clotting factor Xa. Given by SC injection:
  - Prophylaxis: 20–40mg SC enoxaparin od.
  - Treatment: 1.5mg/kg SC od.

Side effects of heparin/LMWH
- Bleeding.
- Thrombocytopaenia (check platelet antibodies if ↓platelets) (📖 p. 100).
- Alopecia.
- Osteoporosis

At-risk groups

Low risk—TEDs only
Day case surgery, minor orthopaedic procedures and surgery where patients mobilize immediately after surgery.

Medium risk—TEDS and prophylactic dose LMWH, IPC boots
E.g. Surgery where mobilization is expected to be slow, abdominal, thoracic, upper limb orthopaedic surgery, or low-risk procedures but with co-morbidity risk factors.

High risk—TEDS and treatment dose LMWH or IV heparin, IPC boots
E.g. Pelvic surgery, major lower limb orthopaedic procedures, surgery for malignancy, or medium-risk procedures with associated co-morbid risk factors.

Thrombolysis

Key facts

- ⚠ *Major surgery within 6 weeks is an absolute contraindication to thrombolysis which could result in catastrophic bleeding.*
- Used in treatment of acute MI, PE, DVT, acute limb ischaemia due to peripheral vascular thrombosis and occasionally blocked dialysis catheters.
- For acute limb ischaemia, usually administered as a low dose intra-arterial infusion or increasingly as an adjunct to surgery intraoperatively.
- Three main agents:
  - *Urokinase:* expensive, rarely used in UK.
  - *Streptokinase:* cheap but has systemic effects and 27-min half life. Has side-effects of anaphylaxis, fever, and antibody resistance limiting repeated use. Widely used for treatment of MI.
  - *Recombinant tPA:* powerful clot affinity, lower systemic effects and bleeding complications and half life <6min.

Regimen

- Administered via arterial catheter and simultaneous heparin via catheter sheath.
- Regular clinical assessment and coagulation checks are needed with clear protocols. Half-hourly, T, PR, and BP as well as foot observations.
- Regular review with angiography (min. 8-hourly).
- ↑complication rate after 24–36h of infusion.

Contraindications

- ↑risk of bleeding (haemorrhagic disorders, peptic ulcer, recent haemorrhagic stroke, recent major surgery or multiple puncture sites).
- Evidence of muscle necrosis as may result in reperfusion syndrome and multi-organ failure.

Complications

- Minor: allergenic, catheter problems (leak, occlusion), bruising, 15% risk of haemorrhage.
- Major: 5% risk of major haemorrhage or stroke.

Respiratory

Arterial blood gas: basics

Indications

- Preoperative evaluation of patient with suspected severe respiratory disease.
- Postoperative diagnosis of respiratory failure.
- Postoperative assessment of *any* critically ill patient.

For definitions of respiratory failure see Box 4.1.

> **Box 4.1 Some useful definitions**
> - *Hypoxaemia:* PaO_2 <11kPa (lower in very elderly).
> - *Hypercapnia:* $PaCO_2$ >6.5kPa.
> - *Hypocapnia:* $PaCO_2$ <3.5kPa.
> - *Type I respiratory failure:* PaO_2 <8.0kPa on *air* (at rest).
> - *Type II respiratory failure:* PaO_2 <8kPa and a $PaCO_2$ >6.5kPa.

Step-by-step interpretation (Box 4.1)

ABG tell you about two things, but *always* take account of the clinical picture and any previous ABG results: normal values are given in Table 4.1.

Respiratory function

- *Look at PaO_2:* <8kPa indicates significant hypoxia (particularly if patient on O_2 therapy), and *defines respiratory failure* (🕮 see p. 180). If this does not fit clinical picture consider if sample is venous or (rarely) if a cardiac right-to-left shunt is present. PaO_2 >15kPa indicates high FiO_2 which is usually unnecessary.
- *Look at $PaCO_2$:* if low, patient hyperventilating, if raised hypoventilating: acutely raised $PaCO_2$>8kPa (60mmHg) can result in coma (🕮 see p. 292). As CO_2 is acidic, this *has an effect* on acid–base status.
- SaO_2 is predicted from PaO_2 (unless the ABG analyser fitted with oximeter). **A pulse oximeter SaO_2 is thus *usually* more accurate than ABG in estimating SaO_2.** Errors in pulse oximetry if: poor peripheral perfusion/badly fitted probe/↑methaemoglobin (SaO_2 falsely low), ↑carboxyhaemoglobin (SaO_2 falsely high).

Acid–base balance

- *Look at pH:* below normal is acidosis, above normal is alkalosis.
- *Look again at $PaCO_2$:* CO_2 is acidic, and acidosis with high $PaCO_2$ or alkalosis with low $PaCO_2$ indicates *respiratory acidosis* or *alkalosis*, respectively.
- *Confirm diagnosis by looking at HCO_3^- and base excess (BE):* $HCO3^-$ and BE are derived values describing the *metabolic* acid–base status of blood. A high HCO_3^- (i.e. a base *excess*) indicates a *metabolic alkalosis*. A low HCO_3^- (or '*negative* base excess') suggests a *metabolic acidosis*.
- In acidotic patients, instead of saying 'the base excess is *minus* 6', many people will say 'the patient has a *base deficit* of 6'. Both are used.

Table 4.1 Normal ABG values

pH	7.35–7.45
PaO$_2$	11–13kPa (83–98 mmHg)
PaCO$_2$	4.8–6.0kPa (36–45 mmHg)
HCO$_3^-$	22–29mmol/L
Base excess	–2 to +2
Haemoglobin O$_2$ saturation	>94%

Box 4.2 Blood gas interpretation in sick surgical patients

1) FIRST look at patient—are they unwell?

2) Look at PaO$_2$: is patient <u>hypoxic</u>?
- Act **now** to prevent respiratory arrest.
- Give high-flow O$_2$ (📖 p.178).
- Call for anaesthetic help.

3) Look at pH: is patient <u>acidotic</u>?
- This is a serious and late sign.

4) Look at PaCO$_2$: is the patient <u>hyperventilating</u>?
- Pulmonary oedema (📖 p.182), PE, (📖 p.194), pneumonia (📖 p.192).

5) Look at PaCO$_2$ again: is the patient hypoventilating i.e. respiratory acidosis?
- Opiate overdose, oversedation, *exhausted*

6) Look at base excess: is there a <u>metabolic</u> acidosis?
- Commonest postoperative causes are:
  • SHOCK (↑lactate) 📖 p.116.
  • DKA (↑glucose) 📖 p.278.
  • Renal failure (↑K+, ↓u/o) 📖 p.212.
  • Metformin, liver failure, ASA rare.

Arterial blood gas: interpretation

Primary and compensatory mechanisms

- Acidosis can be either respiratory (raised $PaCO_2$) or metabolic (low HCO_3^-), or both.
  - In acute *respiratory acidosis* there is no time for metabolic compensation. Thus: low pH, high $PaCO_2$ (and normal HCO_3^-). If metabolic compensation occurs, HCO_3^- will rise.
  - In acute *metabolic acidosis,* there is usually prompt hyperventilation to provide respiratory compensation (this may be only partial i.e. the pH <7.35). Thus: low Ph, low HCO_3^-, (and low $PaCO_2$).
  - A mixed picture acidosis has low Ph, high $PaCO_2$, low HCO_3^-.
- Respiratory alkalosis results from hyperventilation due to hypoxia (e.g. pneumonia, PE) or just hyperventilation alone (anxiety, claustrophobia behind a Hudson mask.
  - Thus: high pH, low CO_2, (and normal HCO_3^-).
  - Gradual compensation by decrease in HCO_3^-.
- Metabolic alkalosis is rare (mild salicylate toxicity, persistent vomiting). As hypoventilation is constrained by our need to maintain PaO_2, respiratory compensation does not really occur: thus high pH, high HCO_3^-, (and normal $PaCO_2$).
- A respiratory acidosis, if acute, is usually due to alveolar hypoventilation (opioids, secretion retention, pain on breathing deeply, etc.). If the pH is normal because of an accompanying metabolic alkalosis, the history will tell you which disturbance came first. Usually chronic CO_2 retention (e.g. COPD) gives rise to a compensatory metabolic alkalosis; it is rarer to see a 1° metabolic alkalosis produce a compensatory CO_2 retention.

Base excess, base deficit, and anion gap

These are derived numbers, calculated by blood-gas analysers, quantifying changes in metabolic or fixed acids but, because they depend on several assumptions, they do not always reflect the true acid–base balance.

- *Base excess* is defined as the mmol per litre of **acid** required to titrate the blood pH back to pH 7.4, if the pCO_2 were normal.
- *Base deficit (–ve base excess)* is defined as the mmol per litre of **base** to titrate the blood pH back to pH 7.4, if the pCO_2 were normal.
- A base deficit is –ve and a base excess is +ve by convention. Normal values are *–2mmol/L to 2mmol/L.* A base deficit greater than this (e.g. –6mmol/L) indicates a metabolic acidosis.
- The *anion gap* is the difference between measured cations and measured anions (= $[K^+ + Na^+] - [Cl^- + HCO_3^-]$). This 'gap' is made up of metabolic acids: ketones, lactate, and phosphates. The anion gap is normally *8–16mmol/L*: an increase in anion gap indicates a metabolic acidosis.

Special circumstances

- CO poisoning: measure blood gases using an analyser with a Co-oximeter to estimate the carboxyhaemoglobin percentage.
- Hypothermia and pyrexia.
- Capillary gases are sometimes used in small children: The PaO_2 is lower than arterial, but other parameters are the same.
- See Box 4.3 for examples.

Box 4.3 Causes of acid-base problems in surgical patients

Metabolic acidosis

Metabolic acidosis due to ↑metabolic acids (i.e. ↑anion gap)

- Lactic acid (global and/or regional hypoperfusion, hypoxia, sepsis, hepatic failure as the liver normally metabolises lactate).
- Uric acid (renal failure).
- Ketones (DKA 📖 p.278, alcoholic and starvation ketoacidosis).
- Drugs/toxins (salicylates, sodium nitroprusside overdose).

Due to loss of bicarbonate or hyperchloraemia (normal anion gap)

- Renal tubular acidosis, e.g. from acetazolamide (loss of bicarbonate).
- Diarrhoea, high output ileostomy (loss of bicarbonate).
- Pancreatic fistulae (loss of bicarbonate).
- Hyperchloraemic acidosis (excessive IV/NS administration).

Metabolic alkalosis

- Loss of H^+ from gut (vomiting, NG tube suction).
- Renal loss of H^+ (diuretics), ↑reabsorption of HCO_3 (↓Cl^-).
- Administration of base ($NaHCO_3$).

Respiratory acidosis

- Any cause of hypoventilation (brain stem lesions, opioid toxicity, high epidural block, motor neurone disease, cervical spinal cord lesion, ankylosing spondylitis, incisional pain in chest/abdominal wall, obstructive sleep apnoea, etc.).
- In patients with hypoxia who have been hyperventilating in order to compensate, the sudden appearance of a respiratory acidosis suggests exhaustion and imminent respiratory arrest.
- ↑production of CO_2 e.g. sepsis, malignant hyperpyrexia.
- Rebreathing CO_2 (circuit misconnections, soda lime exhaustion).

Respiratory alkalosis

Hyperventilation: deliberate, inadvertent, or in non-ventilated patients caused by stroke, anxiety, PE, pneumonia, asthma, pulmonary oedema or any other cause of Type I respiratory failure.

Anion gap in metabolic acidosis

- The anion gap can help determine the cause of metabolic acidosis. It is calculated as $[Na^+] + [K^+] - [Cl^-] - [HCO3^-]$. Normal is 16–18mmol/L.
- An elevated anion gap suggests accumulation of anions; measure these directly in blood to determine diagnosis:
  - Lactic acid (sepsis, shock, hypoxaemia).
  - Ketones (diabetic ketoacidosis, alcohol).
  - Drugs (biguanides, salicylates, ethylene glycol, methanol).
  - Urate (renal failure).
- There are six causes of normal anion gap metabolic acidosis:
  - Renal tubular acidosis, diarrhoea, pancreatic fistula, Addison's disease, acetazolamide, ammonium chloride ingestion.

Respiratory function tests

Indications
- This allows the assessment of lung volume, air flow, lung mechanics, and gas exchange.
- Routinely performed before any lung resection.

Spirometry (Fig 4.1)
This measures expiratory flow and volume over time. Using a variety of measures, obstructive (asthma, COPD) and restrictive (fibrosis) lung defects can be quantified.
- Forced vital capacity (FVC).
- Forced expiratory volume in 1 second (FEV_1).
- FEV_1/FVC ratio (normal is ~75% depending on age, sex, height).
- Peak expiratory flow rate (PEFR, useful in asthmatic patients) (Fig. 4.2).

Obstructive defect
Reduced FEV_1, normal or reduced FVC, FEV_1 reduced more than FVC. FEV_1/FVC <70% due to limitation of peak expiratory flow. Forced expiration is particularly helpful in identifying obstructive disease as many conducting airways that are only just open will be rapidly squeezed shut by the active compression of the lungs.

Restrictive defect:
Reduced FVC, low or normal FEV_1, FEV_1/FVC ≥80%.

Gas transfer tests
These evaluate the integrity of the alveolar capillary membrane and the pulmonary capillary blood volume. They are the best predictor of post operative pulmonary complications. A figure <60% predicted warrants further investigation.

Cardio-pulmonary exercise testing (CPX)
Sometimes used before major (non-cardiac) surgery as a means of estimating operative mortality. The aim is to experimentally determine the patient's anaerobic threshold, i.e. how much work their body can do before their cardiorespiratory system fails to deliver oxygen to the respiring tissues at a sufficient rate. The bigger the operation, the greater the demand on the cardiorespiratory system in the days immediately postoperative, and the greater the risk of death if their cardiopulmonary system has insufficient reserve.

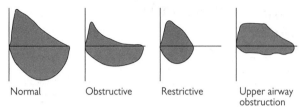

Fig. 4.1 Flow volume loops. Graphical representations of the results with volume on the X-axis and flow rate on the Y-axis. Exhalation is above the line and inhalation below the line. There are four main patterns. Reproduced with permission from Sanders S, Dawson J, Datta S, and Eccles S (2005). *Oxford Handbook for the Foundation Programme*, Oxford University Press, Oxford.

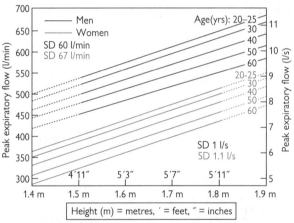

Fig. 4.2 Normal peak expiratory flow values. Reproduced with permission from Sanders S, Dawson J, Datta S, and Eccles S (2005). *Oxford Handbook for the Foundation Programme*, Oxford University Press, Oxford. (2005).

Oxygen administration

Key facts

- O_2 is routinely administered to patients recovering from surgery and anaesthesia. Most require 30–40% O_2 until awake and in control of their airway.
- Indications for extending O_2 administration (24–48h) even in uncomplicated cases, particularly at night when most profound desaturations occur include:
  - Following major surgery (especially thoracic/abdominal surgery from ↓chest excursion due to pain).
  - Patient receiving morphine or other respiratory depressant drugs.
  - Pre-existing respiratory disease (e.g. V/Q mismatch produced by areas of lung atelectasis, COPD, emphysema).
  - Pre-existing ischaemic heart disease.
  - Elderly patients.
- O_2 administered by facemask (24–60%) or nasal cannulae 2–4L/min.
- As with any drug, O_2 should be prescribed in the patient's drug chart.
- Excessive O_2 carries risks of pulmonary toxicity if given for long periods. Administration is best guided by measuring the SpO_2. If the saturation is >98%, reduce the percentage of inspired O_2 a little and reassess the saturations so the patient receives as much O_2 as they require—no more, no less.
- Patients with severe COPD require the hypoxic drive to maintain breathing in the face of chronically elevated $PaCO_2$. High-flow O_2 can be dangerous in this setting resulting in low/normal O_2, but very high $PaCO_2$. Many are poor surgical risk, and require careful management postoperative: give 24% by O_2 Venturi mask (increase to 28% if still hypoxic and alert).

Box 4.4 O_2 for dyspnoeic patients

- Hypoxia will kill a patient by causing cardiac arrest. An alert patient can still be dangerously hypoxic.
- Hypercapnia will make a patient drowsy but only kills if cerebral depression causes the patient to stop breathing and become critically hypoxic. An alert patient cannot possibly have critical hypercapnia.
- **If in doubt give 60%** O_2 via a face mask and check O_2 saturation, or if patient is seriously unwell, blood gases.
- Pulse oximetry is very useful as a saturation of >92% will usually correspond to a PaO_2 >8.0kPa. However, pulse oximetry gives no information about the $PaCO_2$ level. ABGs are essential if you need to know the $PaCO_2$.
- The PaO_2 is affected by the inspired concentration of O_2, the rate of diffusion across the alveolar membrane, and perfusion (V/Q) mismatch within the lungs. The $PaCO_2$ is, essentially, determined by the alveolar ventilation

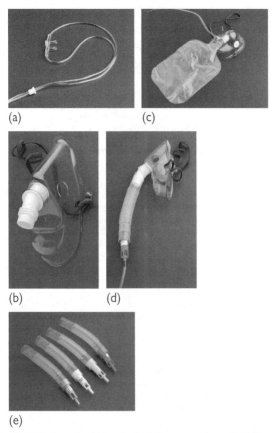

Fig. 4.3 (a) Nasal cannulae. (b) Low flow/ variable concentration mask. (c) Non-rebreath mask FiO_2 = 100%. (d) Mask with venturi valve attached. (e) Venturi apertures. (Reproduced with permission from Thomas J and Monaghan T (2007). *Oxford Handbook of Clinical Examination and Practical Skills*, Oxford University Press, Oxford.)

The breathless patient

Key facts

- It always requires urgent assessment, investigation, and treatment.
- Dyspnoea in a surgical patient is usually caused by hypoxia.
- If the patient is not hypoxic, start looking for metabolic acidosis.

Emergency management

Resuscitate

- Sit patient up and assess airway: remove any obstruction.
- Administer O_2 at high flow rates through a face mask (📖 see p. 178).
- Check that breathing is adequate: assess depth and symmetry of chest excursions, feel position of trachea, listen to percussion note, and the quality and symmetry of breath sounds on auscultation.
- Connect a pulse oximeter: O_2 saturations <95% in a previously fit patient are significant, <90% indicate serious hypoxia.
- Check the circulation. If no pulse, commence chest compressions and call for the cardiac arrest team: 📖 ALS algorithm inside back cover.
- If the situation is life threatening or the conscious level is depressed, immediately contact the anaesthetist on call for ICU.
- Gain IV access.

Establish a diagnosis

- Get a focused history from patient or nursing staff—O_2: Other symptoms (pain, cough, wheeze, bleeding), Onset (sudden/ gradual, triggers).
- *Examine the rest of the patient* including:
  - BP, pulse, and temperature.
  - Conscious level/signs of confusion. Altered conscious level from respiratory failure is critical: it signals impending airway obstruction.
  - Examine the abdomen for distension or tenderness.
- Ask for 12-lead ECG.
  - Look for rhythm changes—fast AF, SVT, bradycardia.
  - Look for ST segment changes—ischaemia or ACS.
- *Request an urgent CXR* on the ward and look for:
  - Pneumothorax (especially COPD/asthma/recent central line/lung biopsy/renal biopsy/liver biopsy).
  - Lobar collapse/consolidation.
  - Haemothorax/pleural effusion.
  - Wedge lucency in acute PE (though usually normal).
- *Measure ABGs* whilst waiting for XR. Look for:
  - Hypoxia: a PaO_2 <8kPa needs urgent treatment. If this is already on high FiO_2, patient may need admission to HDU/ICU. Call them.
  - Hypercarbia: a chronically raised $PaCO_2$ occurs in some patients with underlying chest disease, but may also indicate the patient is tiring and needs assisted ventilation.
  - Acidosis. May be a life-threatening problem: don't miss it. Check whether it is predominantly respiratory or metabolic.
  - Is the patient anaemic? Look at the Hb and transfuse if necessary.

Think about: causes

- Respiratory (pneumonia, pneumothorax, pulmonary oedema, PE, pleural effusion, asthma, ARDS).
- Cardiovascular (acute LV failure, arrhythmia, anaemia), hypovolaemia.
- Other causes (stroke, drug toxicity/withdrawal, anaphylaxis).
- Onset helps differentiate: see Box 4.5.

Box 4.5 Common patterns

Sudden onset
Pulmonary oedema, PE, (tension) pneumothorax, aspiration, cardiogenic, anaphylaxis, panic attack

Onset over a few hours
Atelectasis consolidation, pulmonary oedema, asthma, ARDS

Onset over a few days
Pneumonia, gradual fluid overload

Onset over weeks
Pleural effusion, mass lesions in chest, progressive anaemia.

Ask about: symptoms

Obtain a history:

- Did the dyspnoea follow any specific event, e.g. drug administration (anaphylaxis), eating (aspiration), line insertion (pneumothorax), or transfusion (volume overload or transfusion reaction)?
- Could the dyspnoea be related to the surgical condition or an underlying medical problem?
- Was there any cough, chest pain, haemoptysis, or wheeze?
- A history of bleeding or anaemia? Do they have melaena?
- Ask about onset (see Box 4.5).

Look for: signs

- Respiratory: look for cyanosis, pallor, use of accessory muscles, intercostal recession. Measure respiratory rate. Inspect, palpate, percuss and auscultate the chest—front and back. Is everything normal and symmetrical?
- Circulatory: look for shock—cool peripheries, assess pulse rate and rhythm, BP, assess JVP, auscultate heart sounds, check capillary refill. If they look hypovolaemic, where is the blood? Check wound dressings; look in the bed for melaena, etc.
- Neurological: quickly assess level of consciousness (AVPU) and gross neurology to exclude CVA and assess degree of respiratory compromise.
- Check surgical drains—if the patient has a chest drain check that:
  - It is not kinked or disconnected.
  - It is not displaced so that holes are outside chest wall.
  - If it is attached to suction, that the suction is on.
  - The underwater seal is adequate.
  - It is not full of blood.

Pulmonary oedema

Key facts

- Pulmonary oedema impairs gas exchange causing hypoxia and acute dyspnoea, typically with orthopnoea. The lungs become 'stiff' and expanding them becomes difficult (hence the use of accessory muscles).
- Pulmonary oedema is a symptom, and requires identification of a cause. It is more likely in background chronic LV impairment.
  - Acute deterioration of LV function (AMI, arrhythmia).
  - Other cardiac (severe valvular problem, fulminant myocarditis).
  - Fluid overload especially with chronic LVF (infusion, transfusion).
  - Lung injury (aspiration, contusion, O_2 toxicity).
  - Pulmonary capillary leak (sepsis, ARDS (see 📖 p. 204)).
  - Neurogenic e.g. following head injury.
  - Drug reactions (opioid poisoning, naloxone)

Clinical features

Symptoms
- Breathlessness, may be sudden onset, orthopnoea, wheeze.
- Ask about chest pain, palpitations, previous MI or pulmonary oedema.

Signs
- Cold, clammy, sweating, anxious, cyanosed.
- Pink frothy sputum on coughing if severe.
- Tachycardia, 3rd heart sound.
- Raised JVP, may have peripheral oedema.
- Bilateral lung crackles, sometimes audible wheeze.
- Murmurs if due to valve disease.

Investigations
- CXR shows pulmonary oedema and possibly upper lobe blood diversion (if radiograph taken sitting), enlarged heart on PA film, pleural effusion. Rethink the diagnosis if CXR is clear.
- ECG may be normal or reveal arrhythmia, ischaemia or MI (📖 p. 120).
- ABGs to identify respiratory failure, or metabolic acidosis.
- FBC to check Hb, U&Es to exclude renal failure.

Preoperative care

Pre-assessment clinic
Discuss with general medicine as patient may need acute admission and certainly needs optimizing of current medication.

Day before surgery
- Elective surgery should be deferred for several days until pulmonary and LV function fully optimized: discuss with medical team.
- Emergency patients should be discussed with medical team and ICU.
- 📖 Treatment is described on p. 183.

Discuss with anaesthetist
- Any patient in pulmonary oedema needing emergency surgery: induction of anaesthesia will be hazardous, and an ICU bed will be required.

Postoperative care

The aim is to reduce pulmonary oedema and LV filling pressures.
- Sit the patient up.
- 60% O_2 by face mask. Measure SpO_2 continuously.
- Stop or restrict IV fluids.
- Furosemide 20–40 mg IV.
- Morphine 5mg IV slowly (reduces preload and anxiety), followed by antiemetic (cyclizine 50mg slow IV/IM)
- If patient complains of chest pain GTN spray 1–2 puffs under tongue (unless systolic BP <90mmHg or known AS).
- Treat anaemia logically:
  - Dilutional anaemia due to fluid overload (look for weight gain, peripheral oedema, normocytic anaemia) should **not** be treated by transfusion (adding more volume will only exacerbate the pulmonary oedema). Diuresis is the logical solution.
  - However, anaemia due to blood loss may also worsen dyspnoeic symptoms of heart failure. Here, transfusion of red cells **is** logical, as it will restore both the haemoglobin concentration and the blood volume towards normal.
- If the patient is hypoxic (SpO_2 <92%) and does not improve with these basic measures ask for immediate help either from the on-call medical team who may admit the patient to CCU (vasodilator therapy), or the ICU team (vasodilator, inotropic support, CPAP, or ventilation). If the patient continues to deteriorate, cardiac arrest is likely; delays in therapy may prove fatal.
- Patients in chronic renal failure with pulmonary oedema are less likely to respond to diuretics. If dialysis-dependent, they are unable to excrete fluid so require immediate haemofiltration or haemodialysis. Urgent referral to the renal or ICU team is appropriate.
- If a new murmur is heard, it may show important valve lesion and can qualify LV function. Ask for urgent cardiology advice.

Smoking

Key facts

- Smoking tobacco increases the risks of anaesthesia and many of the risks of surgery. There is a six-fold increase in respiratory complications in patients smoking in excess of 10 cigarettes per day.
- Wound healing is impaired by effects on small vessels, blood viscosity, fibroblasts, and effects listed in the next section. Wound dehiscence is a real risk.
- Long-term smoking is associated with a vast range of problems, including COPD, coronary and peripheral vascular disease, and most cancers.

Effects of smoking

- ↑platelet aggregation (probably explaining the ↑risk of perioperative acute MI and CVA in smokers).
- Raised carboxyhaemoglobin (COHb) levels up to 15% in heavy smokers (which will not be detected by most pulse oximeters).
- COHb reduces the O_2-carrying capacity of blood per unit volume, thus increasing the risk of tissue hypoxia in susceptible organs. The cardiac output required to achieve the normal O_2 delivery to the tissues must therefore rise.
- Reduced mucociliary escalator function.
- Reduced compliance and ↑'closing volume' of small airways increases risk of air trapping, especially whilst supine in postop period.
- Reduction in immune function via reduced neutrophil chemotaxis and reduced natural killer cell efficacy
- The airways are hyper-reactive and hypersecretory, with impaired cell-mediated and humoral immunity: smokers are therefore susceptible to respiratory events during anaesthesia, and postop atelectasis and pneumonia, particularly after abdominal or thoracic surgery.
- This list is not remotely exhaustive: smoking really is not good for your patients!

Stopping smoking preoperatively

- 12h: some benefit as effects of nicotine (activation of the sympatho-adrenergic system with raised coronary vascular resistance) wear off, and COHb falls.
- 48h: some benefit as COHb is cleared from the blood, platelet aggregation begins to return to normal.
- Within 7 days: neutrophil, macrophage, and NK cell function improve.
- Within 6 weeks: upper aerodigestive function returns to baseline level, lung dynamics improve to 'normal' levels (depending on the extent of fixed parenchymal disease).
- 8 weeks: decreases morbidity from respiratory complications after surgery to a rate similar to non-smokers.
- Stopping smoking 6 weeks before surgery is highly recommended. Stopping for a shorter period however (e.g. a few days) can be counterproductive as the airways tend to be hyper-irritable and secretions increase, but the mucociliary escalator has not yet recovered.

Mitigating the effects of smoking in the postoperative period

- Ensure patients remain well hydrated until oral intake is restored.
- Use thromboembolic prophylaxis in most cases.
- Use preoperative chest physiotherapy and education on breathing and coughing techniques.
- Mobilize as soon as possible post operatively.
- Aggressive postoperative physiotherapy, especially if mobilizing slowly.
- Consider the use of epidural analgesia to improve compliance with postoperative physiotherapy.
- Use pre- and postoperative saline nebulizers 5mL qds
- Ensure effective postoperative analgesia to enable mobilization, deep-breathing exercises, and expectoration. Inability to mobilize, or to clear the ↑ secretion burden from the lungs, is likely to end in a postoperative pneumonia, and respiratory failure as a result.

Asthma

Key facts

- Asthma is characterized by, variable, reversible airflow obstruction due to constriction of small-to-medium sized airways in a setting of chronic airway inflammation.
- Bronchoconstriction results from hyperreactivity of smooth muscle, leading to ↓ diameter of the affected airways in response to external triggers (allergens, URTI, exercise, cold air, stress, β-blockers).
- Bronchial inflammation worsens airflow limitation by increasing mucus volume and viscosity.
- ⚠ patients and doctors often underestimate the severity of asthma.

Clinical features

Symptoms

- Symptoms of asthma are usually a combination of shortness of breath (on exertion), wheeze and cough; sputum is less common because of the high viscosity of the mucus.
- In children, non-productive cough may be the only symptom.
- Differentiating asthma from COPD (📖 see also Table 4.2):
  - Presence of childhood symptoms.
  - Cough which wakes the patient at night.
  - Diurnal variation.
  - Specific trigger factors (especially allergic) and history of atopy.
  - Absence of smoking history.
  - Response to previous treatment.
  - 10% of COPD patients have some of the above features, and probably suffer from both diseases.

Signs

- Wheeze, tachypnoea, hyperinflated chest.
- Often there are no signs in well-controlled asthmatics between attacks.
- There is little correlation between the presence or absence of wheeze heard with a stethoscope and the severity of underlying asthma.
- ⚠ *life-threatening asthma is often characterized by a 'silent chest'* (📖 p. 188)

Investigations

- Spirometry:
  - Reduced PEFR compared to predicted for age, sex, height.
  - Reduced FEV_1 and FEV_1/FVC.
  - Reversibility demonstrated by increase in PEFR and FEV_1 after inhaled β-agonists.
  - Airway hyper-responsiveness demonstrated by metacholine challenge (only in supervised conditions with resuscitation facilities).
- CXR usually clear, may show some hyperinflation.
- Skin testing may demonstrate atopy.

Preoperative care

In pre-assessment clinic

- Emphasise the need for good compliance with treatment prior to surgery, and consider doubling dose of inhaled steroids 1 week prior to surgery if experiencing mild symptoms.
- If control is poor (>20% variability in PEFR), consider review by a chest physician and a 1 week course of oral prednisolone 20–40mg od.

In pre-assessment clinic or on ward

- (Re-) assess exercise tolerance (e.g. breathless when climbing stairs, walking on flat, or undressing) and general activity levels.
- Examination is often unremarkable but patients may have a hyper-inflated 'barrel' chest and wheeze.
- A single PEFR reading is helpful (serial measurements better). If reduced, measure response to normal bronchodilators (e.g. inhaled salbutamol).
- Formal spirometry is easy to perform and will give a more accurate assessment if PEFR is reduced.
- Blood gases are usually only necessary in really severe cases (breathless on minimal exertion, persistent symptoms despite optimal therapy) or where the chest signs arise from a different diagnosis.
- Ask if aspirin/NSAIDs induce wheeze as in most cases these are safe (omit from analgesia if known to trigger or patient is unsure)

Discuss with anaesthetist

Tell the anaesthetist about the following patients prior to the list:

- Poorly controlled asthma (frequent courses of oral steroids).
- Frequent hospital admissions.
- Previous HDU/ICU admission.
- Asthmatic patient with recent URTI (↑airway hyper-reactivity).

Changes to medications

- Change to nebulized bronchodilators on admission, and continue until the patient has recovered from surgery and can manage inhalers again.
- Well-controlled asthmatics do not need oral prednisolone routinely.
- Document adverse reactions to aspirin/NSAIDs *if* there are any.

Postoperatively

- Few well-controlled asthmatic patients have respiratory problems with routine surgery. Always request daily chest physiotherapy for asthmatic patients having major surgery.
- If there is increasing SOB and wheeze after surgery consider:
  - Drug reaction (to antibiotics, anaesthetic agent, NSAIDS).
  - Failure/inability to take usual medication (due to sedation, pain).
  - Inadequate bronchodilator therapy. Use nebulized route.
  - Other conditions causing dyspnoea: PE, spontaneous pneumothorax (↑risk in asthma).
  - Aspiration pneumonitis and LVF may also present with bronchospasm.

Acute severe asthma

Key facts

Despite your best efforts, patients may develop acute, severe attacks that can deteriorate rapidly and become life threatening: *if in doubt, get help!*

Clinical features

- Acute onset of breathlessness, wheeze, chest tightness.
- Patients may be unable to complete sentences.
- Symptoms not relieved by inhaled/nebulised β-agonists.
- Tachypnoea, prolonged expiration, use of accessory respiratory muscles, tachycardia, agitation.
- Hyperinflation with polyphonic expiratory wheeze, hyper-resonance. Remember chest may just 'squeak' or even be silent in severe asthma.

Emergency management

Resuscitate

- Assess severity of attack (Box 4.6) but do not delay treatment if patient is obviously unwell.
- Sit patient up. Reassure. 60% O_2 via face mask, humidified if possible.
- Monitor SpO_2 (should be >95% so reduce the FiO_2 if sats >98%).
- Salbutamol 5mg nebulized with O_2 repeated every 15-30 minutes.
- Prednisolone 40–50mg PO/hydrocortisone 100mg IV if unable to take PO.
- If dry, start IV fluids.
- CXR to exclude pneumothorax as invasive ventilation can rapidly turn a simple pneumothorax into a tension pneumothorax.
- Monitor response, *if not improving after 45min, patient tiring, or life-threatening features*:
  - Call for help immediately (medical team, ICU).
  - Salbutamol 5mg nebulized with O_2, repeated every 15–30min.
  - Ipratropium bromide (Atrovent) 0.5mg qds, nebulized with O_2.
  - If still not improving, aminophylline 5mg/kg IV over 20min (omit if on oral theophyllines), followed by aminophylline 0.5mg/kg/h IV.
  - Consider whether the bronchospasm could be part of an anaphylactoid reaction rather than asthma. Look for airway swelling, hypotension, signs of shock, urticaria etc (📖 p. 117)

Establish a diagnosis

- *PEFR*: if able to use, compare with preoperative value.
- *ABG*: if rising $PaCO_2$ or a low PaO_2 request medical/ICU review.
- *CXR*: look for other causes of breathlessness (📖 p. 180), especially pneumothorax (📖 p. 202).

Definitive management

- Consider magnesium infusion and invasive monitoring/management on ICU.
- Once stable, *slowly* wean off above medications, review routine therapy, chest review.

Box 4.6 Assesment of acute asthma severity

- Life-threatening attack:
  - PEFR <33% of normal/predicted.
  - Silent chest, cyanosis, decreasing respiratory effort.
  - Bradycardia, hypotension, exhaustion, coma.
  - ABG: any of high $PaCO_2$ (>5kPa), low PaO_2 (<8kPa), acidosis.
  - Summon help immediately.
- Severe attack:
  - PEFR <50% of normal/predicted.
  - Unable to complete sentences.
  - Respiratory rate >25/min.
  - Pulse >110/min.

Chronic obstructive pulmonary disease

Key facts

- COPD is a disease state with airflow limitation that is not fully reversible. It is characterized by:
  - Chronic bronchitis defined by a productive cough, each morning, for at least 3 months per year, for 2 successive years.
  - Emphysema characterized by destruction of lung parenchyma with reduced elastic recoil leading to dilated alveoli.
  - Small airways disease with chronically narrowed bronchioles.
- The principal problems in chronic bronchitis are bronchoconstriction, mucosal oedema, and mucus hypersecretion, exacerbated by repeated viral and bacterial infections. Progressive airflow obstruction leads to respiratory failure, and may be associated with RV failure (📖 p. 124).
- The majority of patients with COPD (whether predominantly chronic bronchitis *or* emphysema) have been tobacco smokers for many years.
- Many patients have an element of reversible airflow obstruction. If this can be demonstrated it is treated in the same way as asthma (📖 for features distinguishing COPD from asthma see Table 4.2)
- Factors associated with COPD include smoking, occupational exposure to dusts and atmospheric pollution, poor socioeconomic status, repeated viral infections, α_1-antitrypsin deficiency.

Clinical features

Symptoms

- Symptoms of COPD usually start after the age of about 55 years.
- Most common are cough, ↑sputum and breathlessness on exertion.
- Patients frequently give a history of repeated exacerbations of respiratory symptoms during the winter months.
- Mornings are usually worst time for patients with COPD.
- If chronic bronchitis dominates, patient classically cyanosed and easily obtunded by CO_2 retention from hypoventilation ('blue bloater').
- If emphysema dominates, patient typically tachypnoeic with only modest degrees of hypoxia ('pink puffer').
- Rarely, features of RV failure develop (📖 p. 124).

Signs

- Classical picture uncommon, most have combination of these features:
  - 'Pink puffer': thin, tachypnoeic, hypoxaemic; CO_2 retention late or terminal event. Lips often pursed in expiration.
  - 'Blue bloater': overweight, poor respiratory effort, CO_2 retention, (drowsiness), also hypoxaemic (cyanosis).
- Hyperinflated barrel chest, prolonged expiration, wheeze, paradoxical indrawing of rib cage (Hoover's sign), general wasting in end-stage.
- Clubbing and monophonic wheeze not COPD (think lung cancer due to smoking).

Table 4.2 Clinical features distinguishing asthma and COPD

Asthma	COPD
Symptoms present in childhood, resolve in early adult life, and may return later	Unusual for symptoms to start before middle age or later life
May never have smoked	Almost always history of smoking
Woken in early hours of morning by cough and SOB	Sleep generally not disturbed once patient gets off to sleep
History of hay fever or eczema	No history of atopy
Periods with no respiratory symptoms, may improve with increasing age	Decreasing symptom-free periods and progressive loss of exercise tolerance

Preoperative assessment

- Establish exercise tolerance: ask specifically about hills, walking outdoors, climbing stairs, and how many pillows they sleep with.
- Check spirometry (much more informative than PEFR in COPD).
- Check ABG if patient has difficulty climbing 1 flight of stairs, is cyanosed, or has SpO_2 of ≤95% on air.
- Ensure any reversible airflow obstruction is optimally treated:
  - Consider trial of oral prednisolone and medical review.
  - Change to nebulized bronchodilators prior to surgery if reversible obstruction (salbutamol 2.5–5mg qds/ipratropium 0.5mg qds).
- Look for heart failure and, if present, optimize treatment (📖 p. 124).
- If the patient has a very poor exercise tolerance (<1 flight of stairs) and is undergoing a procedure that will make breathing painful or difficult postoperatively, discuss with the anaesthetist whether HDU/ICU care would be appropriate postoperatively. Non-invasive ventilation may have a role.
- Advise to stop smoking!

Postoperative management

- Mobilize early whenever possible. Effective analgesia is vital but patients are very sensitive to respiratory depression from opioids. Use of regional anaesthesia (e.g. epidural) may be able to avoid opioids.
- Regular simple analgesics paracetamol, NSAIDs, (but watch for bronchospasm) often useful. Opioids can be used but great care is required.
- Regular physiotherapy to aid sputum clearance and prevent atelectasis.
- Give O_2 as appropriate (aim for their normal saturation, or 92%, whichever is the *higher*)—see Box 4.4.
- Routine antibiotics are not required.
- If the patient becomes pyrexial with more copious or purulent sputum send a sample for culture and start antibiotic. Oral amoxicillin 500mg tds is usually sufficient for mild exacerbations of COPD. If the patient is seriously unwell, treat as postoperative pneumonia (📖 p. 192).
- Continue nebulized bronchodilators until fully mobile, salbutamol may be given more frequently but there is no benefit from higher doses of ipratropium.
- Change back to inhalers 24h before discharge.

Respiratory infection

Key facts

⚠ Patients who have RTIs producing fever and cough should not undergo elective surgery under GA owing to the ↑risk of major pulmonary complications postoperatively.

- Pulmonary complications occur in 20–40% of patients after upper abdominal operations and in 2–5% after lower abdominal surgery.
- Following GA, lung volumes are reduced, respiration is shallower, and reluctance and inability to cough effectively results in poor basal air entry and sputum retention, causing atelectasis and infection, respectively.
- Effective postoperative analgesia and physiotherapy help prevent this.
- Patients with underlying respiratory disease are at ↑risk of developing problems during, and certainly after, surgery.
- Patients with simple coryza are not at significantly ↑risk of developing postoperative pulmonary problems.

Clinical features

Postoperative pneumonia is more common in patients with serious underlying illness, particularly obesity, prolonged surgery and ventilation, pre-existing respiratory disease, impaired immunity (including diabetes, malignancy, and renal failure), immobility, and prior antibiotics.

Symptoms

- Pneumonia generally develops 36–72h postoperatively.
- General malaise, fevers, sweating, rigors, anorexia.
- There may be pleuritic pain.
- Cough with purulent sputum, occasionally haemoptysis, occurs late.
- Confusion may develop even without hypoxia—especially in the elderly when it can be the only symptom.
- May give history of preoperatively URTI, or postoperatively aspiration.

Signs

- The first signs are generally pyrexia and ↑respiratory rate.
- Tachycardia, hypotension, and new AF may develop.
- Examine for bronchial breath sounds/dull percussion (consolidation).

Investigations

- *CXR*: consolidation is necessary to make the diagnosis of pneumonia.
- Send *FBC, U&E, CRP, LFTs*.
- *Cultures* of blood, wound swabs, urine.
- *Sputum microscopy* (including ZN stain if TB suspected), and *culture* (sometimes only obtainable after physiotherapy), and tracheal suction specimen, if appropriate.

Treatment

- O_2 to maintain saturation >92% (📖 see O_2 therapy p. 178).
- Antibiotics: if the patient has source of sepsis, taking cultures and *giving antibiotics early* have been repeatedly shown to improve survival.
- Antibiotics need to cover the common organisms (Box 4.7). Check with microbiology for local sensitivities, they do vary from place to place.

Box 4.7 Common organisms

- Gram +ve in community acquired pneumonia.
- Gram −ve organisms in hospital acquired pneumonia.
- Commonest gram −ve species are *Ps aeruginosa*, *Klebsiella* and *E. coli*.
- Anaerobes in aspiration pneumonia.
- *S. aureus* accounts for up to 15% of postoperative pneumonia.
- *S. pneumoniae* or *H. influenzae* are common in COPD
- Immunocompromised patients (immunosuppressive therapy, neutropenia, AIDS) may develop opportunist infections (*Pneumocystis*, CMV, fungi, *Pseudomonas*). Always refer these to respiratory physician for further management, likely to include diagnostic broncho-alveolar lavage (BAL)

Preoperative care

- For suspected URTI, check temperature, CRP, WCC early.
- Surgery should be deferred for 4–6 weeks in confirmed cases.
- Prescribe 5–7 day course broad-spectrum antibiotics if community acquired pneumonia (check local sensitivities), and tell patient's GP.

Discuss with anaesthetist
Reserve antibiotics for patients with suspected or proven bacterial infections: most URTIs are viral and antibiotics will not help.

Postoperative care

- Give first dose of antibiotics IV; thereafter, oral route is fine for most patients. If systemically unwell or unable to take orally, continue IV until pyrexia has resolved for at least 24h.
- Once sputum cultures and sensitivities are available, antibiotic therapy should be targeted: try to use an effective drug with the narrowest spectrum of activity to prevent complications such as *C. difficile* enterocolitis or the emergence of resistant organisms.
- Physiotherapy helps mobilize secretions and improve atelectasis.
- Look for hypotension, oliguria: does the patient need IV fluid too?

Complications

- Many patients recover with no complications.
- Respiratory failure (detected clinically or by falling SpO_2 in the face of increasing inspired O_2 concentrations); check blood gases.
- Pleural effusion/empyema may be detected on CXR; differentiate between lung consolidation, effusion and empyema by chest US.
- AF, renal failure (associated with septicaemia, hypotension, aminoglycosides). If in septic shock, notify ICU, even if the patient looks stable at present.

Pulmonary embolism

Key facts
- PE is incorrectly diagnosed in almost 75% of patients as often symptoms are vague.
- The differential diagnosis includes acute MI, aortic dissection, septic shock, chest infection, haemothorax, and pneumothorax.
- Massive PE: resulting in haemodynamic compromise, or compromise of >30% of the pulmonary vasculature.
- Hypoxaemia due to shunting of blood from right to left

Clinical features
Symptoms
- Dyspnoea pleuritic or dull chest pain.
- Haemoptysis.
- May have symptoms of DVT (📖 p. 168): warm, swollen painful leg.
- Risk factors for PE (📖 see p. 168).

Signs
- Tachypnoea, tachycardia, hypotension, elevated JVP.
- AF, RV heave,
- Circulatory collapse in massive PE.

Investigations
- *ECG* usually just shows sinus tachycardia. Right axis deviation, RBBB, RV strain pattern (S1, Q3, T3) is seen rarely, and is not a specific test.
- $\downarrow PaO_2$, $PaCO_2$ is also characteristically low due to hyperventilation to overcome hypoxia.
- *CXR* may show consolidation and effusion early on. Rarely, a 'wedge' of oligaemia or consolidation in massive PE.
- *TTE* may show RV dilatation, TR, and RA or RV thrombus.
- Diagnostic tests include:
  - *CT PA* (almost universally favoured now over VQ lung scans).
  - *VQ lung scanning* with radioactive technetium-labelled microaggregates of albumin (99Tcm MAA).

Complications
- The 30 day mortality of acute massive PE is about 50%.
- About 10% of mortality occurs within the first hour.
- Up to 80% of mortality occurs within the first 2h.
- The mortality of surgical intervention is up to 70% for patients requiring CPR or mechanical circulatory support preoperatively.
- The operative mortality of stable patients is about 30%.

Perioperative care

If the patient is haemodynamically unstable, emergency pulmonary embolectomy should be considered. In patients with large PE and no contraindications (i.e. surgery within 30 days) thrombolysis is the definitive management (ask for specialist help). Otherwise:

- Sit up and give 100% O_2, patient may require intubation.
- Give heparin 75IU/kg loading dose IV, 18IU/kg/h IV maintenance (1000IU per mL N Saline), check APTT 4–6h after starting and every dose change, titrate to APTT 50–70. Daily APTT once stable.
- Once APTT is stabilized APTT should be checked every 24h.
- LMWH e.g. enoxaparin (150IU) has the same efficacy as unfractionated heparin without the requirement for repeated APTT checks.
- Start warfarin.
- Look for causes of PE and correct them if possible.

Fat embolism syndrome

- Fat embolism presents with confusion, coma, dyspnoea, and skin petechiae 24–72h after any major trauma with long bone fractures. Massive fat embolism may resemble thrombotic embolism, but smaller amounts of fat released into the circulation cause little pulmonary distress.
- It may also occur in non-traumatic conditions such as pancreatitis and diabetes.
- Fat that passes through the lungs and occludes small systemic capillaries may cause confusion or other cerebral signs (often disproportionate to the degree of hypoxia), and petechiae (particularly axillary and subconjunctival).
- The diagnosis is usually made clinically and may be difficult to confirm. Fat may be detected in biopsy of petechia, and occasionally fat globules may be present in the urine.
- Treatment is essentially supportive. Assessment by the ICU staff will be required as severe hypoxia due to ARDS may occur. DIC and multi-organ failure may follow immune system activation.
- The incidence of fat embolism syndrome has been reduced by the increasing practice of early long bone fixation.

Bronchiectasis

Key facts

- In bronchiectasis, (sub-) segmental bronchi become permanently abnormally dilated and act as sumps of chronically infected sputum.
- Bronchiectasis may follow pneumonia, airway obstruction, and severe or repeated episodes of chest infection—especially in early childhood.
- Agents often implicated are *S. aureus*, *Klebsiella*, TB; or weakened host defences (HIV, cystic fibrosis [CF], ↓immunoglobulins, ciliary disorders).
- There may be a component of reversible airways obstruction due to the chronic inflammatory changes in the airways.
- Once bacteria have colonized the bronchial tree they are difficult or impossible to eradicate. *Ps. aeruginosa* is common and may be present for many years; also causes intermittent exacerbations of symptoms.
- The mainstay of treatment for bronchiectasis is regular physiotherapy, frequent courses of appropriate antibiotics, and treatment of any asthmatic symptoms.

Clinical features

- Most patients have a chronic productive cough. The volume of sputum that requires clearance in 24h can be impressive, and certainly illustrates the value of physiotherapy.
- Clinical findings similar to COPD, (📖 see p. 190) clubbing.
- May have signs of underlying condition.

Preoperative management

In pre-assessment clinic

- Before elective surgery, aim to get patient as fit as they can be, especially if major surgery which will either inhibit coughing or require a general anaesthetic is planned.
  - Discuss maximizing therapy with the chest physician looking after the patient.
  - Consider course of IV antibiotics and vigorous physiotherapy for 3–10 days immediately prior to surgery.
- In CF, pancreatic insufficiency causes malabsorption, so continuation of an appropriate diet as well as pancreatic supplements is **essential**.

Day before surgery

- Refer patient for respiratory physiotherapy before operation and ensure patient will receive physiotherapy immediately postoperatively if they have severe bronchiectasis.
- Maximize bronchodilatation if reversible airflow limitation:
  - Convert to nebulized bronchodilators (📖 p. 188).
  - Increase prednisolone by 5–10mg/day if on long-term oral steroids.
- Give the patient a sputum pot. Send sputum sample for MC&S before operation so that results will be available if patient needs antibiotics postoperatively (state on request why you are doing this, microbiology may not test sensitivities otherwise).
- Prior to major surgery, consider starting IV antibiotics on admission. Discuss this with chest team/microbiology, use current or most recent sputum culture to guide prescribing.

- It is strongly recommended that antibiotic therapy, including prophylaxis, is discussed with a microbiologist. They will know the local pattern of antibiotic resistance, and taking their advice reduces the risks both of treatment failure and of selecting out a highly resistant bacterial species which will never be eradicable.
- Consider checking spirometry and blood gases.

Discuss with anaesthetists

If patient has more respiratory symptoms than usual before the surgery has even begun, consider postponing elective surgery and ask a chest team to see them.

Postoperatively

- Ensure regular physiotherapy available: three times daily and at night if severely affected.
- It's always better for the patient's sputum to be in a pot than to remain in their lungs. Not only does it make their breathing easier, but sending sputum for culture in the event that the patient deteriorates is also made easy. If they become too tired to cough, the opportunity to obtain a sputum sample is lost.
- Adequate oxygenation; check SpO_2.
- Continue appropriate IV antibiotics for at least 3 days postoperatively or until discharged.
- Maintain adequate nutrition, especially if any malabsorption.
- Refer to chest team early if any deterioration in respiratory symptoms.

Restrictive pulmonary disease

Key facts
- Restrictive pulmonary disease is caused by extrinsic conditions with normal lung parenchyma but failure of the respiratory mechanism to provide adequate ventilation, or by intrinsic parenchymal lung disease.
- All lung volumes are reduced, with (near) normal FEV_1/FVC.
- The ↓ventilation makes pulmonary complications more likely.
- Postoperatively, sputum retention may be a major problem: good physiotherapy and analgesia are vital.

Restrictive pulmonary disease due to extrinsic causes

Key facts
- Extrinsic conditions include those affecting the chest wall (kyphoscoliosis, ankylosing spondylitis, severe obesity, mesothelioma) or abdominal problems (obesity, massive ascites, large pelvic tumours) that cause significant splinting of the diaphragm.
- Spinal disease might preclude certain regional anaesthetic techniques, such as epidural analgesia.
- *In patients who depend on their diaphragm for adequate ventilation because of underlying chest wall disease, a laparotomy may cause respiratory failure in the early postoperative period.*
- △ *Patients may develop respiratory failure with relatively minor postoperative problems and must be assessed regularly.*

Clinical features
- Rapid shallow breaths, splinting of accessory muscles (patient prefers to be in the sitting position), signs of underlying condition.
- ABGs often remain normal until late. CO_2 retention is a later sign than hypoxia and implies advanced disease (or an acute deterioration).
- The severity of the condition may be assessed using spirometry.

Perioperative plan
- Many patients are stable and only slowly deteriorate over years. These patients may tolerate surgery relatively well.
- Check ABGs: a reduced PaO_2 reflects significant disease.
- Obtain lung function tests including spirometry, lung volumes, and gas transfer if these have not been done within previous 6–8 weeks.
- Ask the anaesthetist whether postoperative HDU/ICU admission should be planned.

Postoperative plan
- Vigorous physiotherapy, pre- and postoperatively.
- Ensure adequate additional O_2, maintain SpO_2 >92%.
- Treat any respiratory infection vigorously.
- Consider CPAP or other non-invasive ventilation if insufficient respiratory effort after extubation.
- Early involvement of ICU and chest team if deterioration occurs.

Interstitial lung disease (ILD) and pulmonary fibrosis
Key facts
- Many ILDs progress to pulmonary fibrosis, leaving patients breathless because the lungs are scarred and tough hard to inflate and have impaired ability to take up O_2.
- Initially, inflammation is centred on the alveoli, impairing gas exchange.
- Over time, usually months to years, collagen is deposited around the alveoli causing progressive impairment of gas exchange and smaller, stiffer lungs.
- Pulmonary fibrosis is the final response of the lung to a number of different triggers:
  - Inhaled (in-) organic dusts: asbestos, silica, grain dust (farmer's lung), spores (bird fancier's lung).
  - Autoimmune: rheumatoid arthritis, SLE, systemic sclerosis.
  - Drugs and radiation: amiodarone, bleomycin, paraquat poisoning.
  - Residual ARDS.
- Treatment is aimed at removing trigger; often oral steroids (occasionally other immunosuppressants) are used, with limited success.
- Fit patients with severe fibrosis may be considered for transplantation.
- Congestive (right-sided) heart failure may develop later.

Clinical features
Dyspnoea, tachypnoea, widespread fine inspiratory crackles; late signs are cyanosis and clubbing.

Preoperative plan
- Follow the principles described for extrinsic restriction (see opposite page).
- For those on steroids, increase dose starting with premedication (100–200mg of hydrocortisone) and continuing an extra 5–10mg of prednisolone per day until the patient goes home.
- Inform the anaesthetist.
- Discuss seriously ill patients with chest team.

Postoperative plan
- Ensure adequate additional O_2, maintain SpO_2 >92%.
- Mobilize early, regular physiotherapy.
- Treat any respiratory infection vigorously.
- Ensure patient is continuing to receive steroids in appropriate form, e.g. convert to IV hydrocortisone while NBM.
- Consider CPAP or other non-invasive ventilation if insufficient respiratory effort after extubation.

Sleep apnoea syndrome

Key facts

- Characterized by recurrent apnoea and hypoxaemia during sleep i.e. intermittent respiratory arrest.
- It is caused by occlusion of the upper airway caused by insufficient muscle tone to oppose the −ve pressure during inspiration. Apnoea terminates when patient awakes in response to ensuing hypoxia. This prevents normal sleep, leading to daytime somnolence.
- The patient may develop systemic and pulmonary hypertension, congestive cardiac failure, and respiratory failure with CO_2 retention. Two types of sleep apnoea are recognized:
  - Obstructive sleep apnoea, OSA (obstruction of the upper airway).
  - Central apnoea (due to intermittent loss of respiratory drive).
- Patients are at ↑risk of postoperative airway obstruction.
- ⚠ *Patients are often extremely sensitive to sedative drugs, especially opioid analgesics. The risk of developing respiratory failure or complications after abdominal or thoracic surgery is* **high**.

Clinical features

Symptoms

- Many are obese (BMI >30), middle-aged ♂, who present with snoring (with periods of apnoea), disturbed sleep, and excessive daytime drowsiness.
- Hypothyroidism, acromegaly and short jaw predispose to OSA.
- Collar size >17 is risk factor for OSA.
- Take a history from the patient and their partner. Ask about:
  - Daytime somnolence i.e. how easily they fall asleep when reading, talking to someone, or driving.
  - Snoring and apnoeic spells at night: the patient is not usually aware of these but spouses may be very worried.
- Symptoms of congestive cardiac failure (📖 p. 124)
- Patients may be on home CPAP or BiPAP at night—if so, ask them to bring their unit into hospital with them so they can continue to use it.

Signs

- Obesity (not usually just overweight).
- Signs of congestive cardiac failure.
- Signs of associated conditions.

Investigations

The OSA is diagnosed in a sleep laboratory by monitoring O_2 saturation and nasal airflow. Additional tests (polysomnography) may be required in some patients: these include measurement of respiratory and abdominal muscle activity, EEG, and EMG.

Preoperative management

In pre-assessment clinic

- Weight reduction and management of associated conditions such as airflow obstruction, hypertension, and cardiac failure may help.
- Ensure patient is optimally treated for any associated medical conditions, particularly heart failure and coincidental respiratory conditions.
- Consider postponing severe cases until OSA is treated: severe cases may require surgery to the upper airway to reduce the degree of airway obstruction during sleep.

Day before surgery

- Ensure patient will be able to continue taking usual medication by an appropriate route postoperatively.
- If the patient is receiving CPAP at night, ensure that ward staff are familiar with setting it up.
- Examine the patient: heart failure and peripheral oedema suggests severe OSA.
- Measure pulse oximetry and ABGs to determine the patient's usual O_2 saturation *and* the $PaCO_2$.

Discuss with anaesthetist

- After major surgery some patients may need ventilation for a few hours until they are stable enough to wean from the ventilator, and anaesthetist may want you to book an ICU bed.
- Regional anaesthesia may be preferred to avoid somnolence in the period following GA.
- Regional techniques may also provide effective postoperative analgesia, reducing or avoiding the need for opioids and thereby minimizing their sedative effects.
- NSAIDs assist postoperative analgesia considerably if there is no surgical or medical contraindication.
- Anaesthetist should decide if night sedation is appropriate—it usually isn't.

Postoperative care

- Patients are best managed in the HDU/ICU.
- Continuous pulse oximetry should be used on the ward.
- Nurse the patient sitting up whenever possible.
- Aim to maintain the O_2 saturation that the patient maintained preoperatively, titrating the O_2 to the minimum required.
- A few patients develop CO_2 retention with O_2 therapy. This is detected by blood gas analysis in those patients at risk who become difficult to wake or develop signs of CO_2 retention.
- Most patients benefit from CPAP at night.
- Regular chest physiotherapy.

Pneumothorax

Key facts

- This is the presence of air in the pleural space between the lung and chest wall, with some degree of 2° lung collapse.
- *1° (spontaneous) pneumothorax* is commonly seen in young, tall, ♂ smokers.
  - More common on the right side, <10% are bilateral.
  - Usually caused by rupture of small sub-pleural blebs (bullae <2cm), at the apex of the upper or lower lobe.
- *2° pneumothorax* is associated with established lung disease, or trauma, or both (see Box 4.8).
- Discuss patients at high risk of complications with +ve pressure ventilation with anaesthetist:
  - Very large air leak with failure to adequately ventilate the lungs.
  - COPD/bullous disease.

Clinical features

Symptoms

- May be incidental finding (especially in 1° pneumothorax).
- Sudden onset shortness of breath.
- Pleuritic chest pain.
- Sudden deterioration of asthmatic or COPD patient.
- Hypoxia in ventilated patients.

Signs

- ↓chest expansion on affected side.
- Hyperresonant percussion on affected side.
- ↓breath sounds on affected side.
- May have signs of underlying lung disease.
- Tracheal shift/hypotension are signs of *tension pneumothorax*.

Investigations

- ⚠ **Do not investigate tension pneumothorax, perform needle decompression first (**📖 **see p. 203).**
- PA CXR usually diagnostic, measure the size of the rim of air.
- If PA CXR not diagnostic and high clinical suspicion, get lateral decubitus film or CT (also gives accurate estimate of size and useful for assessing remaining lung parenchyma and contralateral lung).

Preoperative care

- +ve pressure ventilation can convert simple into tension pneumothorax, patients undergoing GA with a pneumothorax not having surgery on the affected lung should have a chest tube connected to an underwater seal. *Do not let anyone clamp the drain tubing.*
- Consider delaying surgery until 6 weeks after complete resolution.
- 📖 Management options for pneumothorax are given on p. 203

Postoperative care

1° pneumothorax

- If rim <2cm and no SOB: observe closely.
- If rim >2cm or SOB: needle aspiration—this can be repeated once.
- If aspiration not successful: intercostal drain (📖 see p. 357).
- Consider surgical pleurodesis after 5 days.
- Always arrange for OPA review after discharge.

2° pneumothorax (Box 4.8)

⚠ *COPD is commonest cause of secondary pneumothorax. Patients often have little pulmonary reserve and may not tolerate surgical repair.*

- If rim <2cm, no SOB, age <50 years: needle aspiration, observe for 24h.
- Any other 2° pneumothorax: intercostal drain (pigtail or large gauge chest drain for large leak 📖 p. 357).
- If no re-expansion, apply suction.
- If no re-expansion, consider surgical pleurodesis (thoracoscopic chemical or abrasive pleurodesis) after 3 days or if:
  - Prolonged air leak, haemothorax, bilateral pneumothoraces, 100% pneumothorax, occupational hazard, underlying giant bulla (i.e. recurrence is inevitable), previous contralateral pneumothorax.
  - Recurrent pneumothorax on same side.
- Remove tube 24h after re-expansion/cessation of air leak.
- Discharge 24h after tube removal with chest OPA review.

Tension pneumothorax

Signs

- Signs of pneumothorax AND
- Mediastinal shift (trachea deviated *away* from side of lesion).
- Respiratory distress, circulatory collapse.

⚠ **Do not waste time with investigations, this is a clinical diagnosis.**

Needle decompression

- Insert 14G venflon into 2nd intercostal space in mid clavicular line.
- Insert chest drain as for 2° pneumothorax once decompressed.

Box 4.8 Causes of 2°pneumothorax (not exhaustive)

- COPD, asthma, bullous disease, cystic fibrosis, ILD.
- Infections including TB, *P. carinii*, bacterial, parasitic, mycotic.
- Malignancy: bronchogenic carcinoma, metastatic lung cancer.
- Marfan's syndrome, Ehlers–Danlos syndrome, scleroderma.
- Trauma: penetrating or blunt (latter associated with rib fractures).
- Iatrogenic e.g. central line, especially subclavian route.
- Think about oesophageal perforation after OGD/TOE.
- Rarely, CO_2 from laparoscopic surgery may enter thorax.
- Catamenial (meaning 'pertaining to menstruation'):
  age 20–30 years. Incidence 3–6%. 2–3 days following onset of menstruation. Right side more common. Often small, with dyspnoea and chest pain. Pathogenesis is unclear.

Acute respiratory distress syndrome

Key facts

- ARDS is a constellation of features representing the severe end of a spectrum of acute lung injury (ALI).
- Non-cardiogenic pulmonary oedema (pulmonary artery wedge pressure (PAWP) <18mmHg), pulmonary infiltrates on CXR, and refractory hypoxia: the PaO_2/FiO_2 ratio <26.6kPa (200mmHg).
- ↑pulmonary capillary permeability develops in response to a variety of direct or indirect insults.
- Non-hydrostatic, proteinaceous pulmonary oedema develops which may resolve with treatment of the underlying problem, but in a few patients progresses rapidly to alveolar fibrosis.
- It is often associated with a generalized capillary leak within the systemic circulation and multiple organ dysfunction or failure.
- The lungs become extremely stiff and difficult to expand. The work of breathing increases enormously and patients often become too exhausted to breathe adequately.
- Risk factors: older patient, chronic EtOH abuse, metabolic acidosis.
- Suspicion is important if ↓SaO_2 and known associated condition (📖 Table 4.3).

Clinical features

Symptoms

- Onset of increasing dyspnoea and exhaustion over 24h.
- Features of underlying condition.

Signs

- Tachypnoea, tachycardia, cyanosis, O_2 sats<90%.
- Use of accessory muscles.
- Usually symmetrical expansion with fine crepitations throughout
- The ventilated patient may require steadily increasing FiO_2 and PEEP to maintain O_2 saturation.
- The diagnosis should be suspected when a surgical patient fails to respond to treatment for pulmonary oedema.

Investigations

- Blood gases demonstrate hypoxia, often with hypocarbia due to hyperventilation. There may be a metabolic acidosis due to the underlying cause of the ARDS, e.g. hypovolaemic shock despite massive transfusion, overwhelming sepsis, major burns
- The CXR may be unimpressive in the early stages but goes on to develop the characteristic ground glass/pulmonary oedema appearance.
- PAWP <18mmHg (classically measured with a pulmonary artery catheter) is part of the diagnosis to underline that the syndrome is different from simple LV failure (with which it can sometimes be confused)

Table 4.3 Conditions commonly associated with ARDS

Direct injury	Indirect injury
Pneumonia	Sepsis
Pulmonary contusion	Pancreatitis
Toxic inhalation	Massive blood transfusion
Aspiration pneumonitis	Cardiopulmonary bypass
	Fat embolism
	Major burn injury

Postoperative care

Care is primarily supportive while an underlying cause is identified and corrected. Mortality is high; 30–60% may die, depending on the underlying cause (Box 4.9). Patients suspected of developing ARDS should always be referred to the ICU team as the management is complex and often requires considerable physiological support. This includes:

- Treatment of the underlying problem (e.g. antibiotics, surgical debridement of necrotic/infected tissue).
- Respiratory support (CPAP/sedation and invasive ventilation).
- Optimization of the circulation with detailed attention to fluid balance and inotropes to ensure adequate O_2 delivery.
- Prophylaxis against VTE, peptic ulcer.
- Haemofiltration if renal failure supervenes—a grave development.
- Steroids are not useful in the early stages.
- Survivors sometimes require many months to fully recover, particularly if long periods of invasive ventilation on ITU were required. Some survivors are left with significant pulmonary fibrosis.
- Early deaths are unusual; non-survivors usually succumb after several days/weeks, with recurrent sepsis and multiple organ failure being the usual mode of death (3 organ failure > 1 week usually fatal).

Box 4.9 Factors associated with poor prognosis in ARDS

- Age >75 vs. <45 years (60% mortality vs. 20%, respectively).
- In ARDS and sepsis: patients >60 years have 3-fold ↑mortality compared with <60 years.
- Pre-existing organ dysfunction from medical conditions (renal failure, cirrhosis, EtOH abuse, immunosuppression).
- Direct lung injury worse than indirect.

Upper airway obstruction

*This is frightening for **everyone**, so keep calm. Summon help and concentrate on oxygenation.*

Key facts

⚠ A noisy airway is *partially obstructed*. A silent airway is *either* wide open *or* totally obstructed.

- Acute upper airway obstruction is an emergency: it is an occasional cause of postoperative respiratory problems.
- It may be 'simple' upper airway obstruction caused by a depressed conscious level, which usually presents in the recovery unit.
- May arise as a complication of a preoperative condition, after surgery/ anaesthesia presenting with acute respiratory distress and stridor.

Features of airway obstruction

Snoring/grunting, stridor, tachypnoea, tachycardia, cyanosis, use of accessory muscles, paradoxical ('see-saw') movement of chest and abdominal walls.

Emergency management

Resuscitation

- 📖 See ALS guidelines, inside cover.
- Give *15L/min* O_2 by face mask and attach a pulse oximeter.
- *Call for help* from anaesthetist on call or ICU staff *immediately* if patient has stridor, or poor respiratory effort, or SaO_2 <85% without an obvious, reversible cause. (If the patient has just undergone ENT/maxillofacial surgery, fast-bleep the appropriate surgeon, too.)
- Sit patient up if conscious/not in shock. Otherwise, recovery position.
- Immediate *airway manoeuvres*—head tilt, chin lift, jaw thrust.
- Clear airway of any visible foreign body, vomit, food.
- *Look, listen, and feel* for air moving through the airway.
- If airway still not adequately patent, an airway *adjunct* (oropharyngeal/ nasopharyngeal airway) helps in most patients—nasal airways are much better tolerated, unless the patient is already unrousable.
- If airway now patent but patient is still hypoxic with very poor respiratory effort, hand-ventilate gently with self-inflating bag.
- If it proves impossible to establish an airway by any of the means above, needle cricothyroidotomy is indicated: feel for cricothyroid membrane which is small flat area *in midline* just between Adam's apple and first tracheal ring—pierce with a grey venflon and connect O_2 tubing until jet insufflation or definitive airway can be performed.

Establish the diagnosis

- Think about precipitants: recent intubation/airway or neck surgery/ food/foreign bodies/opiates or benzodiazepines/recent drugs?
- Assess the face and neck for swelling (haematoma/surgical emphysema/ anaphylaxis); quickly listen for air entry bilaterally.
- *Upper airway obstruction due to decreased conscious level* often sounds like snoring/grunting. Verbal or painful stimuli (to assess conscious level) may improve matters; airway manoeuvres and adjuncts then usually suffice.

- Once a patent airway exists, identify/exclude causes of coma which can be easily reversed:
  - Hypoglycaemia— give IV 50mL 50% glucose IV.
  - Opioid toxicity—give IV naloxone e.g. 400–800mcg repeated to a maximum of 10mg.
  - Benzodiazepines—give IV flumazenil 200mcg.
- *Upper airway obstruction from foreign body/swelling* tends to give *stridor* (crowing/whooping noise on inspiration). This will *not* improve, and may be worsened, by inserting adjuncts: try Heimlich manoeuvre for foreign body, treat swelling with 10mg IV chlorphenamina and 100mg IV hydrocortisone (📖 p. 117) ± intubation.

Further management once stable

- *Laryngoscopy* and flexible bronchoscopy to fully evaluate the airway.
- *PEFR*, if obtainable, is a good measure of the severity of large airway obstruction causing stridor; a peak flow <200L/min is worrying, and <100L/min may indicate critical airway narrowing and asphyxiation.
- *CXR* may show lobar collapse, surgical emphysema.
- *CT* for precise assessment of tracheal lumen and extrinsic compression.

Preoperative care

Discuss with anaesthetist

Try to give anaesthesia as much advance notice as possible of patients with known tracheal narrowing, as specialist techniques e.g. awake fibreoptic intubation/jet ventilation/Heliox may need to be arranged.

Postoperative care

- Trauma to the upper airway following intubation—rare, usually settles spontaneously but the anaesthetist should be informed.
- Following any neck surgery there may be haemorrhage that can extrinsically compress the trachea: *immediately* remove skin staples/sutures and sutures holding strap muscles, to relieve tracheal compression.
- *Tracheomalacia* occurs when a chronic source of tracheal compression (e.g. enlarged thyroid) is removed. The trachea may collapse during rapid inspiration, resulting in stridor. CPAP may help.
- Damage to one or both *recurrent laryngeal nerves*: presents as stridor during rapid inspiration, and a hoarse (bovine) cough. Classically follows thyroid surgery. Diagnosed on flexible laryngoscopy.
- Tumour of upper airway: Swelling may follow biopsy or manipulation. Treatment may include re-intubation and/or tracheostomy.
- Infections: include epiglottitis—this really does require expert input, so if the patient is breathing, call for help and do nothing unless told.
- Heliox is a mixture of 21% O_2 and 79% helium. It has a lower density than air or O_2 and therefore offers less resistance to flow. Although sometimes used to maintain oxygenation in a narrow airway, it is only a temporary measure—a definitive solution to the obstructed airway must still be found.

Ventilation/respiratory support

Invasive methods (intermittent positive pressure ventilation—IPPV)

There are many modes of IPPV but, in the end they all intermittently blow air into the lungs under pressure. This gives rise to predictable adverse effects (on venous return, pulmonary vascular resistance, cardiac output, BP, splanchnic perfusion, cerebral venous drainage, renal blood flow—the list is long). It is *not* a risk-free treatment and can easily render ill patients unstable, or even lead to loss of cardiac output.

Volume control (VC); pressure control (PC) ventilation

Commonly used during routine surgery. A ventilator attached to the anaesthetic machine delivers a preset tidal volume, or a preset increase in airway pressure: air enters the lungs, usually via an endotracheal tube. Expiration occurs when airway pressures are allowed to fall to zero. This is poorly tolerated by awake patients, so in ITU other modes are used.

Synchronized intermittent mandatory ventilation (SIMV)

A variation of IPPV where positive airway pressure may be synchronized with patient-initiated breaths. Mandatory (machine initiated) breaths are given if no spontaneous breaths occur in a preset time.

Mandatory minute ventilation (MMV)

Here the ventilator initiates breaths when patient-initiated breaths falls below a preset minute volume.

Pressure support (PS); assisted spontaneous breathing (ASB); volume support (VS)

The ventilator detects the drop in airway pressures as the patient begins inspiration and assists air inflow to achieve a preset positive pressure, or to achieve a preset tidal volume. The airway pressures are usually lower than in the mandatory modes, as here the patient is making some inspiratory effort.

Positive end-expiratory pressure (PEEP)

If instead of allowing airway pressures to fall to zero, a small +ve airways pressure is maintained throughout expiration, the collapse of small airways and alveoli at the end of expiration is reduced.

- Functional residual capacity, intrapulmonary shunts, lung compliance and PaO_2 are usually improved, and work of breathing becomes easier.
- High levels of PEEP (>15cmH$_2$0) may be necessary in ARDS or to reverse established atelectasis. However, ↑risk of trauma to lungs, and reductions in venous return and cardiac output (even PEEP of 5cmH$_2$0 may cause haemodynamic compromise in patient with poor LV).
- Some patients with COPD purse their lips during expiration, creating their own PEEP, keeping their small airways open in expiration.

Continuous positive airway pressure (CPAP)

In CPAP a continuous airway pressure, constant throughout all phases of respiration, is applied to the endotracheal tube. It is also commonly used in the extubated patient via a tight-fitting facemask or transparent full-head helmet. (📖 see p. 209).

Non-invasive methods

Non-invasive intermittent positive pressure ventilation (NIPPV)

This is IPPV delivered by face, or more commonly, nasal mask. The patient must be co-operative in order to remain calm and synchronize breaths with the ventilator. It may be used in the tiring COPD patient.

Continuous positive airway pressure (CPAP)

Delivered via a tight-fitting face mask, a transparent hood/helmet, or via a tracheal tube.

- This results in a kind of non-invasive PEEP, where additional alveoli are recruited with the benefits described on the previous page.
- CPAP is a useful adjunct in the extubated patient with COPD, atelectasis, pulmonary oedema, or ARDS.
- CPAP *cannot* produce ventilation by itself, and it has same risks as any form of IPPV.

Biphasic positive pressure ventilation (BiPAP)

BiPAP is a solution to the problem of air trapping that can occur in patients, particularly those with COPD, on CPAP. Airway pressure is cycled at preset rates between high and low levels. This contributes significantly to ventilation so is often used in those with severe CO_2 retention.

High flow (Venturi) face mask (fixed performance) (see Fig.4.3)

The key part of the Venturi facemask is the Venturi valve, which draws in large flows of air through calibrated inlets, which mix with the O_2 flowing into the valve, before entering the mask together.

- Oxygen-enriched air is delivered into the mask faster than the patient can use it. The excess mixture escapes safely though holes in the mask.
- The FiO_2 is set by the choice of valve, and the flowrate of O_2 *must be correct* (it is written on the coloured Venturi valve if you're unsure).
- The FiO_2 is not affected by the patient's breathing pattern, hence the term 'fixed performance'. The maximum FiO_2 that can be delivered by a Venturi mask is about 60%.

Low flow (Hudson) face mask (variable performance)

Oxygen flows at a set rate (e.g. 2L/min) into the mask (☐ see Fig. 4.3). However, this is diluted by the air drawn into the mask during inspiration. Since inspiratory flow can briefly touch 30L/min, a tachypnoeic patient will actually receive a lower FiO_2 than a patient with a slow and comfortable breathing pattern (hence 'variable performance' masks).

- The FiO_2 achieved depends primarily on the patient, and the delivery system should not be used if accurate control of FiO_2 is required.
- The maximum FiO_2 that can reliably be delivered is about 30%.
- Use of non-rebreathing mask and reservoir bag (into which high flow O_2 is pushed during expiration before being inhaled) increases FiO_2 up to 60%: reservoir bag must be filled with O_2 *before* the patient uses it.

Nasal prongs

Nasal prongs deliver FiO_2 that is determined primarily by the patient, as in a low flow mask, but they are less obtrusive, allowing the patient to expectorate and eat. They increase tracheal FiO_2 to barely more than room air levels, particularly if the patient breathes through their mouth.

Renal and urological

Acute renal dysfunction/failure

⚠️↑K$^+$ >6.0mmol/L needs urgent treatment (📖 see p. 234).

Key facts

- Acute renal failure may be oliguric or polyuric.
- Occult renal impairment is very common in elderly patients undergoing surgery and is a significant risk for postoperative renal failure.
- Renal dysfunction (Box 5.1) is associated with life-threatening sequelae:
  - Hyperkalemia.
  - Acidaemia.
  - Pulmonary oedema.
- *Think*: risk factors for acute renal failure: elderly, DM, chronic ↑BP, arteriopaths, emergency, hypovolaemia, dehydration, chronic renal insufficiency.

Box 5.1 Renal dysfunction

- Creatinine >73–126µmol/L in ♂; >55–102 in ♀.
- Urea >2.5–7.0mmol/L.
- Creatinine clearance <90–130mL/min.

Diagnosis

Think about causes (Box 5.2)

- Look for sepsis, recent hypotension, dehydration, massive tissue injury.
- Recent drugs: NSAIDs, aminoglycosides, ACE-inhibitors, IV contrast.

Ask about symptoms

- Usually asymptomatic in early stages.
- May notice change in frequency of voiding.
- Tachypnoea e.g. from acidaemia, pulmonary oedema, underlying sepsis.

Look for signs, causes, and indications for dialysis

- Oliguria (📖 see p. 214)/polyuria: look at fluid balance chart, place/change a Foley catheter to exclude urinary obstruction in anuric patient.
- Try to decide if patient dehydrated, euvolaemic, overloaded (📖 see p. 65).
- Look for signs of complications: hyperkalaemia, arrhythmias, pulmonary oedema, fluid overload, confusion are late, worrying signs act quickly.

Establish a diagnosis

- *U&E*: raised and rising creatinine diagnostic. If ↑urea only, suggests dehydration, GI bleed, steroid use.
- *FBC* (GI bleed may cause ureamia), LFT, ESR. Blood catheters.
- *Urinalysis*: Na$^+$, urea, creatinine, osmolality, cells, casts. Urine for M, C&S.
- *12-lead ECG*: changes of hyperkalaemia (peaked T, flat P, ↑P–R, wide QRS) mandates emergency management of hyperkalaemia (📖 see p. 234).
- *CXR*: look for evidence pulmonary oedema, pleural/pericardial effusions, infection.
- *Renal US* to identify renal artery stenosis/hydronephrosis.

Preoperative management

- Get specialist help if renal function not responding to simple measures.
- For elective surgery, defer the procedure until renal function stabilized or corrected, and cause identified.
- In emergency surgery, minimize further renal deterioration by identifying factors which can be modified to allow recovery to take place.
- Hypovolaemia will make matters even worse: the intravascular space must be reasonably filled, use judicious IV NS.
- Identify other modifiable contributory factors:
  - Relieve post-renal urinary obstruction (urinary catheter, nephrostomy).
  - Stop nephrotoxic drugs where possible, especially NSAIDs, ACE inhibitors, any antihypertensives in hypotensive patient.
  - If toxic levels of gentamicin, omit next dose (get advice).
  - Control sepsis with antibiotics, and surgery if necessary.
- Ensuring euvolaemia and avoiding further renal insults are usually all that is needed in most cases, though recovery takes days.
- If creatinine has doubled preoperatively, notify ITU that the patient's renal function is deteriorating. Discuss admission pre- or postoperatively both for optimization of haemodynamics and for haemofiltration if necessary.
- ☞ Diuretics do not prevent acute renal failure or speed recovery, but may make the situation simpler to manage.
  - Many teams still use furosemide, as fluid balance and electrolytes are easier to manage if some urine continues to flow.
  - With or without furosemide, it is important to avoid hypovolaemia.
  - Furosemide in large doses is associated with significant side effects, including ototoxicity.
  - Clearly, if the patient remains anuric despite adequate filling, good BP, no further renal insults, and large doses of loop diuretic, there is no point in continuing to give furosemide stop it.

Box 5.2 Aetiology of postoperative renal failure

- Intraoperative risk factors: cardiac, aortic, biliary, emergency surgery; intraoperative hypotension, hypovolaemia, or both.
- Postoperative risk factors:
  - *Pre-renal:* shock (hypovolaemic, septic, cardiogenic 📖 see p. 116), especially in setting of renal artery stenosis.
  - *Renal:* diabetes, ATN from sepsis, hypoxia, contrast, drugs (NSAIDs, gentamicin, vancomycin, teicoplanin), haemoglobinuria, myoglobinuria, rhabdomyolysis (tissue necrosis, crush injury, or compartment syndrome).
  - *Post-renal:* obstructive uropathy, obstructed Foley catheter, ureteric damage after pelvic surgery or fracture.

Oliguria

Key facts

- The usual physiological response to surgery is oliguria, due to ↑secretion of antidiuretic hormone, cortisol, and a degree of hypovolaemia.
- Normal urine output ranges from 0.5–1mL/kg/h depending on hydration: urine output <400mL/day or <30mL/h for 3 consecutive hours is usually abnormal and may herald renal failure if not treated.
- Management of oliguria depends on the answers to three questions:
  - *Is the patient really oliguric?* Check bladder, fluid balance.
  - If so, *is the patient euvolaemic?* Hypovolaemia needs fluid, hypervolaemia diuretics. Beware the patient with chronic oedema who is, infact, hypovolaemic.
  - *Is the patient in established renal failure?* This requires urgent investigation, avoidance of further renal insults, and specialist help.

Diagnosis

Think about: causes

- Is it oliguria, urinary retention, or incontinence? Is the Foley catheter blocked, kinked, or malpositioned? Did urine stop suddenly?
- Is it hypovolaemia? (Dark urine, obvious haemorrhage /dehydration.)
- Is the patient hypotensive? And is there evidence of a cause? (Sepsis, haemorrhage, dehydration, cardiogenic shock, drug toxicity.)
- Is the patient in established oliguric acute renal failure and steadily becoming volume overloaded? (Hypertensive, raised JVP, pulmonary oedema, rising creatinine and urea, metabolic acidosis on ABG.)

Ask about: symptoms

- Does the patient feel a need to void, or have bladder distension?
- Have they been incontinent, or disposing of urine before it's charted?
- Is the patient thirsty? This strongly suggests hypovolaemia.
- Do they have any signs of fluid retention, breathlessness?
- Any symptoms of sepsis: chills, rigors, wound infection, dysuria?
- Look through the notes for evidence of and risks for acute renal failure: preoperative renal insufficiency, hypotension, shock, sepsis, NSAIDs, aminogycosides, ↑creatinine.
- Is patient normally on diuretics, and have they actually been given?

Look for: signs (Table 5.1)

- Measure BP and if patient is hypotensive treat this first (📖 see p. 116).
- Assess fluid status (↓skin turgor, dry mucous membranes, tachycardia, low JVP, ↓weight) suggest dehydration; ↑oedema, new respiratory crepitations, ↑JVP, ↑weight suggests fluid overload.
- Palpate and percuss the suprapubic area for a distended bladder.
- Look for sepsis: chest, wound, urinary, skin, cannula/drain sites.
- Review the patient's fluid balance chart and work out daily fluid intake and output for the last 48h, including surgical drains.
- Check U&E and FBC.
- Consider ABG to look for acidosis and hyperkalaemia patients in whom you suspect acute renal failure.

Management

- Kidneys need adequate blood *pressure*, adequate blood *flow*, and (sometimes) an additional stimulus with diuretic. Diuretics in the face of a low blood volume low BP and low cardiac output just make matters worse.
- Pass a urethral catheter (flush or change an existing one): if there is a large residual the patient may simply be in urinary retention (📖 see p. 216).
- Postoperative patients are often hypovolaemic: restriction of oral intake preoperatively, 3rd space sequestration, blood loss, sepsis.
  - Give rapid fluid challenge with 500mL fluid (crystalloid or colloid) over 15–30min. In hypovolaemia, BP and urine flow will increase.
  - If there is a good BP response, start 1L NS over 4–6h to maintain euvolaemia. If BP improvement is only transient, repeat bolus.
  - If BP fails to improve despite IV fluid, look for other causes of hypotension and treat aggressively (📖 see p. 116).
  - If urine output fails to improve with adequate BP and hydration, look for intrinsic renal failure and post-renal obstruction.
- A minority of patients may be fluid overloaded (patients with established oliguric renal failure, or poor left ventricular function).
  - If ⬇⬇BP, get help as inotropic support/invasive monitoring of CVP and arterial pressure on HDU/ICU may be necessary.
  - Get an urgent CXR to look for pulmonary oedema and ECG to look for signs of ACS.
  - If BP adequate give 20–40mg IV furosemide.

Table 5.1 Biochemistry in oliguric states—in ATN note that the characteristic change is the loss of concentrating ability

Test	Dehydration/ hypotension	ATN
Serum urea	Raised disproportionately to creatinine	Raised proportionately to creatinine
Serum creatinine	Normal or slightly raised	Raised proportionately to urea
Urinary Na$^+$ (mmol/L)	<20	>40
Urine osmolality (mosmol/kg)	>500	<350
Urine: serum urea	>8	<3
Urine: serum creatinine ratio*	>40	<20

* NB urine creatinine in mmol/L, serum creatinine in μmol/L.

Urinary retention

Key facts
- Common postoperatively in ♂ particularly after removal of Foley catheter, or after groin surgery e.g. inguinal hernia repair.
- Previous prostatism frequently identified retrospectively.

Clinical features
Defined as a painful inability to pass urine.

Local causes
- Prostatic enlargement (BPH or carcinoma)—often acute on chronic retention.
- Post-urological surgery e.g. post-TURP, clot impaction.
- Bladder or urethral stone impaction.
- Pressure on bladder e.g. late pregnancy, faecal impaction.
- Urinary tract infection.

General causes
- Pharmacological e.g.:
  - Anti-cholinergic side effects of many drugs.
  - Opioids.
  - Alcohol intoxication.
  - α sympatheticomimetics (e.g. ephedrine, some glaucoma drops).
- Post non-urological surgery:
  - Precipitated by recent catheterization.
  - Abdominal surgery with lower abdominal pain.
  - Epidural or spinal anaesthesia/analgesia.
- Loss of normal neurological control (neurogenic bladder):
  - Spinal injury e.g. trauma, 'slipped disc', neurological disease.
  - Epidural/spinal anaesthesia.
  - Spinal cord compression (medical emergency).

Symptoms
- Suprapubic pain, inability to pass urine despite desire.
- May dribble urine in small volumes especially if there is underlying chronic retention.

Signs
- Palpable/percussible bladder strongly suggests pre-existing chronic retention/lower urinary tract disease.
- Prostatic enlargement on PR examination.
- Check for other neurological deficits. Is there a spinal level?

Emergency management
Resuscitation
- Give analgesia (e.g. morphine 5–10mg IV). It will also help relaxation which may aid spontaneous micturition.
- Encourage patient to stand, walk around, ensure private toilet.
- Run taps.
- Treat constipation.
- A warm bath may aid micturition in drug-induced retention.

- Catheterize (📖 see p. 360) if retention persists. Seek senior advice before starting if there are concerns about local pathology as a cause or if there is a history of previous surgical instrumentation of the urethra.
- Suprapubic catheterization may be required for known or suspected urethral disease or failed urethral catheterization (📖 see p. 362).
- Document initial urine volume passed after catheter inserted—large volumes suggest underlying chronic retention.
- Send urine for MC&S.
- Send blood for FBC (Hb, WCC), U+E (Na$^+$, K$^+$), creatinine.

Establish a diagnosis
- Check medications especially recent changes, and ensure any preoperative prostatic medication has been restarted if discontinued.
- Cystoscopy may be required.
- Review full clinical examination including neurological findings and rectal examination.

Early treatment
- Monitor renal function especially if there is underlying chronic retention—renal function may deteriorate even after relief of the obstruction.
- Monitor fluid balance in first 48h if there is associated chronic retention—a 2° diuresis often occurs.
- Start antibiotics if there is evidence of a UTI.

Definitive management
Prostatic disease
- TURP may be required.
- α blocker may enable successful trial of voiding.

Box 5.3 Troubleshooting Foley catheters

No drainage
Flush with 10mL NS (should flush and aspirate flush without difficulty), use 2mL syringe to aspirate urine from Foley: if still unstable to aspirate sit patient up, change Foley, give fluid challenge, investigate and treat for oliguria (📖 p. 214).

Excessive pain
- History and exam: is pain from bladder (catheter may be blocked, UTI, renal colic, Foley under traction), penis (check foreskin for paraphimosis which *must* be reduced to avoid gangrene of penile tip—call urology if in doubt); urethral ulceration (which may respond to topical lidocaine gel, or reducing excessive traction on the Foley), scrotal (oedema, ulceration), or vulvul (ulceration, Foley under traction)?
- Can Foley be removed?

Haematuria

Causes and features

May be microscopic or macroscopic.

- Common after instrumentation of urological tract (e.g. post-TURP, post-cystoscopy, post-catheterization).
- Urinary tract infection: usually associated with lower urinary tract symptoms, particularly dysuria.
- Renal stones: often associated with pain (renal colic).
- Other rare causes rare: malignancy (transitional cell tumour, renal cell carcinoma, prostate adenocarcinoma)—most likely to be macroscopic, often with few other acute symptoms. Renal disease (e.g. glomerulonephritis, vasculitis) usually causes microscopic haematuria, is often asymptomatic and rarely presents as an emergency.

Complications

- Suprapubic colicky pain or acute retention of urine suggests clots in the bladder/urethra.
- Haemodynamic compromise is very unlikely, even in anticoagulated patients.

Emergency management

Resuscitation

- Establish large calibre IV access if the bleed is large: give crystalloid fluid up to 1000mL if tachycardic or hypotensive. To some extent, higher urine flows might offer a degree of protection against clot formation/ infarction even if cardiovasularly stable.
- **Do not** catheterize without seeking senior advice if there is any suggestion of lower urinary tract pathology or post-interventional bleeding.
- Irrigation ('3-way') catheters may be used to relief acute symptoms of clot colic or clot retention but should be placed by experienced staff
- Send blood for FBC (Hb, WCC), U+E (Na^+, K^+), G+S, clotting.

Establish a diagnosis

- Full clinical examination: particularly check the prostate or PR exam.
- US kidney: to identify renal tumours, cysts and exclude hydronephrosis.
- Cystoscopy (usually rigid, may be flexible): to identify bladder tumours.
- CT scan abdomen if renal tumour is suspected.

Early treatment

- Ensure all clotting abnormalities are corrected.
- Ensure fluid balance is correct: promote an active diuresis to prevent clot formation and retention.
- Transfuse blood only if Hb <8g/dL or the patient is symptomatic or high risk.
- Start antibiotics according to local protocol if infection is suspected (before cultures are available).

Definitive management

Post-interventional

- Flexible cystoscopy may be required.

Renal stones

- May pass spontaneously.
- May need endoscopic removal, lithotripsy or percutaneous treatment.

Chronic renal failure

Key facts

- Renal impairment covers a spectrum of patients: from sub-clinical dysfunction (with normal serum creatinine and urea, borderline creatinine clearance) to patients with end-stage renal failure.
- In terms of management patients fall into two groups:
  - Patients with chronic renal impairment (↑creatinine).
  - Dialysis dependent patients (📖 p. 224).
- Renal impairment is very common in elderly patients undergoing surgery and is a significant risk for postoperative renal failure when one or more additional renal insults coincide.
- Common complications: hyperkalemia, acidaemia, pulmonary oedema.

Clinical features

Symptoms

- Reduced exercise tolerance: may be caused by anaemia, ischaemic heart disease, pulmonary oedema, uraemia.
- Reduced appetite and nausea, the patient may be malnourished.
- Fluid retention.
- Dialysis history (📖 see p. 224).

Signs

- Look for signs of fluid overload including:
  - Hypertension or (in extreme cases) hypotension.
  - Peripheral oedema (check ankles, calves, sacrum, elbows).
  - Elevated JVP: it is more important to establish if JVP is elevated than accurately measure its height.
  - Pulmonary oedema: ↑respiratory rate, widespread crepitations, orthopnoea, SaO_2 <95% on room air.
- Look for signs of dehydration:
  - Check for postural hypotension: >20mmHg fall in systolic BP on moving from supine to standing.
  - Relative tachycardia: pulse >90bpm at rest.
  - Reduced JVP.
  - Reduced skin turgor: gently pinch a skin fold on the forearm and let go, the fold should disappear almost instantly.
  - Oedema is unusual in dehydration, but not impossible if serum albumin very low (nephrotic syndrome 📖 see p. 226).
  - Oedematous patients can still become acutely dehydrated/hypovolaemic.

Investigations

- *Serum creatinine* is the key measure of renal function. Kidney function is not the sole determinant of serum creatinine: it also depends upon muscle bulk, body weight, age, and sex.
- The *glomerular filtration rate* (GFR) can be estimated by the Cockroft–Gault formula (normal range: ♂ 97–137mL/min; ♀ 88–1284mL/min; decrease 1%/year over 40 yrs).
  - GFR=[(140–age) × weight × constant]/creatinine.
  - Constant: ♂ 1.23; ♀ 1.04; age: years, weight: kg, creatinine: µmol/L.

Dialysis patients

Key facts (Box 5.4)

• Two main techniques of renal replacement therapy are used in acute settings in ICU: *haemodialysis* (HD) and *haemofiltration* (HF). In both, access to the circulation is required and blood passes through an extra-corporeal circuit that includes either a dialyser or a haemofilter.
  • HF is continuous, avoiding large swings in fluid balance and electrolytes so is good for unstable patients.
  • HD can result in large swings in electrolytes and fluids, removes large molecules (heparin, insulin, vancomycin).
  • HF may be combined with dialysis.
  • Vascular access may be arteriovenous or venovenous (see Box 5.5).
• *Peritoneal dialysis* (PD) can be done at home: dialysis fluid is instilled into the peritoneal cavity via a Tenchkoff catheter, allowing the peritoneum to act as a dialysis membrane, before withdrawal of the fluid

---

Box 5.4 Life-threatening states needing urgent dialysis

• Hyperkalemia, acidosis, drug toxicity.
• Pulmonary oedema, fluid overload.
• Uraemia + pericarditis, encephalopathy, seizures, coagulopathy.

Clinical features

History
• Ask about dialysis frequency and timing of most recent dialysis.
• Ask about bleeding, sepsis, poor wound healing, malnutrition (📖 see p. 246).
• Ask how much urine they make per day (the answer may be 'none').

Examination
Look for sepsis, peripheral and pulmonary oedema. Find their AV shunt and feel for thrill (if AV shunt) but **never take blood from it.**

Investigation
• FBC, U&E, LFTs, clotting, bleeding time if bleeding history.
• 12-lead ECG and CXR.

Perioperative management
Management of patients with end-stage renal disease has a slightly different emphasis than management of patient with renal dysfunction, where the aim is to prevent further deterioration in renal function.

Pre-assessment clinic
• Ensure that the patient is scheduled for dialysis on day before surgery.
• Patient should not undergo PD for several weeks after abdominal surgery—you will need to liaise with the renal team who may need a temporary dialysis catheter inserted at the time of surgery to allow PD postoperatively.
• If patient nephrotic syndrome (📖 see p. 226) try to postpone

---

• EDTA measurements of GFR are more accurate, but time consuming.
• *Serum urea* is of limited help in assessing renal function. Urea rises in dehydration, GI bleeding, sepsis, steroid use, catabolism. Urea falls in malnutrition and starvation. A disproportionate rise or fall in urea relative to creatinine suggests these problems.
• *Electrolytes:* Na^+ normal or low; $\downarrow\uparrow K^+$; $\downarrow Ca^{2+}$; $\downarrow HCO_3^-$.
• *Serum HCO_3^-* (or pH/standard HCO_3^-): acidosis common in renal failure. It aggravates hyperkalaemia and may cause tachypnoea.
• *Hb* low in advanced renal failure due to $\downarrow$ erythropoietin release.
• $\downarrow$*albumin* due to poor nutrition even if no urinary loss of protein.
• *Renal US:* obstruction (hydronephrosis, dilated collecting system) must never be missed. It is easy to identify with US and readily treatable by removing or bypassing the obstruction.

Preoperative preparation

Pre-assessment clinic
• Check if ACE-inhibitors/aspirin can be withheld before surgery.
• Inform GP if new diagnosis of renal dysfunction, get renal artery US.
• Check BP and inform GP if >150mmHg systolic so this can be rechecked, and treated if appropriate.

Day before surgery
• BP should be 110–170 systolic and 70–95 diastolic.
• Fluid balance should be near normal.
  • A slightly 'wet' patient is safer than a dehydrated one: significant dehydration may result in reduction in renal blood flow and a further deterioration in renal function. Avoid this at all times.
  • A central line will help where clinical assessment is difficult.
  • Start IV NS infusion of 1L over 12h while NBM.
• Consider transfusion if Hb <9g/dL and major surgery is planned. Transfuse at a higher level if there is co-existing cardiorespiratory disease.
• Beware of inducing fluid overload when giving blood to a euvolaemic patient who cannot mount a diuresis to excrete the additional volume.
• Defer surgery if K^+ >6.0mmol/L. K^+ 5.5–6.0mmol/L is usually manageable but the anaesthetist must be notified.
• *In emergencies, lower K^+ with infusion of 15units actrapid in 50mL 50% glucose or with nebulized β-agonist (e.g. salbutamol 2.5mg). Cardiac protection with 10% $CaCl_2$ 10mL IV (📖 see p. 234 for full management).*
• Insert Foley catheter after induction if not already present.

Discuss with anaesthetist
• *Biliary surgery and jaundice:* the risk of postoperative renal failure is very high, consider deferring elective surgery.
• *Emergency surgery, aortic surgery, emergency abdominal surgery,* or any surgery in the presence of sepsis: accurate fluid resuscitation is key; consider preoperative insertion of central line, and invasive arterial monitoring to guide fluid resuscitation and inotropic support.
• All of these patients may need an HDU/ICU bed postoperatively.

Postoperative care

- Avoid NSAIDs which increase risk of acute-on-chronic renal failure.
- Care with all doses of opioids: metabolites of morphine that are both sedative and depress respiration may accumulate in renal failure. Doses may need to be reduced, and/or the interval between doses increased.
- PCA morphine or regional analgesia are often the best regimens following major surgery (see Pain control 📖 p. 78).
- Maintain hourly fluid balance chart: aim for u/o >0.5mL/kg/h (📖 see p. 214)
- A CVP line will help correct fluid status: aim for CVP 12–16mmHg.
- Replace fluid losses carefully and give normal maintenance requirements based around the normal daily urine output of the patient.
- Do not allow patient to become dehydrated as permanent deterioration of existing renal function may occur, accelerating need for dialysis.
- Daily creatinine, electrolytes, K^+, Ca^{2+}, Mg^{2+} until stable.

Management of established renal failure

There should be collaboration from the medical or nephrology team. Dialysis may not be required, particularly if you adapt your management to avoid potentially life-threatening complications:
- Avoid routine infusion of fluids; they will result in pulmonary oedema.
- Minimize or avoid giving K^+ in diet or infusions.
- Check biochemistry daily and ensure K^+ remains <5.0mmol/L.
- Modify the doses of drugs that are renally excreted (Table 5.2).
- Avoid additional insults, e.g. NSAIDs, aminoglycosides, ACE inhibitors.
- Beware of the accumulation of opioid metabolites that cause respiratory depression and prolonged sedation. This becomes progressively more likely as time goes by: the opioids accumulate with each administered dose, while the pain they are intended to alleviate reduces with each passing day. Keep analgesic prescriptions under twice daily review.

Specialist referral

Indications for emergency dialysis/filtration are discussed on 📖 p. 224.
Contact ICU (for the unstable patient) or the renal unit for:
- Hyperkalaemia >6.5mmol/L refractory to medical management (📖 see p. 234)
- Acidosis with pH <7.1.
- Pulmonary oedema.
- Oliguria preventing adequate enteral or parenteral nutrition.
- Rapidly rising urea >30mmol/L and creatinine >500µmol/L.
- Clinical uraemic features—vomiting, drowsiness, confusion, pericarditis—are late features of renal failure.

Table 5.2 Perioperative prescribing in renal failure (a

Drugs	Convert to IV	Give normal dose	Reduce dose
Diuretics	✓	✓	
Heparin			✓
Opiates			✓
NSAIDs			
β-blockers		✓	
Aminoglycosides			✓
Other antibiotics			✓
ACE-inhibitors			✓
Vasodilators			✓
Immunosuppression		✓ (ciclosporin check levels)	

Box 5.5 Vascular access in dialysis patients

- *Never cannulate an AV fistula*: infusing drugs may cause arterial compromise, and infection or thrombosis will destroy the fistula.
- Do not use long-term lines for routine IV access, to minimize risk of line infection.
- *HD patients* depend on good vascular access for their survival; PD patients may need HD in the future. Preserve large forearm veins during surgery/anaesthesia (cannulating these veins may result in their loss and prejudice long-term renal care for the patient).
- Use veins on back of hand/ulnar aspect of forearm (rarely used for dialysis).
- *During surgery* lightly wrap arm with fistula in soft gauze/cotton wool and place without compromising blood flow.
- Take BP in arm opposite to fistula.
- Arterial cannulae should be placed in the contralateral radial artery, and only inserted if strictly necessary.

Night before surgery

- HD patients: dialyse the patient a few hours preoperatively, so K^+ is in normal range (dialysis patients often have K^+ 5.5–6.5mmol/L before dialysis). Blood transfusion/suxamethonium ↑K^+ by up to 1mmol/L.
- Continue PD right up to surgery, but drain peritoneal cavity preoperatively for optimal respiratory function.

Discuss with anaesthesia

If period of temporary HD is planned postoperatively, ask anaesthetist to place a temporary central venous dialysis line under GA.

Postoperative management

- Monitor K^+ daily: *do not overload with K^+.*
- Monitor daily fluid balance, weight, *do not give 'routine' IV fluids.*
- Anuric patients do not require a Foley catheter.
- Delay PD for 4–6 weeks after abdominal surgery, use HD: start this 24–48h after surgery to prevent heparin-induced bleeding.
- *Drugs:* 📖 see Table 5.2.
- *Bleeding:* platelet function in renal failure may be impaired. Correct ↑APTT with FFP. Improve platelet dysfunction with IV desmopressin 0.3mcg/kg in 50mL NS given IV over 30min.
- *Perioperative fluids:* maintenance fluids are only 500–750mL/day including oral intake. If passing urine, allow a little extra intake to compensate for this. Make allowance for sweating, diarrhoea, etc. (📖 p. 64).
- *Third space losses* (wound oedema, paralytic ileus) need to be replaced with IV NS in short term to maintain circulating volume.
  - Subsequently, this fluid is reabsorbed and in anuric patients this may precipitate intravascular fluid overload.
  - Fluid removal by dialysis must therefore match reabsorption of sequestrated fluid.

Nephrotic syndrome

Key facts

- Syndrome defined by a triad of heavy proteinuria (>3g/24h), hypoalbuminaemia (<30g/L), oedema.
- It is commonly due to glomerulonephritis, but occasionally SLE, amyloid, diabetes.
- Often associated hyperlipidaemia: The physiological disturbances relevant to surgery include:
  - Malnutrition and muscle wasting 2° to protein loss.
  - Intravascular volume depletion from diuretics + hypoalbuminaemia.
  - Blood hypercoagulability due to ↑platelet stickiness, loss of anti-thrombin-III in the urine, and volume depletion.
  - Skin fragility due to malnutrition, oedema, ± steroid therapy directed at underlying cause.
  - ↑risk of infection due to loss of immunoglobulins in the urine, malnutrition, ±steroid therapy.
  - Poor wound healing.
  - Problems from associated systemic disease (amyloid, SLE, DM).

Clinical features

Symptoms

- Marked oedema, weight loss, poor wound healing, infections.
- Ask about steroid use and immunosuppression.

Signs

- *Fluid overload:* oedema is part of the nephrotic syndrome, so it is useless as a sign of intravascular volume overload. The only reliable sign of fluid overload in nephrotic syndrome is elevation of the JVP (or CVP if a line is present) as ↑BP can also occur in the face of intravascular volume depletion.
- *Dehydration:* check for postural hypotension (>20mmHg fall in supine systolic BP on standing) and reduced skin turgor over the clavicles. The classic sign of intravascular volume depletion in nephrotic syndrome is the combination of an apparently dry upper part of the body with soggy legs—reduced turgor over the clavicles together with massive leg oedema.

Investigations

- Serum creatinine to assess renal function.
- Electrolytes: Na^+ often low in nephrotic syndrome, especially if over-diuresed. Hypokalaemia may occur with high-dose diuretics.
- Total calcium may be low, but most labs correct for albumin—if not: $Ca_{corr} = Ca_{measured} + (40 - albumin) \times 0.02$.
- Albumin: patients with levels of >25g/L are not at major risk, but extreme protein loss will result in serum albumin levels <20g/L. At this level complications as already outlined are likely.

Preoperative preparation

Pre-assessment clinic

- Avoid surgery in patients with nephrotic syndrome if possible.
  - Remission, with or without the use of immunosuppressive therapy, occurs, and provides a more favourable state for surgery.
  - Other patients will progress to renal failure, but without heavy protein loss and oedema. Surgery is then less hazardous as serum albumin levels are usually normal, volume status normal or ↑, and blood coagulability normal or reduced.
- Assess for malnutrition and treat this (📖 p. 244).

Day before surgery

- BP should be 110–170 systolic and 70–95 diastolic.
- Intravascular fluid balance should be near normal. A slightly 'wet' patient is safer than a dehydrated one.
- DVT prophylaxis is mandatory, adjust dose to the degree of renal failure if present (📖 p. 168).
- Start pressure sore prevention preoperatively.
- Pharmacokinetics: changes in albumin and volume of distribution can alter bioavailability of drugs, for example:
  - Benzodiazepines are strongly albumin bound and therefore have a greater effect in nephrotic patients due to the low level of albumin.
  - Aminoglycosides have lower blood levels for any given dose due to the ↑volume of distribution.
  - Think of this mechanism if unexpected consequences of standard drugs, check *BNF*.

Discuss with anaesthetist

- In hypotensive, septic or unstable patients it may be sensible to place a central line preoperatively to guide fluid resuscitation.
- Consider use of 4.5% human albumin solution if serum albumin <20g/L, though the heavy proteinuria makes its effects short-lived.
- Patients with chronic nephrotic syndrome often on ACE inhibitors (↓proteinuria); discuss perioperative use.

Postoperative care

- Perioperative fluid replacement should be with colloid.
- Restrict salt intake, total body Na^+ already high.
- Avoid malnutrition: early parenteral nutrition may be needed.
- In addition to complications of surgery already outlined, recovery from abdominal and chest surgery may be influenced by accumulation of ascites/pleural effusions.
- Sutures may need leaving in place longer than usual because of delayed wound healing.
- Monitor urine output and renal function closely. The risk of postoperative renal failure is high.

Hyponatraemia

Key facts

⚠ *↓Na⁺ <120mmol/L with mental status changes is a medical emergency:*
- Normal Na^+ is 135–145mmol/L.
- $↓Na^+$ is common and potentially fatal (depending on level):
  - ↓plasma osmolality causes cerebral oedema, the patient is at risk of obtundation/confusion/seizures/coma.
  - $↓Na^+$ >125mmol/L suggests underlying disorder, but is generally well tolerated.
  - Acute $↓Na^+$ much more likely to cause fatal cerebral oedema. Rate of change of serum Na+ of more importance than actual level.
- Preoperative $↓Na^+$ may be acute or chronic which affects the urgency and type of therapy. Significant preoperative $↓Na^+$ should be corrected.
- 📖 See Box 5.6 for causes of hyponatraemia.

Box 5.6 Causes of hyponatraemia

Artifact: if blood is taken close to an IV infusion of hypotonic fluid.

Preoperative hyponatraemia
- Dehydration: GI loss e.g vomiting, diarrhoea, high-output stoma.
- Long-term diuretic therapy may lead to chronic $↓Na^+$.
- Oedematous states (heart failure, liver failure, nephrotic syndrome) often result in $↓Na^+$.
- Adrenal insufficiency in patients on long-term steroids is an uncommon cause of hyponatraemia (📖 for prevention see p. 281).

Postoperative hyponatraemia
- Usually due to excessive IV 5% glucose, especially in elderly patients who cannot excrete free water as effectively.
- Major surgery, pain, hypotension, nausea, pneumonia, drugs, cancer can cause syndrome of inappropriate anti-diuretic hormone (SIADH), decreasing free water excretion by the kidney.
- Post-TURP, 1.5% glycine irrigating solution may be absorbed through raw prostatic bed; causes cerebral irritability, confusion, seizures, coma.

Clinical features

Normovolaemic hyponatraemia

Dilutional state with normal circulating volume. No oedema and BP is normal. This is the commonest clinical setting for postoperative $↓Na^+$ and is usually due to inappropriate therapy with 5% glucose or glucose/saline, which should be stopped.

Hyponatraemia with volume depletion

There will be evidence of GI losses. Skin turgor reduced, tongue dry. BP may be low, if normal it may show a postural drop.

Hyponatraemia with fluid overload

Peripheral or pulmonary oedema, ↑JVP. Cardiac failure is the likeliest cause, also renal or hepatic failure, nephrotic syndrome.

Management (Box 5.7)

Management of acute hyponatraemia with neurological changes

- Apply standard resuscitation measures for coma (📖 see p. 293): check airway, give O_2, and monitor O_2 saturation; check BP; check BM stick.
- Call senior help and consider admission to ICU.
- Subsequent therapy will depend on volume status of patient:
  - *Volume depletion*: give IV NS as fast as necessary to restore circulating volume to normal, ideally guided by CVP
  - *Normovolaemia*: give NS (see Box 5.8).
  - *Volume overload* (or cardiac failure): give normal or hypertonic saline (see Box 5.8) with IV loop diuretics. Place urinary catheter, give repeated 20–40mg furosemide IV to establish diuresis to remove hourly intake, plus estimated volume overload.

Management of asymptomatic or chronic hyponatraemia

- Exclude SIADH if not oedematous/hypovolaemic/on diuretics
  - 24h urine: osmolality >500mmosm/L, Na^+ >20mmol/L with concomitant serum Na^+ <125mmol/L or osmolality <260mosm/L.
  - If SIADH, look for causes, treat as chronic hyponatraemia.
- Give 0.9% saline if volume depleted.
- If not volume depleted, restrict fluid intake to 1L per 24h, for 3–4 days, and monitor Na^+, K^+, and creatinine daily.
- Consider demeclocycline in resistant cases.

Box 5.7 General principles of managing hyponatraemia

⚠ *Aggressive therapy of asymptomatic ↓Na^+ may do more harm than good: tardy therapy of acute severe ↓Na^+ can be fatal.*

- Either give salt (as saline solution), or restrict water intake.
- If you know ↓Na^+ is of acute onset (24–36 h), or if the patient has neurological changes, then rapid correction is necessary.
- Otherwise, act more slowly, as the syndrome of central pontine myelinolysis (bulbar palsy, long-tract signs) can be caused by rapid correction of chronic (>2–3 days) hyponatraemia.
- Do not use hypertonic saline. In hyponatraemia NS is already hypertonic and will increase serum Na^+.

Hypernatraemia

Key facts

⚠ *In acute, severe hypernatraemia (>155mmol/L) cellular dehydration and osmolar shrinkage of brain cells can cause confusion and coma. Venous rupture and subarachnoid haemorrhage can occur as a consequence.*

- Normal Na^+ is 135–145mmol/L.
- Hypernatraemia is due to ↑total body Na^+, water deficiency, or both.
- In a surgical setting water loss in excess of Na^+ loss is typical, but if water intake is deficient, hypernatraemia also results:
  - Loss of normal thirst from postoperative sedation.
  - Patient is NBM.
  - Repeated administration of Na^+ load (e.g. NS, multiple antibiotics— usually sodium salts).
- A lesser degree of hypernatraemia is not itself usually a hazard, but the underlying water deficiency and hypovolaemia may cause vascular complications due to a sluggish circulation of hyperviscous blood.
- Cerebral and coronary insufficiency are most likely, with renal failure possible if circulating volume is not rapidly restored.
- 📖 See Box 5.8 for causes of hyperatraemia.

Box 5.8 Causes of hypernatraemia

Preoperatively
- Dehydration with water losses exceeding Na^+ losses, e.g. GI losses (vomiting, diarrhoea, stoma, burns) without fluid intake.
- Uncontrolled DM causing osmotic diuresis.
- Rare: 1° hyperaldosteronism, diabetes insipidus (may follow neurosurgery or brain trauma).

Postoperatively
- Incorrect IV fluid replacement with 0.9% saline in excess of Na^+ losses. Many fluid losses—diarrhoea, intestinal contents, burns—are hypo-osmolar, and in the absence of normal thirst or oral intake fluid replacement with NS alone is inappropriate.
- Patients who have received large volumes of IV fluid containing saline (colloids, NS) and who have been given diuretics for oedema.
- Nephrogenic diabetes insipidus after relief of chronic urinary obstruction. Renal tubular function is damaged by chronic obstruction and urinary concentrating ability is lost. Disproportionate loss of water leads to ↑Na^+ if insufficient water intake.
- Patients recovering from acute renal dysfunctioon may, in the polyuric phase, excrete water disproportionately in the same way and ↑Na^+ may occur, accompanied by hypovolaemia.
- Patients recovering from major surgery or critical illness sometimes excrete vast volumes of tissue oedema as urine, with similar results.

Clinical features

Symptoms
- Ask about history of vomiting, diarrhoea, DM, recent relief obstructive uropathy, ↓ fluid intake, lengthy periods of NBM.
- Check IV prescription sheet for excess NaCl prescribing.

Signs
- Look for any evidence of neurological deficit.
- Assess fluid status (oedema, skin turgor, JVP 📖 see p. 64).

Perioperative management
- Treat hypernatraemia by replacing the estimated body water deficit.
- If hypernatraemia is chronic, correction should be slow. As with hyponatraemia, *rapid correction can do more harm than the physiological derangement* itself.
  - Hypernatraemia initially causes brain shrinkage, but after 1–3 days brain volume is restored by uptake of solutes. If water is given rapidly, cerebral oedema can occur, with seizures, permanent neurological damage, and death.
  - In a surgical setting, if *hypernatraemia can be shown to be acute* (<24h), it can be corrected more rapidly. Aim to lower the serum Na^+ by 0.5mmol/L per hour, to approximately 145mmol/L.
- Aim to correct hypernatraemia by giving 25–50mL/hr of free water (orally or via NGT or PEG, or it as 5% glucose) *in addition* to the patients' standard fluid balance
- In the example in Box 5.10, the 28mmol/L Na^+ excess should be corrected by providing the necessary 4.8L of water over 56h (86mL/h). In addition, insensible losses are ~40mL/h and urinary water loss will be another 40mL/h, so water can be given in this example at 160mL/h.
- If the patient can drink, give water orally, or give 5% glucose IV.
- Monitor hourly urine output via a bladder catheter, aim for >30mL/h.
- Check serum Na^+ 6-hourly: ensure rate of fall is <0.5mmol/L per hour.
- Resume normal fluid replacement when serum Na^+ is <145mmol/L.

Hypokalaemia

Key facts

⚠ *K⁺ <2.5mmol/L can cause lethal cardiac arrhythmias, and needs urgent treatment before anaesthesia and surgery.*

- Normal K^+ is 3.5 – 5.0mmol/L
- Hypokalaemia is common in surgical patients.
- Other problems include paralytic ileus, muscle weakness, and cramps.
- A deficit of 200–400mmol is necessary to lower the K^+ from 4.0 to 3.0mmol/L, and a similar deficit lowers the K^+ from 3.0 to 2.0mmol/L.
- KCl is normally used to replace K^+ deficiency, as there is normally Cl^- deficiency in addition.
- 📖 See Box 5.9 for causes of hypokalaemia.

Box 5.9 Causes of hypokalaemia

Decreased intake

Normal K^+ intake is 40–120mmol/day. This is commonly reduced in surgical patients who are anorexic.

Increased entry into cells

- Alkalosis, excess insulin, β-agonists, stress, hypothermia all cause a shift of K^+ into cells.
- There is no true state of K^+ deficiency if this is the sole cause of low serum K^+

GI losses

- Vomiting, diarrhoea, tube/stoma /fistula drainage are common causes after abdominal surgery.
- Villous adenoma of the rectum can cause ↓K^+ preoperatively.
- Laxative abuse is a common cause in the elderly or in younger patients with eating disorders.

Urinary losses

- Diuretics, low Mg^{2+}, mineralocorticoid excess cause urinary K^+ wasting.
- Loss of gastric secretions (mechanism of hypokalaemia in gastric fluid loss is complex).
  - When excess gastric fluid is lost (by vomiting or via NG tube), loss of hydrochloric acid leaves the patient alkalotic.
  - Na^+ is reabsorbed from the distal renal convoluted tubule in exchange for K^+ instead of for H^+ (which would worsen the metabolic alkalaemia) and a consequential increase in K^+ loss is seen.
  - The renal loss of K^+ in response to severe vomiting is the major factor causing hypokalaemia; little K^+ is present in gastric secretions.
- Metabolic acidosis:
  - ↑tubular delivery of H^+.
  - H^+ preferentially exchanged for Na^+, so urinary K^+ increases.

Increased sweating

- This can exacerbate hypokalaemia.

Clinical features

Symptoms
- History usually identifies the causal factor(s): vomiting, diarrhoea, stoma output, urinary output, diuretics, laxatives.
- Ask about palpitations, muscle weakness, and cramps.

Signs
- Tachyarrhythmias e.g AF, VT, VF.
- ↓power and muscle tone.

Investigations
Serum K^+ and ABG (look for ↑pH), ECG.

Perioperative management
- Oral therapy with K^+ salts is appropriate if there is time for correction and clinical manifestations are absent. Most cause a degree of nausea. Preparations include:
  - Sando K® effervescent tablets containing 12mmol K®: prescribe 2–3 tablets 8–12-hourly for 48h, check K^+ daily.
  - Kay-Cee-L® syrup has 1mmol K^+/mL.
    Slow K® is sugar coated and contains 8mmol KCl.
  - Oral $KHCO_3$ and potassium citrate preparations are also available
  - Foods that are particularly rich in K^+ include baked potatoes, dried apricots, bananas, spinach, prunes, and raisins.
- Give KCl IV (see below) if patient has severe hypokalaemia and is unable to eat or tolerate oral preparations (which can cause nausea/ vomiting).
- If chronic diarrhoea is the cause, $KHCO_3$ or potassium citrate may be more appropriate than KCl
- Replacement of 40–60mmol K^+ leads to a rise of 1–1.5mmol/L in the serum K^+, but this is transient as K^+ is shifted back into cells. Regular monitoring of serum K^+ is necessary to ensure full correction of deficit.

Giving IV potassium
- General rule: no more concentrated than 40mmol KCl per litre, and no faster than 40mmol in 6–8h (unless emergency via central line).
- Use manufactured prepacks, rather than adding KCL by hand, 40mmol K^+/L should be the standard IV K^+ replacement fluid.
- If you do add KCl to an IV infusion, *check the dose with another doctor as well as the nurse who will administer the infusion.*
- Use saline: giving glucose K^+ leads to a transient fall in serum K^+ due to stimulation of insulin release by glucose.
- Large volumes of saline may cause fluid overload: if severe cardiac arrhythmia is present, then a more concentrated K^+ solution (10–20mmol KCl in 100mL NS can be given slowly through a central venous line with ECG monitoring. Regular monitoring of serum K^+ is vital.
- A concentration >60mmol/L through a peripheral vein should avoided as pain and sclerosis of the vein are likely.

Hyperkalaemia

Key facts

⚠ *K+ > 6.6mmol/L needs rapid correction, do not wait for an ECG before starting treatment: by the time ECG changes cardiac arrest is imminent*

- Normal K^+ is 3.5 – 5.0mmol/L
- This is a tiny proportion of total body K^+, the rest of which is intracellular.
- A serum K^+ above the normal range but <6.5mmol/L is not in itself a medical emergency but the underlying cause may be (⬚ see Box 5.10).
- By the time you get a lab result of ↑K^+ the situation will have changed: *always repeat the blood test at the same time as starting therapy.*
- The risk of cardiac arrest relates to the degree of ↑K^+ *and* acidosis, hypoxia, hypocalcaemia, and sympathetic overactivity (due to pain or shock). Cardiac arrest is rare with K^+ <7mmol/L unless other factors are present. Above that level K^+ alone is sufficient to cause arrest.

Box 5.10 Causes of ↑K^+ (ABC)

- *Artifact:* old sample or difficult venepuncture cause haemolysis.
- *Acidosis causes a shift of K^+ from cells to plasma.* Typical causes include diabetic ketoacidosis, renal impairment, or any shock state.
- *Acute/chronic renal failure,* particularly if acidosis.
- *ACE*-inhibitors, NSAIDs, K^+-sparing diuretics (amiloride, spironolactone).
- *Adrenal insufficiency.*
- *Blood transfusion (massive):* K^+ leaks from cells when blood is stored. A massive transfusion may deliver K^+ load beyond rate of renal excretion, this is commoner in the acidotic, shocked patient.
- *Burns:* leads to release of intracellular K^+.
- *Necrosis:* leads to release of intracellular K^+ (crush injury, ischaemia, infection, tumour lysis, compartment syndrome).

Emergency management

Resuscitation (⬚ see also Box 5.11)

- In unresponsive patient start ALS protocol (⬚ see inside cover).
- Get IV access, send urgent blood sample to recheck K^+, and request pH, HCO_3, blood glucose—in an emergency ward blood gas analysers provide rapid results, but lab will be more accurate.
- Request continuous ECG monitoring but do not delay treatment.
- Give 10mL calcium gluconate 10% IV over 1–2min.
- Give 15 units insulin in 50mL 50% glucose IV slow push.
- If difficult IV access give 5mg nebulized salbutamol while cannulating.
- If persistent ECG changes, repeat insulin/glucose and calcium gluconate.
- Check BM and treat hypo/hyperglycaemia appropriately (⬚ see p. 278).
- Give calcium resonium 15g PO or 30g PR.
- In refractory hyperkalaemia consider dialysis (⬚ p. 224).

Establish a diagnosis

- Send blood for U&E, FBC, ABG. Look for:
  - ↑Cr confirms renal failure (⬚ see p. 220).
  - ↓Na^+ suggests adrenal insufficiency, particularly if ↓BP and ↓glucose.

- ↑WCC suggests sepsis, ischaemia, necrosis.
- Isolated ↑K^+ suggests iatrogenic cause: drugs/supplements.

Think about: causes

- Was there pre-existing renal impairment preoperatively?
  - Has ↓BP/drugs/sepsis precipitated acute renal failure? (📖 p. 214)
  - Has ↑K^+ been precipitated by acidosis, abnormal K^+ load, or use of a drug inhibiting K^+ excretion? (📖 see Box 5.12)
- Check drug chart for infusions, K^+-sparing drugs, blood transfusions.
- Is the patient at risk of sepsis, tissue ischaemia, necrosis?

Ask about: symptoms

- Dehydration, infection.
- Limb pain and pressure areas (ischaemia, compartment syndrome).
- Changes to drug regimens, particularly diuretics, K^+ supplements.

Look for signs

- Evidence of sepsis? (📖 see p. 90); ischaemia/necrosis? (📖 see p. 156)
- ECG: peaked T, flat P, wide QRS (Fig. 12.9).
- Has the patient developed diabetic ketoacidosis? Check a bedside blood glucose.
- Is adrenal insufficiency possible? Look for low Na^+ and low BP. Is the patient at risk of adrenal suppression from previous steroid therapy?

Box 5.11 Principles of treating ↑K^+

- Block the direct cardiac effects of K^+:
  - Ca^{2+} blocks the effect of K^+ on the heart, it does not lower K^+.
  - Give 10mL calcium gluconate 10% IV over 1–2min. This is entirely safe and can be repeated every 5min for 4 doses if the ECG continues to show features of hyperkalaemia.
- Lower K^+: 5 drugs lower K^+ by different mechanisms: insulin, β-agonists such as salbutamol, $NaHCO_3$, calcium resonium, furosemide.
  - Insulin moves K^+ into cells: 15 units soluble insulin should be given by bolus in 50mL of 50% glucose (to prevent hypoglycaemia) unless the patient is hyperglycaemic. This should lower K^+ within 30min, lasting for several hours. It can be followed by an infusion
  - Salbutamol (β-agonist) lowers K^+ by about 1mmol/L: give 5mg by nebulizer.
  - $NaHCO_3$ may help correct acidosis and lowers K^+ by causing movement of K^+ into cells: give 50mL IV slow push. $NaHCO_3$ is very damaging on extravasation–be sure your venous access is safe.
  - Calcium resonium is a chelator that binds K^+: give 15g 6-hourly PO or 30g twice daily PR to deplete total body K^+.
  - Furosemide results in a diuresis in *euvolaemic* patient with normal renal function that may reduce K^+: give 10–40mg IV.
- Treat the causes of hyperkalaemia (📖 see Box 5.13).
- Dialysis (📖 see p. 224).

Hypercalcaemia

Key facts

⚠ *Severe hypercalcaemia (>3mmol/L) can cause cardiac arrhythmias, and coma, it is usually accompanied by severe dehydration.*

- Normal Ca^{2+}: 2.12–2.65mmol/L (all values in this chapter are corrected).
- Correct for albumin $Ca_{corr} = Ca_{measured} + (40 - albumin) \times 0.02$
- Modest hypercalcaemia (<3mmol/L) rarely causes clinical problems beyond thirst, polyuria, and modest dehydration, but may be aggravated by dehydration and immobilization.
- 1° hyperparathyroidism is the commonest cause of a slightly elevated Ca^{2+} in an otherwise fit patient. Malignancy is a common cause. 📖 See Box 5.12.

Box 5.12 Causes of hypercalcaemia

- 1° hyperparathyroidism.
- Bony metastases from lung, breast, prostate, renal, thyroid cancer, primary bone tumours.
- Myeloma.
- Iatrogenic: vitamin D or derivative (alfacalcidol, calcitriol); milk-alkali syndrome is excessively rare.
- Sarcoid (rare), thyrotoxicosis (very rare).

Emergency management

- Give 1L NS over 1h (depending on cardiac and renal function).
- Once adequate urine flow has been established, give pamidronate 60mg IV in 500mL NS over 3h (the Ca^{2+} will fall over 2 days except when 1° hyperparathyroidism is the cause).
- Continue IV fluids until the patient is normovolaemic:
  - CVP and Foley catheter to guide IV fluid replacement (hourly urine output).
  - Typically 4–6L are required over the next 24h.
- Stop thiazides and NSAID as they impair calcium excretion.
- Repeat pamidronate if no marked improvement in Ca^{2+} after 48–72h.
- In patients with marked hypercalcaemia *and* life-threatening features (e.g. coma, cardiac irritability) consider adding calcitonin 8 units/kg IM every 6h to the above management.

Clinical features

'Bones, stones, abdominal groans and psychic moans'

May be detected for first time preoperatively, be cause of presenting symptoms, or consequence of 1° surgical problem, particularly in malignant disease. Often it is an unrelated finding (1° hyperparathyroidism).

Symptoms

- Abdominal pain, nausea, vomiting, constipation, anorexia, weight loss.
- Kidney stones, polyuria.
- Tiredness, weakness, depression.

Signs
- Dehydration, hypotension.
- Altered mental state (drowsiness, confusion).
- Cardiac arrhythmia.

Investigations
- Na^+, K^+, urea, creatinine, Ca^{2+}, phosphate (low in 1° hyperparathyroidism), albumin (may be low in malignancy remember to correct Ca^{++} for this), alkaline phosphatase (raised in bone metastases, sarcoid, thyrotoxicosis).
- PTH (raised in hyperparathyroidism, suppressed in other causes).
- ECG: bradycardia, AV block, short QT.
- Look for malignancy (see Box 5.14).
  - Prostate specific antigen in ♂ >40 years.
  - Myeloma: ESR, serum protein electrophoresis, ±bone marrow.
  - CT thorax, abdomen, pelvis, bone scan if primary hyperparathyroidism excluded biochemically.

Perioperative management
- Ideally hypercalcaemia should be diagnosed and corrected preoperatively.
- The risks of surgery in mild hypercalcaemia are modest. Simply ensure adequate hydration with IV NS administered during preoperative fasting and continued postoperatively.
- Elective surgery should be deferred if Ca^{2+} >3mmol/L.
- Emergency or urgent surgery in the face of severe hypercalcaemia should be postponed until Ca^{2+} has been corrected.
- Hypercalcaemia may appear or increase postoperatively due to dehydration, and immobilization, typically in the elderly. Treatment is rehydration with close monitoring of renal function.

Hypocalcaemia

Key facts

⚠ *Severe hypocalcaemia can cause cardiac arrhythmias, tetany, fits.*
- Normal Ca^{2+}: 2.12–2.65mmol/L (all values in this chapter are corrected)
- Correct for albumin $Ca_{corr} = Ca_{measured} + (40 - albumin) \times 0.02$.
- The ionized Ca^{2+} is again a more direct way of assessing the true impact of a low Ca^{2+}. Blood gas analysers often measure the ionized Ca^{2+}, the normal range being 1.07–1.27mmol/L.
- Hypocalcaemia is dangerous if the total Ca^{2+} is <2.0mmol/L or the ionized Ca^{2+} <0.9mmol/L.
  - ↑neuromuscular excitability predisposes to tetany, fits, broncho- and laryngospasm.
  - Prolonged QT interval on ECG predisposes to VT.
  - Rare postoperatively unless the patient has had thyroid or parathyroid surgery. It may arise as a complication of acute renal failure, pancreatitis, or crush injury syndrome.
- 📖 See Box 5.13 for causes of hypocalcaemia.

Box 5.13 Causes of hypocalcaemia

If phosphate raised
- Thyroid or parathyroid surgery (loss of parathormone).
- Chronic renal failure due to insufficient vitamin D conversion to calcitriol.
- Hypoparathyroidism, pseudohypoparathyroidism (but not pseudop-seudohypoparathyroidism which has normal chemistry).
- Rhabdomyolysis.

If phosphate normal or low
- Overhydration.
- Pancreatitis.
- Osteomalacia.
- Hyperventilation (anxiety, introgenic)

Clinical features

Symptoms
Tetany, depression, perioral parasthesia.

Signs
- Chvostek's sign: tapping over facial nerve causes facial muscles to twitch (neuromuscular excitability).
- Carpo-pedal spasm, may be worse if BP cuff occludes brachial artery (Trousseau's sign).
- Cataract in chronic hypocalcaemia.

Investigations
- Ca^{2+}, phophate, Mg^{2+}, alkaline phosphate (high in osteomalacia), PTH (low in hypoparathyroidism, but not pseudohypoparathyroidism).
- Albumin (low if hypoalbuminaemia is cause of spurious low Ca^{2+}).
- ECG may show prolonged QT interval.

Management
- If due to hyperventilation, correct this.
- If Ca^{2+} >2mmol/L (or ionized Ca^{2+} >0.9mmol/L), give oral Ca^{2+} supplements and monitor Ca^{2+} daily.
- If Ca^{2+} <2mmol/L (or ionized Ca^{2+} <0.9mmol/L), give:
  - 10mL 10% calcium gluconate IV over 30min, faster if cardiac arrhythmia (e.g. 1–3min).
  - Calcitriol 0.25–2mcg PO od (ask medical team for advice, usually only required in hypoparathyroidism or CRF).
  - Check Ca^{2+} 4h later: if not rising, start 10% calcium gluconate continuous infusion of 2–5mL/h using a syringe driver.
  - Correct hypomagnesaemia if present.
- Recheck Ca^{2+} daily.
- Temporary overcorrection of hypocalcaemia is not harmful.

Magnesium and phosphate

Hypophosphataemia

Key facts

- Phosphate is involved in all processes of life, as a component of structural proteins/bone, enzymes, kinases, cell signalling, and energy stores.
- 10–15% of hospital inpatients have low serum phosphate (<0.8mmol/L). A smaller proportion has profound hypophosphataemia (<0.3mmol/L).
- The biochemical impact of phosphate depletion on cellular metabolism is potentially dangerous in surgical patients (the chronic effects of low serum phosphate on bone metabolism are irrelevant in acute situation).
  - Red cell 2,3-DPG (diphosphoglycerate) levels fall causing reduced tissue O_2 delivery.
  - Intracellular ATP levels fall and cellular functions involving energy-rich phosphate compounds may be affected.
- 📖 See Box 5.14 for causes of hypophosphataemia.

Box 5.14 Causes of low hypophosphataemia

Decreased absorption (usually well compensated)
- Malnutrition, antacids (bind phosphate), malabsorption syndromes e.g. Crohn's disease.
- Reduced intake of phosphate does not cause hypophosphataemia as cell catabolism releases phosphate from cells and renal retention of phosphate can compensate for reduced intake.

Increased loss
Diuretics, steroids, alcohol abuse, hyperparathyroidism, volume expansion, metabolic acidosis, pancreatitis, burns, diarrhoea.

Redistribution
- *Insulin secretion during re-feeding.* Glycogen synthesis promotes the phosphorylation of carbohydrates in the liver and skeletal muscle with a consequent rapid fall in the serum phosphate. This is particularly likely in malnourished or alcoholic patients, or in patients receiving TPN.
- *Respiratory alkalosis* (for example in ventilated patients) causes a rise in intracellular pH that leads to enhanced glycolysis. Alkalosis is the most common cause of hypophosphataemia in hospitalized patients.

Clinical features
- *Nervous system:* metabolic encephalopathy can occur leading to irritability and confusion or even delirium and coma.
- *Heart:* may impair myocardial contractility with reduced cardiac output.
- *Respiration* may be impaired due to weakness of the diaphragm.
- *Muscle function:* proximal myopathy, dysphagia, and ileus can occur. Rhabdomyolysis is a risk in alcoholic patients with hypophosphataemia.
- *Red cells:* ↑risk of haemolysis, rare with hypophosphataemia alone.
- *White cells:* severe deficiency can impair phagocytosis and chemotaxis.
- *Platelet numbers* and function may be diminished.

Management

- The treatment of hypophosphataemia is predominantly the treatment of the underlying cause. Oral supplementation is inappropriate except for those with chronic untreatable urinary losses.
- IV phosphate supplementation is usual in all patients receiving TPN, and a phosphate infusion is occasionally needed in alcoholic patients who are at risk of rhabdomyolysis from hypophosphataemia.
- The IV dose of phosphate should not exceed 0.08mmol/kg body weight over 6h. IV phosphate is potentially dangerous and can cause cardiac arrhythmias.

Hypomagnesaemia

Key facts

- Estimated to affect 7% of inpatients, but many of these are asymptomatic, and do not need aggressive therapy.
- Frequently associated with both hypocalcaemia and hypokalaemia. Always check Mg^{2+} levels if Ca^{2+} or K^+ levels are low.
- Common in surgical patients: reduced food intake, ↑GI losses from diarrhoea, vomiting, or intestinal fistulae.
- Other high-risk patients include chronic alcoholics and patients on chronic diuretic therapy.

Clinical features

- Fits, tetany, irritability, delirium, psychosis.
- Ventricular arrhythmias if Mg^{2+} <0.5mmol/L.

Management

- Monitor Mg^{2+} 3 × a week in high-risk patients.
- Replace or prevent deficiency with Mg^{2+} salts added to enteral or parenteral nutrition.
- Give a Mg^{2+} infusion in symptomatic patients: 8mmol Mg^{2+} (4mL of 50% Mg^{2+} solution) over 10–15min.

Gastrointestinal

Nutrition

Key facts

- Surgical patients have markedly ↑energy requirement, from surgery itself and also from associated conditions (fractures, infection).
- Food intake is often reduced and utilization of energy sources impaired, leading to an imbalance between energy supply and demand.
- Malnutrition increases the risk of postoperative infection, the length of hospital stay, and mortality.
- Appropriate nutritional support can reduce mortality in severe illness, speed the rate of recovery, and reduce complications.
- For those where full recovery is not anticipated, the aim of nutritional support is to improve duration and quality of life.

Basic principles

- Nutritional management begins as you take the Hx and examine the patient: nutritional status, risk, and need for intervention are based on simple clinical assessment without special tests or formulae.
- The approach to nutritional requirements is threefold:
  - *Recognize* and understand the problem of nutrition.
  - *Refer early* when necessary to the ward dietician or hospital nutritional support team; nutritional support is highly cost-effective as it reduces the incidence of major complications.
  - *Reassess* your patient regularly (📖 p. 246).

Physiology of nutrition in surgical patients

- During starvation of a healthy patient, endogenous fuels are utilized to meet daily energy requirements.
- Liver and muscle glycogen stores are small——approximately 150g—and are exhausted within 24h.
- After this, structural protein and lipid are mobilized. During each of the first few days of starvation, around 75g of protein from skeletal muscle and around 160g of adipose tissue are broken down, providing 1800kcal (7500k).
- Glucogenic amino acids are converted to glucose for obligate glucose-using tissues such as the CNS. Nitrogenous residues are lost from the body, resulting in an initial –ve nitrogen balance of about 12g/day.
- Adaptive processes then place in an increasing reliance on lipid stores, reducing gluconeogenesis from protein (nitrogen sparing). After 7–10 days of fasting, daily nitrogen loss is down to 2–3g/day.
- Surgery and sepsis increase protein breakdown in proportion to the degree of stress, leading to hypercatabolism (switch from 'structural support' to 'energy generation').
- The nitrogen-conserving response is rapidly overwhelmed, with a marked increase in skeletal muscle protein breakdown, whole body protein turnover, and a net nitrogen-losing state. The nitrogen loss is about 5–10g/day after elective surgery; 10–15g/day in sepsis, 15–20g/day in trauma with sepsis; and can be as high as 30g/day in major burns.
- *The daily nitrogen loss in major burns will result in a loss of >50% of body cell mass over 2.5 weeks.*

Box 6.1 Patients at high risk of malnutrition

- Already *undernourished* on admission to hospital:
  - Elderly, unsupported, poor, self-caring people are fine.
  - Chronic infection or alcohol dependency.
  - Anorexia.
  - Prolonged nausea or vomiting, dysphagia.
- Conditions associated with massive metabolic deficit:
  - Systemic sepsis.
  - Major trauma, burns, surgery.
  - Advanced malignancy.

Nutritional requirements

Energy

- Most patients should receive a maximum of 25kcal/kg per day—approximately 2000kcal (8400k) in a 75kg individual. (Protein calories are not included in calculating energy requirement.) This is provided in standard feed formulae as 1kcal/mL so enteral or parenteral feed should therefore be prescribed at 75–100mL/h in most patients.
- Avoid excess calories that can lead to hyperglycaemia, ↑risk of infection, ↑CO_2 production, and fatty liver change.
- The maximum glucose oxidation rate in health is 4mg/kg per min. In illness, the body may not assimilate or utilize the energy supplied.

Nitrogen

- Requirements are 0.15–0.25g/kg per day of estimated lean body mass (ideal weight). The higher value reflects extreme catabolic states e.g. burns and sepsis where –ve nitrogen balance develops rapidly.
- Standard amino acid solutions contain 6–12g nitrogen/L. TPN mixtures typically contain either 9g or 14g nitrogen/2.5L bag, as amino acids.
- 1g nitrogen equates to 6.25g protein.
- Excessive nitrogen load may precipitate renal and hepatic impairment.

Water

NB include the volume of feed in the patient's total fluid intake.

Other nutrients

- Vitamins (water- and fat-soluble), minerals (e.g. phosphate), electrolytes, and at least seven trace elements including Fe are now added routinely to feed solutions either in manufacture or at the pharmacy stage. Many of these compounds are now recognized to be essential in the prevention of specific nutritional deficiencies which have a profound effect on recovery from surgery.
- Arginine and glutamine are important in immune function, metabolic regulation, gut protection, and alternative substrate provision. Both become severely depleted early in serious illness. Supplementation may improve immune response and reduce length of hospital stay.
- Omega-3 polyunsaturated fatty and ribonucleic acid may have beneficial effects on organ function and immunity independent of their general nutritional value.

Nutritional assessment

Identifying need for nutritional support

Clinical indices

- Perioperative history and examination (📖 see Box 2.2)
- A nutritional assessment tool (e.g. BAPEN) may be recorded during the nursing admission procedure. This stratifies the patient into low, moderate, and high risk of nutritional deficiency according to five readily observable parameters as shown in Table 6.1.

Laboratory indices

- *Serum albumin:* a normal albumin on admission to hospital indicates good nutritional status. It is a sensitive but non-specific nutritional marker, a level <35g/L being associated with increasing morbidity, longer hospital stay, higher costs, greater use of antibiotics, greater duration of mechanical ventilation, and ↑mortality. However, the albumin level falls rapidly following surgery with large fluid shifts and is not a reliable marker of nutritional status at that time. Once illness or injury is underway, albumin *reflects* the patients condition; it is not *responsible* for it.
- *Haematological indices:* Hb, lymphocyte count, haematinics, and biochemical variables have some value in further quantifying general nutritional status or identifying areas of specific nutritional deficiency.
- Anthropometry and biochemical calculations are beyond the scope of this book.

Monitoring nutritional status

Clinical

- Weight:
  - Daily weight changes reflect fluid balance.
  - Rapid weight gain results from fluid gain and may lead to overload, as feeding after chronic malnutrition triggers SIADH-like status.
  - Early weight loss may reflect diuresis: malnutrition is characterized by an expanded ECF volume which reverts to normal as nutrition improves.
- Strict fluid input/output measurement should be maintained throughout any nutritional intervention plus an estimate of insensible losses.
- Signs of infection (may indicate ↑metabolic rate/requirements, parenteral feeding associated with line sepsis):
  - Fever.
  - Local signs at site (PEG or CVP line).
  - Hyperalimentation can cause pyrexia.
- Rehabilitation:
  - Well-being.
  - Appetite.
  - Muscle strength and mobility (objective/subjective).

Laboratory

- FBC (for Hb and WCC—evidence of infection): every 3rd day.
- Clotting (hepatic synthetic function): every 3rd day.
- B_{12}, folate, Fe parameters: baseline then fortnightly.
- U&E, glucose: at least once daily if fed by NGT or IV fluid/feed.
- LFTs, albumin: every 3rd day.

- Ca^{2+}, Mg^{2+}, PO_4^- – every 3rd day.
- Trace metals (zinc, copper, selenium): baseline, then if indicated.
- CRP for infection if indicated.
- 24h urine collection for urinary electrolytes and urea.
- Nitrogen input should equal or exceed losses:
  - Urinary nitrogen output (g) = [24h urinary urea (mmol) $\times$ 0.035] + [24h urine protein (g) /6.25]
  - Total nitrogen loss (g) = [urinary nitrogen (as above)] + [Change in blood urea $\times$ body weight (kg) $\times$ 0.017] + [sweat loss: 1.6g/day (normothermia) + 0.8g/day/°C of fever] + [stool loss: 2–4g/L] (if not measured).
- All clinical and laboratory measurements should be entered on a flow chart kept at the patient's bedside.

Table 6.1 Preliminary assessment of nutritional status/risk of elderly patients

Assessment parameter	Low risk	Moderate risk	High risk
Body weight for height	Normal BMI* (20–25)	Underweight but stable	Severely underweight or actively losing weight
Appetite	Good: eats all meals	Poor: eats part of meals	Eats very little; or IV only; or NBM for >2 days
Ability to eat	Fully independent	Needs help choosing menu; some feeding or swallowing difficulty	Dependent on others for feeding or severe swallowing difficulty
Psychological state	Fully alert	Mildly confused	Disorientated or depressed
Skin condition	Healthy	Dry or flaky	Broken or with pressure sores

From British Association of Parenteral and Enteral Nutrition (1998). *Standards and guidelines for nutritional support of patients in hospital.* * Body mass index = weight (kg)/height^2 (metres).

Nutritional support

Key facts

- The majority of patients undergoing surgery regain their ability to eat normally in a few days and don't need specialized nutritional support.
- High-risk patients (📖 see p. 247) require close nutritional support; the vast majority can be fed enterally and TPN will be required for only a few.
- *Always consider enteral feeding if at all achievable.*

Box 6.2 Advantages of enteral (GI) over parenteral (IV) route

- Supports and promotes gut function.
- Protects the gut from breakdown of its barrier function.
- Reduces the risk of sepsis.
- Lower rate of serious complications than parenteral nutrition.
- Is technically easier to manage.
- Is approximately 1/10th the cost of parenteral nutrition.

Basic principles

Stratify patient risk of malnutrition (📖 see p. 247)

- *Low risk*: review weekly or when clinical course changes.
- *Moderate risk*: provide advice with food choice, assistance with eating, and record food intake, refer to ward dietician for review.
- *High-risk*: refer to dietician or nutritional support team for detailed assessment of the level of nutritional support to be offered. Typical interventions include nasogastric, percutaneous endoscopic gastrostomy (PEG) or jejunostomy tube siting, TPN prescribing, and line insertion.

Enteral support

The concept of bowel rest following anastomotic bowel surgery and pancreatitis is outmoded. Enteral feeding is often feasible and beneficial.

Basic principles

- Gastric stasis is common perioperatively, but not always accompanied by small-bowel ileus. These patients can be fed via the small bowel, even when gastric aspirates are significant.
- Jejunal feeding reduces the risk of aspiration in patients with reflux or unprotected airways.
- Restoration of gastric emptying may be promoted by prokinetic drugs e.g. metoclopramide (10mg IV q8h) or erythromycin (250mg IV q8h).

Routes

- Consider the appropriate site to deliver the feed:
  - Is the stomach emptying adequately?
  - Is there evidence of significant gastro-oesophageal reflux or impaired airway protective reflexes?
  - Decide whether gastric or postgastric tube siting would be best.

- NG feeding is simplest as the tube can be sited on the general ward.
- Percutaneous and transnasal distal techniques need an appropriately trained surgeon, gastroenterologist, or radiologist.
- Insertion of a feeding jejunostomy or nasoenteral feeding tubes during GI surgery (e.g. oesophagogastrectomy) is strongly recommended.

Complications
- Aspiration pneumonia, feed-associated diarrhoea, and tube dislodgement. Confirm correct placement before infusing feed.
- ⚠ *Never re-insert NGT in recent oesophagectomy/gastrectomy patient—you may cause perforation at the anastomosis.*

Parenteral nutritional support
TPN is a complex treatment that is often inappropriately used. Most hospitals have recommended TPN regimens and many have a clinical team running the service locally. Liaise closely with these experts when considering the use of TPN. It should *never* be given in situations where it will only be used for 1–2 days.

Indications for parenteral nutrition
- Concern about distal bowel anastomosis.
- Severe exacerbations of inflammatory bowel disease.
- High-output proximal small-bowel stoma.
- Enterocutaneous fistulae.
- Critical illness states with failing alimentary tract.

Routes
- Central venous access is necessary for TPN in most patients.
- An appropriate feed can be supplied by the pharmacy for short-term peripheral venous administration.
- The site of feeding lines should be determined by a nutrition team who provide a dedicated service.
- TPN and other therapy may be safely delivered for a week or more via a non-tunnelled multi-lumen central line with a *dedicated delivery port* if aseptic precautions are meticulously adhered to.

Complications
- *The major complication of TPN is infection:*
    - Peripherally-inserted central catheters (PICC lines) have low incidence of infective and thrombotic complications in medium term.
    - For IV feeding over the longer term (greater than 2 weeks duration) subcutaneously tunnelled central lines are preferred.
- Fatty change and cholestasis are common in patients receiving TPN. Changes in LFTs (e.g. alkaline phosphatase) may occur after 2–3 weeks of TPN, and jaundice occasionally accompanies this.
- TPN promotes intestinal bacterial overgrowth, which promotes cholestasis by bacterial sepsis, and ↑production of 2° bile acids.
- TPN also contributes to cholestasis by the increase in biliary sludge that occurs after 6 weeks of TPN.

Acute abdominal pain

Key facts

- Take a careful Hx and examination with the aim of deciding if the patient has peritonitis (which may be local or widespread) or not.
- Resuscitate the patient properly and give adequate analgesia—this can improve the quality of the history and localize pain on examination, and it won't hide true signs of peritonism

Clinical features

Think about: causes (Fig. 6.1)

- Viscera are often mobile and pain may radiate, but location gives a clue.
- Timing is key: septic causes of abdominal pain are unusual before day 3 postoperatively, obstruction is a late complication of GI surgery.
- Constipation presents with severe pain can present tenderness in any quadrant.

Right lower lobe pneumonia/embolism Cholecystitis/biliary leak or colic Sub-diaphragmatic collection	MI/oesophagitis/ gastritis/Peptic ulcer Pancreatitis /biliary colic Anastomotic leak	Left lower lobe pneumonia/embolism Large bowel obstruction Anastomotic leak (upper GI surgery)
Renal colic Appendicitis Retroperitoneal bleeding Paracolic collection	Small bowel obstruction Intestinal ischaemia Aortic aneurysm Gastroenteritis Crohn's disease	Renal colic Large bowel obstruction Retroperitoneal bleeding Paracolic collection
Appendicitis Right tubo-ovarian pathology Incarcerated inguinal hernia	Cystitis Urinary retention Dysmenorrhoea Endometriosis	Sigmoid diverticulitis Left tubo-ovarian pathology Incarcerated inguinal hernia

Fig. 6.1 Causes of pain by area (not exhaustive or always diagnostic)

Ask about

- SOCRATES: Site/ Onset/ Character/ Radiation/ Associated symptoms/ Timing/ Exacerbating factors/ Surgery.
- Constant pain, gradual in onset but progressively worsening suggests an underlying inflammatory/infective cause.
- Anorexia, fever and general malaise suggest sepsis/peritonitis.
- Poorly localised, intermittent pain suggests visceral colic.
- Severe constant pain out of proportion to the clinical signs suggests ischaemic bowel until proven otherwise.
- Pain in the loin or back arises from (at least partially) retroperitoneal structures—consider the pancreas, renal tract, and aorta.
- Well localized pain worse on movement suggests wound or drain pain or other abdominal wall pathology.

Look for

- Signs of systemic illness: hypotension, tachycardia, pyrexia.
- Examine chest, auscultate for bronchial breath sounds: postoperative chest infection is common and can mimic an acute abdomen.
- Take off dressings: assess wounds for cellulitis, abscess, haematoma.
- Inspect/palpate hernia sites on coughing, gently try to localize pain if possible, carefully assess rebound/percussion tenderness, guarding.
- Send blood for FBC (Hb, WCC), U+E, glucose, amylase, LFTs, CRP, G&S: these investigations are very rarely diagnostic, but help indicate presence of sepsis. Diabetes occasionally presents with abdominal pain.
- Serum amylase more than 3 × normal is suggestive of acute pancreatitis.
- Send blood, urine, and stool for culture if pyrexial.
- Plain AXR are very rarely diagnostic (📖 see p. 416).
- Always request a plain erect CXR—it is the first-line test of choice for free abdominal air.
- Upper abdominal US is good for suspected hepatobiliary pathology.
- Pelvic US (transabdominal or transvaginal) is a good test for suspected tubo-ovarian disease.
- CT scanning is a good 'general survey 'of the abdomen but exposes the patient to significant radiation (roughly 100 AXRs).

Perioperative care

- IV access and fluid resuscitation; maintenance fluids.
- Keep patient NBM if uncertain of diagnosis.
- Adequate analgesia: give 2.5–5mg morphine IM/IV, with antiemetic. Avoid NSAIDS if hypovolaemic/dehydrated, previous peptic ulcer, or renal impairment (or asthma with documented NSAID intolerance).

Constipation
📖 See p. 254.

Small bowel obstruction
- May resolve with NBM, NGT, and IV fluids ('drip and suck').
- Patients can become very unwell due to large fluid shifts and malnutrition, so discuss early with surgeon if this is suspected.

Incarcerated hernia
- Make one gentle attempt to reduce.
- Discuss with general surgeons: may need exploration, open reduction and repair.
- Increasing pain suggests **strangulation** and constitutes an emergency.
- Remember femoral hemae occur to.

Anastomotic leak
📖 see p. 262.

Intra-abdominal abscess
- Radiologically guided drainage of non-loculated collections (by US or CT scanning) *may* be possible depending on location.
- Otherwise open surgical drainage is indicated, particularly if surgery is required anyway to deal with the underlying problem e.g. anastomotic leak.

Irritable bowel syndrome
Very common, but always a diagnosis of exclusion.

Nausea and vomiting

Key facts

For many patients this is worse than pain. Try hard to relieve it.

- Nausea and vomiting is common in surgical patients.
- Vomiting can lead to ↑pain, risk of bleeding, ↓absorption of oral medication, ↓nutrition and hydration, ↓K^+, risks incisional hernias and aspiration pneumonitis.
- Nausea and vomiting are mediated through central and peripheral pathways; a number of neurotransmitters are involved.
  - Central structures: the chemoreceptor trigger zone (CTZ) lies outside the blood–brain barrier. The nucleus of tractus solitarius and vagus connect with CTZ. Neurotransmitters include serotonin/5-HT, dopamine, noradrenaline and acetylcholine. Further input is from cranial nerves, hypothalamus, cortex, vestibular system.
  - Peripheral structures include the mechanoreceptors in the muscular wall of the distal stomach and proximal duodenum, and the chemoreceptors in the mucosa of the upper small bowel. Both serotonin and cholinergic pathways are involved.
  - Patient factors (strong history of PONV, motion sickness) are also important as are higher brain centres (disgust, anxiety, etc.).

Clinical features

- Think about causes (Box 6.3) particularly gastric stasis, ulcer disease, sepsis.
- Ask about postoperative course: could a complication be brewing?
- Other symptoms: new abdominal/chest pain, fevers?

Box 6.3 Risk factors for postoperative nausea and vomiting (PONV)

- Patient factors: children >adults >elderly; ♀ >♂; non-smokers > smokers.
- Surgery: prolonged; bowel, middle ear, pelvic and gynae.
- Severe pain, hypotension, hypoxia, dehydration.
- Drugs e.g. opioids, etomidate, N_2O, ketamine, antibiotics chemotherapy.
- Gut: gastric distension, bowel obstruction, ileus, constipation.
- Blood in stomach: bleeding ulcer/varices; pharyngeal/nasal surgery.
- Comorbidity (pancreatitis, cancer, ↑Ca^{2+}, angina/MI, dyspepsia).
- Obesity: gastro-oesophageal reflux, hiatus hernia.
- Sepsis.
- Hyponatraemia.
- Raised ICP (in head trauma, stroke).

Perioperative care

- Treat underlying cause, e.g. NGT to decompress stomach.
- Adjust opioid dosing. Could the patient use PCA?
- Avoid oral route for antiemetics. Consider combinations of antiemetics or regular prescriptions if nausea and vomiting persist.
- Keep patient well-hydrated.

Antiemetic drugs

These only relieve the symptoms: try to correct the cause. In severe cases, two agents acting at different sites may be needed. Do not combine cyclizine and metoclopramide (↑↑extrapyramidal side effects).

Antihistamines

Cyclizine 50mg IM or *slow* IV (painful on injection) is helpful for opioid-induced or postoperative nausea and vomiting. It can be very sedating.

Anti-dopaminergic agents

- *Substituted benzamides* are relatively inactive in PONV, though metoclopramide (10mg IV/IM/PO tds) acts as a prokinetic agent for the gut. Extrapyramidal side effects e.g. oculogyric crises—especially in young ♀ and the very old. (See below)
- *Phenothiazines*: e.g. prochlorperazine (12.5mg IM) can reduce opioid-induced emesis but are sedative, also risk extrapyramidal side effects.
- *Substituted butyrophenones* e.g. domperidone (10–20mg PO qds/60mg PR bd) do not cross blood–brain barrier so avoid some side effects.
- *Butyrophenones* e.g. haloperidol are neuroleptic drugs, in small doses (1.5mg PO bd) retain antiemetic effect but can cause dysphoria, oversedation, extrapyramidal symptoms.
- *Centrally acting dopamine antagonists are likely to significantly worsen movement disorders such as Parkinson's disease.*

$5HT_3$-antagonists

- *Ondansetron* (4–8mg IM/slow IV 8-hourly) is less impressive in PONV than chemotherapy-induced emesis (↓dose in hepatic impairment).
- In paediatric practice, ondansetron (0.1mg/kg by slow IV injection, max 4mg) is drug of choice. Side effects include headache and constipation.

Steroids

Dexamethasone (4–8mg PO/slow IV 8 hourly) good with chemotherapy, also stimulates appetite which may be helpful. Commonly used to reduce swelling, e.g. in airway surgery. Side effects include euphoria (avoid after 4pm), psychosis ('roid rage'), Na^+ and fluid retention.

Anticholinergics

Hyoscine hydrobromide 0.3–0.6mg SC/IM is used in motion sickness, opioid-induced vomiting, but rarely in PONV. Adverse effects: sedation, confusion, urinary retention, dry mouth. ↓ respiratory secretions may be desired.

Other drugs

- *Benzodiazepines* may help if nausea and vomiting is induced by higher centres in the brain (e.g. anticipatory vomiting before chemotherapy).
- *Neurokinin-1 receptor antagonist* (aprepitant) and *cannabinoids* (nabilone) only used for chemotherapy-induced emesis.
- *Ginger root* used in alternative remedies, and may help some patients.

Treatment of oculogyric crisis and acute dystonia

- Signs include muscle rigidity, involuntary jaw or eye movements, can be generalized. Treat with procyclidine, 5–10mg by slow IV injection. The response is usually rapid.

Diarrhoea and constipation

Key facts

- Diarrhoea is common in hospital.
- It consumes many hours of nursing time, puts patients at risk of fluid and electrolyte loss, and predisposes to pressure sores.
- Diarrhoea is technically the passage of >300mL stool daily: patients may refer to diarrhoea when they simply have frequent stools but it is the volume and consistency of a diarrhoeal stool that matters.
- Infection control measures (e.g. hand washing, gloves, aprons) are important. Follow them for your own protection and everybody else's.

Clinical features

Think about
- Does the patient need IV fluids or nutritional support?
- Possible causes are listed in Table 6.2.

Ask about
- Onset, frequency, relation to meals.
- Associated symptoms e.g. abdominal pain, nausea, vomiting.
- Blood in stool suggests infection, malignancy or IBD; mucus suggests impaction/IBD (can occur in malignant/infection).
- Floating, offensive stool: steatorrhoea due to loss of bile.
- Drugs: sensitivities, recent changes, laxatives, antibiotics.
- PMHx: IBD, coeliac disease, IBS, previous surgery abdominal.

Look for
- Dehydration: thirst, tachycardia, low BP, oliguria, dry skin and mucosa, falling daily weight.
- Sepsis: pyrexia, abdominal tenderness, warm peripheries.
- Malnutrition: pressure sores, glossitis, stomatitis.
- Examine the abdomen *including PR* to look for constipation/faecal impaction/palpable rectal tumour/blood.

Investigations
- *C. difficile* needs to be excluded in all cases by stool culture and assay of stool for *C. difficile* toxin.
- The endocrine causes of diarrhoea can be diagnosed by the appropriate blood tests: glucose, cortisol, thyroxine, Ca^{2+}.
- Colonoscopy can be used to diagnose mesenteric ischaemia, pseudomembranous colitis, IBD, and rare infective causes.

Management of postoperative diarrhoea

- Exclude faecal impaction with a PR examination.
- Exclude *C. difficile* if patient has recently had antibiotics: cefuroxime and ciprofloxacin are particular culprits.
- Fluid and electrolyte replacement e.g. Hartmann's solution at 2mL/kg per hour if clinically indicated.
- The simplest anti-motility agents are codeine phosphate 15–30mg 4–6-hourly or loperamide 4–8mg initially followed by 2–4mg bd.
- Avoid anti-motility agents in febrile, bloody diarrhoea as they may prolong or exacerbate diarrhoea.
- Increase pressure sore care.
- Encourage continuing nutrition

Constipation

Common and exacerbated by immobility, lack of privacy, pain (wounds/anal fissures), dehydration, ↓dietary fibre, opioids, Fe supplements. Careful history and examination to differentiate from ileus (📖 see p. 256) and bowel obstruction (📖 see p. 256) *includes a PR.*

- *Bulking agents:* e.g. Fybogel® 1 sachet PO bd.
- *Stool softeners:* e.g. sodium docusate 100mg PO bd–tds.
- *Osmotic agents:* e.g. lactulose 15mL bd.
- *Stimulants:* e.g. Senna 1–2 tabs bd, bisacodyl 5–10mg at night PO.
- *Enemas:* e.g. sodium phosphate.

Table 6.2 Causes of postoperative diarrhoea

Spurious	Faecal impaction with overflow: common in elderly. Caused by opioids, low-fibre diet, immobility, dehydration
Drug-induced	Laxatives, antacids (e.g. Mg^{2+} salts)
	Enteral tube feeding (use low-volume, high-strength feed)
	Many other agents: always check side effects in *BNF*
Antibiotics	Simple bacterial overgrowth
Infective	*C. difficile:* pseudomembranous colitis
	Salmonella, Shigella, Campylobacter
	Pathogenic *E. coli* (e.g. *E. coli* O157)
	Viruses (e.g. rota, noro, Norwalk)
	Parasites
	Cryptosporidium/CMV colitis in immunosuppressed
After GI surgery	Lactose intolerance (after small bowel resection)
	Bile acid loss (after cholecystectomy)
	Dumping (after vagotomy/pyloroplasty)
Endocrine	Diabetes
	Hypoadrenalism
	Thyrotoxicosis
	Hypocalcaemia
Vascular	Mesenteric ischaemia
	Melaena/frank blood
Pre-existing conditions	Inflammatory bowel disease
	Coeliac disease
	Irritable bowel syndrome
	Bowel malignancy

Paralytic ileus/Obstruction

Key facts
- Paralytic ileus is the cessation of GI tract motility.
- See Box 6.4.

> ### Box 6.4 Causes of postoperative ileus
> - Prolonged surgery and handling of the bowel.
> - Localized or generalized peritonitis (usually slightly later presentation).
> - Abdominal trauma.
> - Electrolyte disturbances (most can affect GI function!).
> - Anticholinergic agents, opioids.
> - Prolonged hypotension, hypoxia.
> - Immobilization
> - Pain
> - Critical illness.

Clinical features
Symptoms
- Abdominal discomfort and bloating.
- Nausea, vomiting and hiccoughs.

Signs
- Abdominal distension, tympanic or dull on percussion.
- Absent bowel sounds.

Investigation
Air/fluid filled loops of small and/or large bowel on AXR.

Postoperative care
- Pass NGT to empty the stomach of fluid and gas if the patient is nauseated or vomiting. Small volumes of oral intake are better tolerated and may help a mild ileus to resolve.
- Ensure adequate hydration by IV infusion ('drip and suck').
- Maintain normal electrolytes and fluid balance. The gut will continue to secrete significant volumes of fluid and electrolytes but is failing to reabsorb them. Be prepared to give extra fluid and electrolytes intravenously until the ileus resolves.
- Reduce/stop opioid analgesia if possible, and encourage the patient to mobilize.
- After 5–7 days, look for other causes and consider nutritional status.

Postoperative mechanical bowel obstruction
It is important to distinguish between this and ileus since management is different.

Causes
- Early adhesions (usually self limiting).
- Internal, external, parastomal, or wound herniation.

Clinical features
- Nausea and vomiting.
- Colicky abdominal pain.
- Abdominal distension, tympanic on percussion.
- Examine hernial orifices, and stoma if any, for incarcerated hernias. Remember to examine for a femoral hernia—it's easy to miss this.
- High-pitched 'tinkling' bowel sounds (borborygmi).
- Dilated loops of small bowel (relative paucity of gas in colon).

Treatment
- Resuscitation as for paralytic ileus, with strict bowel rest.
- CT scan to define level of the obstruction.
- Consider surgical exploration if incarcerated hernia or very occasionally for adhesional obstruction which fails to resolve with non-operative management.

Peptic ulcer disease & reflux

Key facts

- Peptic ulceration develops when a breakdown in the mucosal defence of the lower oesophagus, stomach, or duodenum leads to a mucosal breach, usually due to gastric acid.
- May be acute and transient (e.g. 'stress', 'and/or *H. pylori*' or 'Cushing's' ulcer after surgery, trauma, critical illness).
- If the repair system fails to deal with the breakdown of the mucosa, it may become chronic.
- >90% of gastric and duodenal ulceration is associated causally with *Helicobacter pylori*; many patients will have undergone triple therapy to eradicate the organism. Accordingly, most patients take acid-suppressing therapy for acid reflux/dyspepsia, not for 'ulcers'.
- Other risk factors include chronic NSAID use, smoking, heavy alcohol intake, steroids, ♂ sex. Gastrinoma (Zollinger–Ellison syndrome) is rare.
- Main risks are acute ulceration after major surgery, and brisk haemorrhage.

Clinical features

Symptoms

- Epigastric pain: take careful history to avoid mistaking angina for peptic ulcer disease (and *vice versa*) as picture can be similar.
- Duodenal ulceration typified by hunger pains with central back pain *relieved by food*. Pain is often cyclical and occurs in the early hours of the morning.
- Gastric ulceration typified by *pain precipitated by food* with associated weight loss and anorexia. Pain less cyclical.
- Nausea, vomiting, and upper abdominal distension suggest gastric outlet obstruction (⊞ see also Complications below).
- Haematemesis and/or melaena severe haemorrhage.

Signs

- Usually normal abdominal examination, but patients may have epigastric tenderness: peritonism suggests perforation.
- Distension and succussion splash (>3h after last meal) suggests gastric outlet obstruction.

Investigations

- *Gastroscopy:* this is the commonest diagnostic (and occasionally therapeutic) test.
- *Barium meal:* may be used if gastroscopy contra-indicated.
- *Urease testing:* to assess for presence of *H. pylori* can be performed on antral biopsies from gastroscopy, or as a breath test.

Complications

- Acute upper GI bleed (⊞ see p. 260).
- Fe deficiency anaemia 2° to chronic low-level bleeding.
- Perforation (⊞ see p. 262).
- Gastric outlet obstruction due to scarring around pylorus.

Preoperative care

Pre-assessment clinic

If patients have poor symptom control, treat risk factors (advise on stopping smoking, reduce alcohol, stop NSAIDs, convert aspirin to enteric coated) and start omeprazole 20mg PO od if not on PPI.

Day before surgery (Table 6.3)

- For patients with gastro-oesophageal reflux, preoperative therapy to reduce risks of regurgitation during anaesthesia (prophylaxis of acid aspiration). Omeprazole 20–40mg od for 3 days preoperatively results in maximal acid suppression. Omeprazole 40mg on the preceding evening then 40mg 2–6 h before surgery (as recommended in the *BNF*) is almost as effective. Some anaesthetists use ranitidine preoperatively and sodium citrate 30mL just before induction.
- Antacids: continue current formulation or change to oral sodium citrate 30mL qds.
- H_2 receptor antagonists: change to ranitidine 50mg IV tds if unable to take H_2 receptor antagonist orally.
- PPIs: continue on oral therapy if possible (open and dissolve capsule contents in water and give via NGT). Pantoprazole 40mg can be given by slow IV injection over >2min.

Discuss with anaesthetist

Or record in notes a history of reflux/peptic ulcer disease. The anaesthetist might need to manage the patient differently in theatre and avoid prescribing regular NSAIDs for postoperative analgesia, for example.

Postoperative care

- In patients with active peptic ulceration document NSAIDs as drugs to avoid (in notes and on drug chart).
- In lower risk patients with poor pain control on non-NSAID analgesia:
  - Prescribe a NSAID for breakthrough pain prn, but not regularly.
  - Consider cover with regular PPI as already discussed.
  - Ibuprofen said to cause fewer gastric side effects than diclofenac.
  - Review the need for the prescription at 48–72h.
  - Never discharge a patient with a new, open-ended prescription for regular NSAIDs. Their GP may mistakenly think you want them to continue this.

Table 6.3 Perioperative therapy for patients with peptic ulcer disease

NSAIDs and aspirin	Stop
Steroids	Switch to IV, 🕮 see p. 281
Antacids	Change to oral sodium citrate 30mL qds
PPI	Continue oral therapy if possible. Consider pantoprazole 40mg IV
H_2 receptor antagonists	Ranitidine 50mg IV tds until able to take PO or change to IV pantoprazole.

Gastrointestinal bleed

Key facts

- *Haematemesis* is vomiting blood, usually due to bleed proximal to duo-denojejunal junction (upper GI).
- *Melaena* is the passage of altered blood (dark purple, pitch black or 'tarry') again usually from upper GI bleeding.
- Melaena often presents (or continues) several days after an upper GI bleed, due to ↓gut motility.
- *Haematochezia* is bright rectal bleeding (usually lower GI, or occasionally torrential upper GI).
- 📖 See Box 6.5 for causes.

Emergency management

Resuscitation

- Check airway is patent and that patient is breathing.
- Lay the patient in the recovery position; give 15L/min O_2 via mask.
- Assess SaO_2, pulse, BP, capillary refill, conscious level (AVPU).
- Establish *large* calibre IV access in both antecubital fossae with 14G (brown/orange) or 16G (grey) cannula; 18G (green) is insufficient.
- FBC, clotting, U&E, LFTs; XM 3U of red cells.
- In known or suspected liver disease, consider vitamin K and/or FFP to correct clotting (FFP better if synthetic hepatic function impaired).
- Give crystalloid fluid up to 2000mL if persistently tachycardic or hypotensive, until cross-matched blood arrives, then give 2U blood.
- If pulse, BP, and conscious level have not responded, alert a general surgeon and an anaesthetist—surgery is likely.
- Catheterize, and commence fluid balance chart. Consider requesting HDU/ITU bed if very unwell.
- Insertion of a Sengstaken–Blakemore gastro-oesophageal tube may be a life-saving resuscitation manoeuvre.
- Stop all NSAIDS. Give IV PPI (e.g. omeprazole 40mg IV).
- Surgery—may be required if:
  - Massive haemorrhage requiring ongoing resuscitation.
  - Failed endoscopic treatment with ongoing bleeding.
  - Rebleeding not suitable for repeated endoscopic treatment.

Establish a diagnosis

Get help from appropriate specialist for further management:

- Urgent OGD is the investigation of choice for upper GI bleeding (at least within 24h):
  - May require ongoing resuscitation with anaesthetist present.
  - Allows diagnosis and biopsy if appropriate.
  - May allow therapeutic interventions including adrenaline injection, heater probe coagulation, banding of varices.
- Rectal examination (haemorrhoids), proctoscopy or sigmoidoscopy for lower GI bleeding.
- Angiography:
  - Rarely suitable for active bleeding as time-consuming and done in radiology department.
  - May allow selective embolization in some patients with recurrent bleeding inaccessible to endoscope e.g. angiodysplasia.

Definitive management

Varices (📖 see also p. 264)
- Endoscopic coagulation or banding/interventional radiology/surgery.
- IV vasopressin or somatostatin analogues.

Gastric/duodenal ulcer
- Endoscopic coagulation or injection, may be repeated if suitable ulcer.
- Surgery for failed 1° management or re-bleeding which is unsuitable for attempted repeat endoscopic treatment.
- *H. pylori* eradication with triple therapy for one week, e.g: omeprazole 20mg bd + clarithromycin 250mg +metronidazole 400mg bd.
- Remove triggers and modify risk factors (📖 see p. 258).

Gastric carcinoma
- Endoscopic treatment often not effective.
- Partial or subtotal gastrectomy (often palliative, rarely curative).

Oesophageal trauma
Oral antacids, occasionally surgical resection.

Aortoenteric fistula
Surgery, if the patient survives beyond diagnosis.

Anastomotic bleed
Correct any coagulopathy, may require repeat laparotomy.

Haemorrhoids
Injection/banding/laxative.

Box 6.5 Causes of postoperative GI bleeding

Upper GI bleed
- Peptic ulcer pre-existing/triggered by surgery; (📖 see p. 258).
  - Fresh red blood with clots, occasionally mixed with food.
- Oesophageal ulceration e.g. after NGT/TOE.
- Mallory–Weiss tear: bleed preceded by violent or prolonged vomiting or retching.
- Oesophageal varices/arterial malformation/malignancy.
- Anastomotic bleed.
- Aortoenteric fistula (late complication of aortic surgery): copious bright red blood (often rapidly fatal).
- Over-anticoagulation.
- False +ve: $FeSO_4$ therapy makes stool dark grey and FOB +ve.

Lower GI bleed
- Haemorrhoids.
- Bleeding from low anastomosis (e.g. sigmoid colectomy).
- Mucosal trauma from instrumentation.
- Diverticular disease
- Malignancy

Postoperative anastomotic leak

Key facts
- Any intra-abdominal anastomosis may leak.
- Highest risk of leak occurs with oesophageal and rectal anastomosis and lowest with small bowel anastomosis (Table 6.4).
- Clinical picture depends on location of leak.

Table 6.4 Risk factors associated with ↑risk of leak

Patient factors	Disease factors	Operative factors
Chronic malnutrition	Unprepared bowel (e.g. obstruction)	Poor blood supply to bowel ends
Immunosuppression	Local or generalized sepsis	Tension on bowel ends
High-dose steroid use	Metastatic malignancy	Under-resuscitated patient, emergency operation
DM		

Clinical features
Anastomotic leakage may present as one of several clinical pictures:

Peritonitis
- Acute, severe generalized abdominal pain with guarding and rigidity.
- Fever, tachycardia, and tachypnoea are common.
- Diagnosis is usually clinical but may require CT scanning if unsure.

Intra-abdominal abscess
- Swinging fever and tachycardia, commonly around 5–7 days postoperatively.
- Localized tenderness related to the anastomosis may be present.
- Diagnosis should be sought by CT scanning.
- 📖 see p. 263

Enteric fistula
- Any fistula between the anastomosis and the wound or another organ.
- Usually occurs as a result of a subclinical leak and abscess formation which discharges through a pathway of low resistance.
- Often presents late as an apparent wound infection which discharges with enteric content.
- Diagnosis made by CT scanning or occasionally fistulography if presenting very late.

Acute physiological disturbance
- Sepsis originating from an initially subclinical leak may present with cardiovascular abnormalities (e.g. sinus tachycardia, AF/supraventricular tachycardia, chest pain).
- *Any acute postoperative disturbance of physiology in a patient with an intraabdominal anastomosis is due to leak until proven otherwise.*

Emergency management

Resuscitation

- Establish large calibre IV access: send FBC, clotting, U&E, LFTs, G&S.
- Give crystalloid fluid up to 2000mL if tachycardic or hypotensive.
- Catheterize and place on a fluid balance chart.
- ABGs.
- Ensure appropriate analgesia. If the patient is hypotensive and an epidural infusion is running, stop it. Additional opioids may not be safe so *ask an anaesthetist for advice.*

Establish a diagnosis

- Acute peritonitis needs no diagnostic investigation. Emergency re-look laparotomy should be organized immediately.
- CT scanning with IV and oral contrast is the investigation of choice for all other suspected leaks.
- For rectal anastomoses, water soluble contrast may delineate leak.

Early treatment

- Give IV antibiotics (e.g. cefuroxime 750mg IV tds and metronidazole 500mg IV tds)
- Monitor fluid balance hourly: urine output should be at least 0.5mL/kg/h.

Definitive management

Peritonitis

Always requires surgical intervention unless the patient is deemed unfit.

- Prepare for theatre: ensure blood results from resuscitation are written clearly in the notes.
- Once the leak has been identified options for management include:
  - Dividing the anastomosis, closing the distal end, and forming the proximal end into a stoma (do not waste time getting stoma team involved before emergency surgery).
  - Emptying the bowel (lavage) and forming a proximal defunctioning stoma.
  - Reforming/repairing the anastomosis (only suitable for fit patients with minimal contamination and an otherwise healthy anastomosis).
  - Placing a large drain(s) next to the anastomosis

Intra-abdominal abscess

- Radiological guided drainage and antibiotics provided patient does not become peritonitic or show signs of 2° complications.
- Open surgical drainage if inaccessible or unresponsive to radiological drainage.

Enteric fistula

- Usually managed by antibiotics and may close spontaneously. If it fails to close, surgical repair may be required.
- Treat for abscess or peritonitis if either develops.

Hepatic disease and failure

- A few patients with hepatic disease may need surgery for problems directly related to their liver disease e.g. GI bleeding, while many more with compensated chronic liver disease present for unrelated surgery.
- In ALD, there may be other problems, e.g. Korsakoff's psychosis, withdrawal delirium (📖 see p. 295); fits (📖 see p. 306), neuropathy; malnutrition (📖 see p. 246); pancreatitis, varices (📖 see p. 260); anaemia (📖 see p. 100).
- Chronic liver damage results in cell necrosis, fibrosis, and cell regeneration. In the early stages the liver is enlarged, but later becomes small, hard and shrunken as cirrhosis progresses. Fibrosis causes portal hypertension, and repeated cell necrosis eventually leads to liver failure.

Box 6.6 Causes of liver failure ± jaundice in surgical patients

- Acute hepatocellular injury due to injury by viruses or toxins (usually drugs). Cholestasis may also be a feature.
  - Hepatitis A or B.
  - Alcohol, paracetamol overdose.
  - Hepatic vein thrombosis (Budd–Chiari syndrome).
- Chronic liver disease from alcohol, hepatitis B and C, right heart failure, 1° biliary cirrhosis, haemochromatosis, Wilson's.
- Sepsis, hypotension, burns, trauma, metastases, renal failure can cause acute decompensation.
- Acute jaundice, especially postoperatively, may be caused by additional mechanisms (📖 see p. 266).

Clinical features

Think about
- Problems due to the hepatic dysfunction e.g. coagulopathy, jaundice (📖 see p. 266), encephalopathy.
- Problems due to the underlying cause of hepatic dysfunction.

Ask about
- Previous symptoms of upper GI bleeding, ulcers, past intervention (ulcer surgery, sclerotherapy, surgical portal shunt/TIPSS).
- Nutrition, alcohol intake.
- Diagnosis of/risk factors for HIV, hepatitis (📖 see p. 92).

Look for
- Spider naevi, gynaecomastia, palmar erythema, ascites, jaundice.
- Assess conscious level, and nutritional state (📖 see p. 246).

Investigations
- Serology for hepatitis viruses A, B, and C, consider HIV.
- FBC, clotting (including fibrinogen), U&E, glucose, LFTs.

Child–Pugh classification of cirrhosis (points for bilirubin, albumin, PT, ascites, hepatic encephalopathy): Child–Pugh score 5–6 (A) is low risk—30-day mortality 12%; Child–Pugh score 7–9 (B) is medium risk—30-day mortality 40%; Child–Pugh score ≥10 (C) is high risk—30-day mortality 74%.

Preoperative care

⚠ *Severe hepatic impairment is not trivial. If in doubt, get expert help*, although many patients with liver disease have sufficient hepatic reserve and require little specialist precautions (especially if not cirrhotic).

- Remember universal precautions against BBVs. Alert staff if +ve.
- Admit 2–3 days preoperatively with HDU/ICU postoperatively for Child-Pugh B/C cirrhosis.
- Adjust medications for hepatic impairment, continue vitamins IV.
- Encourage abstinence from alcohol, stop hepatotoxic drugs.

Haemostasis

- XM blood and FFP as appropriate to procedure (NB portal hypertension increases blood loss from all abdominal surgery).
- Correct coagulopathy with vitamin K, consider FFP (📖 see p. 68).

Management of ascites

- Massive ascites may need paracentesis—but first check FBC and clotting.
- Ensure bladder is empty. Use Bonano catheter, insert 5–10cm below umbilicus in midline (📖 see p. 364). Send ascites for MC&S *and* cytology.
- Give colloid to maintain intravascular volume: albumin 20% solution 100ml IV with every 3rd litre of ascites drained.
- Change diuretics to IV for perioperative period.

Fluid and electrolyte imbalance

- Strict fluid balance. Hyponatraemia (📖 see p. 228) is common in failure. Avoid NS: total body Na^+ already high (with fluid overload).
- ↑K^+ may be from spironolactone or renal failure.
- Consider switching to loop diuretics if K^+ >5.0mmol/L.
- Renal impairment is serious: contact renal physician or ICU.
- If unable to take oral fluids, insert IV line: use glucose saline 2000 mL/ day, add K^+ if serum K^+ <4.0mmol/L. Beware fluid overload and worsening hyponatraemia. Monitor serum Na^+ twice daily.
- Hypoglycaemia: consider glucose 20% at 50–100mL/h. Monitor levels.

Postoperative care

- Reduce morphine doses (in liver disease ↑half-life and ↑sedative effect).
- Request low protein, low Na^+ diet.
- Monitor renal function: hourly urine output, daily weight (ascites).
- Hypotension or hypoxia may result in severe hepatic decompensation.
- Constipation can precipitate encephalopathy in cirrhotic patients, use regular lactulose (10mL bd PO) to achieve 2–3 soft stools/day.
- Drowsiness may represent hepatic encephalopathy, without classical signs. Seek expert advice from a gastroenterologist.
- Following major surgery a daily coagulation screen should be performed. An ↑PT is a very sensitive indicator of ↓liver synthetic function. Frequent bedside blood glucose tests whilst stable.
- Patients prone to sepsis, often without signs. Have low threshold for:
  - Cultures, seeking microbiological advice, imaging.
  - Diagnostic ascitic tap (green needle, send 10–20mL for MC&S): *spontaneous bacterial peritonitis in patients with ascites is serious.*
- GI bleed may precipitate worsening liver function in patients with chronic liver disease. If multi-organ failure develops, mortality >50%.

Diagnosis of postop jaundice

The priority is to exclude obstruction/dilatation of the biliary tree: request an urgent abdominal US scan.

- Postoperative jaundice results from an accumulation of bilirubin.
  - This is often related to the nature of the surgery performed and resulting hepatobiliary problems: obstruction usually after biliary, hepatic, or pancreatic surgery.
  - Jaundice may also develop after non-biliary surgery, and is often multifactorial in origin.
- Although jaundice itself may be relatively benign, it should always be investigated as it may be a sign of a serious underlying problem.
- Patients who *in addition* have postoperative hepatocellular dysfunction have a poor prognosis and need urgent investigation and management.

Box 6.7 Causes of postoperative jaundice

- *Biliary obstruction* after hepatobiliary surgery.
- *Cardiac failure* is one of the commonest causes of mild jaundice and deranged LFTs postoperatively.
- *Drugs* can cause cholestatic (co-amoxiclav, erythromycin, OCP, phenothiazines, *TCA*, oral hypoglycaemics) and hepatocellular (statins, anti-TB, halothane, antifungals) jaundice.
- *Hepatic decompensation in chronic liver disease* after surgery, particularly if complicated by sepsis, shock, or an acute GI bleed (jaundice combines with deranged LFTs and ↑PT).
- *Haemolysis* (infection, cold agglutinins, transfusion reaction), or resorption of haematoma.
- *Sepsis, hypotension, hypoxia.*
- *TPN* (📖 see p. 248).
- *Gilbert's syndrome* (or other congenital bilirubin metabolism disorders) may become apparent postoperatively.

Think about:

Hypotension and hypoxia

- Cholestasis is a common reaction to a low perfusion state of the liver (haemorrhagic/hypovolaemic/septic shock, heart failure).
- Clinical picture: raised AST/ALT, less commonly jaundice and ↑PT. If shock state is promptly corrected, the liver abnormalities usually resolve over a few days.

Sepsis

- Both bacterial sepsis, and the drugs used to treat it can lead to cholestatic jaundice ± deranged LFT.
- Hepatic insults include hypotension and bacterial endotoxins.

Chronic liver disease

Jaundice may develop (or worsen) after any surgery in patients with chronic liver disease (📖 see p. 264)

Haematoma

- Macrophages degrade haem in phagocytosed blood to bilirubin. Serum unconjugated bilirubin can rise to ~60mmol/L, without ↑AST/ALT.
- Urinary urobilinogen is elevated.
- Tests for haemolysis are –ve, reticulocytosis may be seen in response to blood loss.

Infective

Viral hepatitis (hepatitis A/B/C) should be excluded by serology; until this is done take precautions as described, 📖 see p. 92.

Gilbert's syndrome

- Gilbert's syndrome (↑unconjugated bilirubin) is a benign inherited disorder of bilirubin metabolism leading to fluctuating low-grade hyper-bilirubinaemia, often worse in starvation, infection, or after surgery.
- Other LFTs are normal.
- The diagnosis is based on Hx (previous episodes after typical triggers), and exclusion of other causes (e.g. haemolysis).

TPN

- 📖 See p. 248.

Ask about

- *Biliary surgery:* if the patient has had hepatobiliary surgery, then surgery needs to be excluded as the cause of postoperative jaundice.
- *Shock:* is there a recent history of sepsis, hypotension, or hypoxia?
- *Haematomas:* has the patient a large collection of extravasated blood, e.g. after pelvic fracture or ruptured aortic aneurysm?
- *Drugs/TPN:* has the patient been exposed to hepatotoxins?
- *Chronic liver disease:* was this present preoperatively? Perhaps the patient was alcoholic, but not recognized to have liver disease?
- *Heart failure:* may be the sole cause.

Look for

- *Sepsis* is the most important causal factor to consider. Regard jaundice as a marker of potential infection, and initiate a sepsis screen.
- LFTs, coagulation screen (PT is the most sensitive test of liver synthetic function), glucose (patients may become hypoglycaemic due to impairment of gluconeogenesis in the liver), U&E. The serum urea is typically low in liver failure.
- Haemolysis is characterized by anaemia, unconjugated hyperbilirubi-naemia, ↑urinary urobilinogen, reticulocytosis, reduced haptoglobin, elevated LDH, and a *blood film* shows reticulocytes, polychromasia, spherocytes, and red cell fragments.

Perioperative care

- Problems associated with hepatic dysfunction are described on 📖 p. 264
- Management of postoperative jaundice is described on 📖 p. 268

Management of jaundice

- Jaundice may be a sign of serious pathology (📖 see p. 266) and associated with major morbidity and mortality if not adequately managed.
- 📖 See Box 6.8 for perioperative risks.

Preoperative care

Day before surgery

- Consider requesting HDU bed.
- Avoid morphine as it constricts the sphincter of Oddi. Use pethidine.
- Hydration is key. Give 1000mL 0.9% saline/Hartmann's solution IV over 6–12h before induction of anaesthesia (unless severe LVF/hepatic failure).
- Insert urinary catheter and monitor hourly fluid balance.
- Consider 500mL 10% mannitol over 20–30min either an hour before, or following induction of anaesthesia to maintain urine flow.
- Correct coagulation with FFP p. 68, give prophylactic antibiotics (📖 see p. 60).
- If possible, standard practice is to decompress a potentially infected biliary tree by ERCP before any definitive surgery to reduce perioperative morbidity and mortality, but they remain high.

Discuss with anaesthetist

- Would patient benefit from invasive monitoring on HDU?
- Anaesthetist may elect to insert CVP ± arterial line during GA.

Box 6.8 Perioperative risks of jaundice

- *Sepsis* may be the cause of jaundice, but may also be triggered through bacteraemia after operation on an infected biliary tree. Sepsis and jaundice may lead to multiorgan failure.
- *Bleeding:* ↓vitamin K absorption (dependent on on bile salts in gut) leads to ↑PT. In addition, platelet count may be low from septicaemia.
- *ARF:* bilirubin can be toxic to kidneys; ARF complicates liver failure in 10% of patients (hepatorenal syndrome).
- *High mortality* in cholangitis, the presence of three or more of the following factors predicts a mortality as high as 50%:
  - Major cardiorespiratory disease.
  - pH <7.4.
  - Bilirubin >90mmol/L.
  - Platelet count <150 × 10^9/L.
  - Albumin <30g/L.

Postoperative care

- Protect renal function; renal failure is avoidable! (See Box 6.9.)
  - Monitor volume status carefully: hourly urine output, careful fluid balance, use a CVP line if necessary to assess filling status.
  - If urine output <50mL/h for 2 consecutive hours, give 100mL mannitol 10% over 15min.
  - Avoid additional nephrotoxic insults (hypotension, hypoxia, sepsis, drugs, especially NSAIDs).
  - Diuretics have only a limited role in preventing renal failure, liaise with renal team early.
- Check U&E, LFTs, PT, glucose daily.
- Meticulous aseptic precautions, low threshold for septic screen (📖 see p. 90).

Box 6.9 Avoiding renal failure in jaundice

The best way to keep the kidneys working is to ensure that they are continuously well-perfused with oxygenated blood at a pressure they are used to. If for whatever reason this has been interrupted, it becomes critical to quickly eliminate additional renal insults: avoiding nephrotoxins, hypovolaemia, hypotension, hypoxia and treating sepsis promptly and aggressively. *However, nothing protects the kidneys better than adequate blood volume, BP, and blood flow and only when volume resuscitation is complete may diuretics have any role.* Even then furosemide and mannitol are not without risks, some of them serious, and neither drug prevents renal failure.

Inflammatory bowel disease

Key facts

- Chronic, episodic inflammatory condition affecting whole GI tract
  (Crohn's disease) or large bowel (ulcerative colitis), with continuum
  between the two in colon: a clear diagnosis is not always possible.
- Hallmark of Crohn's: transmural, granulomatous inflammation leading
  to fissures and strictures—may spare intervening sections (skip lesions).
- Patients may require surgery for IBD, or unrelated conditions.
- The main risks of surgery result from the following factors:
  - Immunosuppressive therapy leads to poor wound healing, ↑infection
    rate, pressure sores, easy bruising.
  - Anaemia, malnutrition (see p. 246) electrolyte imbalance, dehy-
    dration.
- It follows that surgery has least risk when the patient is on minimal
  immunosuppressive therapy together with minimal disease activity.

Clinical features

- Diarrhoea (may be bloody), abdominal pain, fever, malaise, weight loss.
- Abdominal tenderness, tachycardia, fever during active disease phase.
- In Crohn's, look for fistulae, anal abscesses, RIF mass, aphthous ulcers.
- Non-GI signs: clubbing, ocular inflammation, large joint arthritis, ery-
  thema nodosum, pyoderma gangrenosum.
- Anaemia, ↑WCC, ↑ESR, ↑CRP, evidence of poor nutrition.
- AXR: toxic megacolon requires urgent intervention/surgery.

Preoperative care

Pre-assessment clinic

- Assess disease activity: weight gain/loss, blood in stool, pain, frequency
  of opening bowels.
- Identify complications, e.g. fistulae, abscesses, strictures, stoma.
- Assess nutritional state (see p. 246).
- If stoma a possibility, contact stoma team to counsel patient
  preoperatively.
- Defer non-urgent surgery until the patient is in best possible condition.

Day before elective surgery

- Send blood for FBC, ESR, U&E, LFTs, XM, stool for MC&S.
- Correct K^+ <4.0mmol/L (see p. 232). In severe diarrhoea,
  >30mmol K^+/day may be required.
- Hb <9g/dL should be transfused; this can be done intraoperatively.
- ESR >30mm/h and active rectal bleeding usually indicates active disease:
  liaise with senior surgical and medical staff.
- Albumin <30g/L requires intensive nutritional support (see p. 248).

Emergency presentation of IBD

- Severe acute colitis may present with shock; resuscitation should be
  immediate (see p. 116). Urgent surgery may be required.
- Pain requires opioids: pethidine causes less smooth muscle spasm, morphine is a superior analgesic. The patient may have a clear preference
  and PCA probably provides the best pain control (p. 78).
- Bowel perforation or toxic bowel dilatation necessitates emergency
  surgery, and the risks are always high.

Postoperative care
- As for major bowel surgery.
- In patients on steroids and other immunosuppresants, postoperative anastomotic breakdown and other septic complications may occur with *no* specific signs (📖 see p. 90).
- Enteral nutrition may be delayed for some days: consider TPN via a dedicated feeding line (📖 see p. 248).
- Check Hb, U&E, and CRP daily.
- Restart oral medication as soon as able to tolerate oral intake.

Table 6.5 Perioperative prescribing in IBD

Rectal steroids	Replace with IV hydrocortisone prior to surgery (and afterwards too if colostomy is performed)
Oral steroids	Replace with IV hydrocortisone while patient is NBM (📖 see p. 281)
Sulfasalazine	Continue up to day of operation
NSAIDs	*Avoid*, because of risks to upper GI tract, renal function, and platelet aggregation

Endocrine and metabolic

Diabetes mellitus

Key facts

- Affects 3% of population in UK, incidence increasing with age and obesity (Table 7.1).
- Underlies 1 in 6 vascular admissions, so always look for it.
- Main problems are control of blood glucose and complications: retinopathy, nephropathy, ischaemic heart disease, peripheral vascular disease, CVA/TIA, somatic/autonomic neuropathy, ↑risk of infection.

Clinical features

History

- Previous episodes of uncontrolled hyperglycaemia and their trigger.
- Ask how patient assesses diabetic control and their insulin regimen.
- Ask for symptoms of IHD: angina, dyspnoea, previous MI, PCI.
- Ask for symptoms of autonomic neuropathy: postural hypotension, gastric distension, diarrhoea, excessive sweating, urinary retention.

Examination

- BP is elevated in many type 2 diabetics. Aim for 160/90 or less before elective surgery, long-term <145/90.
- Postural hypotension may be a sign of autonomic neuropathy if the patient is normally hydrated.
- Look for diabetic foot ulcers; assess the vascular/neurological supply of feet—if either is compromised, then high risk of developing ulcers.
- Check pressure areas in elderly patients for decubitus ulceration.
- Fundoscopy only if new symptoms (retinopathy can lead to blindness).

Investigations

- *Blood glucose:* aim for glucose in the range 6–10mmol/L. 📖 see Box 7.1.
- *U&E:* renal impairment affects 30% of diabetics at some point in their life (if in doubt, formal assessment of renal function 📖 p. 212).
- *HbA$_{1C}$* indicates level of long-term glycaemic control.
- *Urine analysis for ketones and proteinuria:* if ketones are present check blood gases and/or HCO$_3^-$ to exclude ketoacidosis. Proteinuric diabetic patients are at ↑risk of postoperative renal failure.
- *ECG (if >30 yrs):* ↑risk of ischaemic heart disease, possibly 'silent' i.e. without overt angina.

Perioperative management (📖 see also Box 7.1)

- If unable to eat normal diet (NBM, anorexia, vomiting, stroke), or unwell (sepsis, haemodynamically unstable), start insulin sliding scale (📖 see Insulin sliding scale p. 276). Consider how you will provide full nutritional support.
- In most patients, combination of diet, oral hypoglycaemic agents and/or SC insulin can usually achieve good glucose control.
- Switch patients to their normal regimen as soon as they are eating and drinking normally.
- Most hospitals will have a diabetes specialist nurse who can advise on insulin regimens and has access to a diabetologist if needed.
- Treat invasive investigations (e.g. barium enema, OGD) as minor operations. Radiological contrast agents can precipitate lactic acidosis

in patients on metformin; discontinue drug at time of contrast radiographic procedure and re-start 2 days later.
- IV contrast agents in fasted (i.e. dehydrated) patients with nephropathy can precipitate acute renal failure. Encourage oral intake or give IV fluids. Consider giving N-acetyl cysteine and explore whether non-contrast imaging (e.g. US, MRI) is an acceptable alternative.

Table 7.1 Classification of DM

Type 1	Type 2
Always require insulin for glucose control	Not insulin dependent, but often will require insulin later on (and may have absolute requirement for insulin)
Prevalence: 5/1000	Prevalence: 25/1000, + 10/1000 undiagnosed
More commonly juvenile onset	More commonly adult onset
Autoimmune B-cell destruction	Insulin resistance
Insufficient insulin quickly leads to ketoacidosis	Insufficient hypoglycaemic leads to ↑glucose and dehydration

Box 7.1 Principles of perioperative management of DM

Aims of management
- Aim to maintain blood glucose 6–10mmol/L.
- Avoid hypoglycaemia: aggression, confusion, drowsiness, seizures.
- Avoid profound hyperglycaemia: it causes electrolyte disturbances, osmotic diuresis leading to dehydration, and may cause ketosis.
- Avoid dehydration: it exacerbates poor blood sugar control.

Management principles
- If in any doubt, contact anaesthetist.
- Put diabetic patients *first* on theatre list if possible.
- Take medication as normal until midnight before surgery, except long-acting insulin—stop this the night before.
- Do not give oral hypoglycaemics on morning of surgery, but give short-acting insulin if procedure in the afternoon in type 1 DM.
- Start insulin sliding scale (☐ see Insulin sliding scale p. 276) on morning of surgery in type1 DM if facing lengthy fast, start IV fluids to avoid dehydration.
- If sepsis, emergency, poorly controlled type 2 give IV insulin via sliding scale preoperatively.
- Except in cardiac surgery, tight glycaemic control is unnecessary.
- It is better to have slightly high blood sugar (rather than low) during GA when patients cannot report symptoms of hypoglycaemia.
- K^+ should be added to the glucose unless the patient has renal impairment, since insulin facilitates intracellular K^+ uptake.
- Use separate cannulae for each of the infusions, to ensure each solution is delivered reliably. Whenever possible use a syringe driver for the insulin and an infusion pump for the glucose. Do not be tempted to use a 3-way tap; if infusions are given using the same cannula a non-return valve *must* be incorporated into the maintenance fluid tubing.

Insulin sliding scales and regimens

Insulin sliding scales (Table 7.2)

- Add soluble insulin (e.g. Actrapid®) 50U to 50mL 0.9% (normal) NaCl and infuse by syringe pump according to Table 7.2.
- *IV sliding scale* (preferred method in all patients requiring sliding scale):
  - Check blood glucose every hour (every 2–4h if stable).
  - Give IV 5% glucose with 20mmol KCl at 125mL/h.
- *SC sliding scale* is a useful alternative in patients with poor IV access.
  - Short-acting SC insulin allows rapid alterations of glucose levels. It has a peak action at 2–3h with little effect after 6h.
  - When using a SC sliding scale blood glucose should only be measured before meals.

Table 7.2 Insulin sliding scale

Blood glucose (mmol/L)	IV insulin	SC insulin
<3	No insulin, give glucose IV or PO (GlucoGel®, Lucozade®)	
3–5	0.5U/h	No insulin
6–10	1U/h	2U/h
11–15	2U/h	5U/h
16–20	4U/h	7U/h
>20	6U/h	10U/h

In patients who normally take insulin >0.75U/kg/day, double IV insulin dose (for glucose 6–10mmol/L, infuse 2U/h, 11–15mmol/L infuse 4U/h, etc.).

Commence infusions early on the morning of surgery.

Measure blood glucose hourly using glucose reagent sticks and an electronic meter.

Postoperatively, check blood glucose 1-hourly initially, then 4-hourly once good control has been established.

This regimen may be different from that used in your hospital. Use local regimen if available.

Insulin-treated diabetes (type 1 and 2)

- Stop long-acting insulin the night before surgery.
- Only give short-acting insulin on morning of surgery if not NBM and procedure in afternoon.
- Start an IV insulin sliding scale (rather than giving normal SC insulin) if:
  - Patient septic or shocked.
  - Preoperative patients need to fast longer than just overnight.
  - Postoperative patients not able to tolerate normal diet.
  - Poor blood sugar control (fasting glucose >10mmol/L).
- **A rough guide to anticipated hourly insulin requirements is to divide the total normal daily insulin requirement by 24.**
- Schedule insulin-treated diabetics first on the operating list to minimize catabolism during fasting, and allow early resumption of oral feeding.

Non insulin treated diabetes (always type 2)

- Patients with diet-controlled diabetes require no special preparation, if their glucose and electrolytes are normal.
- Insulin and glucose infusions can be instituted if blood glucose levels become consistently raised above 10–15mmol/L in the perioperative period.
- Discontinue long-acting hypoglycaemics (chlorpropamide, glibenclamide) 24–48h prior to surgery.
- Discontinue metformin as rarely this can cause a lactate acidosis
- Omit oral hypoglycaemic drugs on the day of surgery.
- If patients are having minor surgery, and will be eating and drinking soon after their procedure, no further special preparation is necessary.
- If poor glycaemic control (glucose >10mmol/L) monitor levels 2-hourly.
- If more major surgery is planned, or if diabetes is not well controlled on drugs, manage in the same way as insulin-treated diabetics, with insulin and glucose infusions.

Types of insulin

- Ultrafast acting: e.g. insulin aspart glulisine or lispro (inject SC immediately after or at start of meal).
- Fast: soluble insulin e.g. Actrapid®, Humulin S® or Insuman® Rapid (inject SC 15–30min before meals) can be infused IV for rapid perioperative control of hyperglycaemia.
- Intermediate: SC e.g. biphasic isophane insulin (NPH), biphasic insulin aspart or lispro.
- Long-acting: SC e.g. insulin zinc suspension, insulin determir or glargine.
- Premixed combinations of long and shorter acting insulins increase compliance, usually at the expense of tighter glycaemic control.

Increased insulin requirements and resistance

- Several factors can cause elevation in insulin requirement. Adjust prescription according to blood glucose levels.
  - Major surgery.
  - Sepsis.
  - Obesity.
  - TB drugs.
  - Renal failure.
- For the following, also get specialist advice:
  - Cushing's disease.
  - Pregnancy.

Dynamic algorithm

In some units, a treatment flowchart allows insulin infusions to be titrated up or down in response to measured blood glucose, without the need to rewrite the sliding scale prescription. Such an algorithm is capable of matching treatment to the patient's needs, despite the huge variation in insulin requirements between individuals, or even in the same individual at different times.

Diabetic emergencies

Diabetic ketoacidosis (DKA)

Key facts

- ⚠ *Medical emergency:* the associated dehydration is more life threatening than hyperglycaemia, fluid resuscitate first, then correct hyperglycaemia.
- Ketoacidosis: acidosis (pH <7.2 or HCO^-_3 <15mmol/L) **and** ketosis (at least ++ ketones in urine). It may occur with only relatively minor elevation of glucose (if due to insufficient insulin, rather than none).
- Hyperglycaemia up to 25–30mmol/L without ketoacidosis or dehydration is not a medical emergency.
  - High levels lead to thirst, dehydration, impaired wound healing
  - Reduce slowly, give additional small dose (4–8U) of SC insulin.

Emergency resuscitation

- Assess consciousness and ability to protect airway (📖 see p. 292). Consider ITU/HDU if unconscious.
- Sit responsive patients up, give O_2 by face mask.
- IV access, give NS 1L bolus (only add K^+ if known to be <3.0mmol/L).
- Give 4–8U Actrapid® IV if glucose >20mmol/L, start IV sliding scale (📖 see p. 276).
- ABG for acidosis (and pO_2), urine for ketones (and MC&S).
- Check U&E, glucose, HCO_3^-, osmolality, FBC, blood cultures.
- NGT if vomiting.
- Replace K^+ with each of the subsequent bags of IV fluid (see Table 7.3).
- Continue fluid replacement: 1L over 1h, then 1L over 2h, then 1L over 4h, then 1L over 6h, continue at 4L/24h. Switch to 5% dextrose when glucose <15mmol/L (slower rate if poor LV or elderly).
- Hourly glucose, K^+ and ABG (until acidosis corrected).
- Add long-acting SC insulin once glucose stable and patient eating (continue sliding scale to cover variation for 24h, decrease rate of infusion in anticipation of effect of long-acting insulin).

Table 7.3 K^+ replacement in DKA

Serum K^+ [mmol/L]	Add K^+ to each litre of IV fluid
<3	40mmol/L
3–4	30
4–5	20

Establish a diagnosis

- *Look for causes:* infection, breaks in skin (check between toes) insulin resistance, poor compliance.
- *Ask about* fevers, chills and rigors, symptoms of chest infection, urinary tract infection, wound infection, cutaneous abscesses.
- *Look for* pyrexia, and localizing signs of sepsis: auscultate chest, look at surgical wounds, drain and all line sites.
- *Request* blood and urine cultures, CXR.

Hypoglycaemia

- Hypoglycaemia (blood glucose <3.0mmol/L) is often rapid in onset and associated with feeling faint, sweating, tremor, feeling hungry, but also disorientation, aggression, and can lead to convulsions, unconsciousness, and permanent cerebral dysfunction if not rapidly treated.
- In conscious patient give a sweet drink (e.g. sugary tea, non-diet lemonade, Lucozade®, Coca-Cola®) followed by biscuits or sandwiches.
- If unable to eat, give 50mL of 50% glucose IV: can be an irritant to veins and should be given slowly via a large-bore cannula.
- If venous access is not possible give glucagon 1U IM or rub glucose gel (e.g. GlucoGel®) on the gums.
- Think about causes (usually excess insulin or oral hypoglycaemics, but also from liver disease, insulinoma, Addison's disease, pituitary insufficiency)

Hyperosmolar non-ketotic coma (HONK)

- In type 2 DM, relative insulin deficiency and inadequate fluid intake lead to hyperglycaemia and dehydration, exacerbated by osmotic diuresis of glucose.
- Surgical stress or intercurrent illness can precipitate HONK, which usually develops over a period of days (or weeks in the community).
- Typically, the glucose levels are very high (>35mmol/L), and the patient is very dehydrated.
- There is no acidosis and no urinary ketones as there has been no switch to ketone metabolism
- Treat with IV fluid (half the rate used in ketoacidosis 📖 see p. 278). If Na^+ >150mmol/L (see 📖 p. 230) use 0.45% saline (if elderly patient, more cautious fluids).
- Re-assess blood glucose after first litre of NS, if still >20mmol/L, give bolus Actrapid® (8U), followed by sliding scale (📖 p. 276).
- Anticoagulate as high risk of DVT/PE (📖 p. 194).
- If this develops on the ward, you have not done your job looking after the patient!

Steroid therapy

Key facts

- Chronic steroid therapy may cause depression of adrenal axis: the normal steroid response to stress is blunted and patients may become very unwell after major surgery, sepsis or trauma.
- Patients taking long-term steroids (Box 7.2) should have supplemental steroid therapy given after major surgery (PO or IV if NBM). Taper additional steroid rapidly as they suppress wound healing/response to infection (📖 see Table 7.4).
- Glucocorticoid drugs are prescribed for two main reasons:
  - Most commonly anti-inflammatory or immunosuppression: including asthma, rheumatoid arthritis, polymyalgia, temporal arteritis, skin disorders, connective tissue diseases, hypersensitivity states.
  - Replacement therapy for adrenal or pituitary disease.
- Failure to give steroid perioperatively can lead to adrenal insufficiency.

Acute adrenal insufficiency

Key facts

- Adrenocortical suppression results in blunted response to any stress.
- Surgery, anaesthesia, underlying illness, sudden withdrawal of steroid after prolonged therapy can precipitate acute adrenal insufficiency.
- Cover all surgical procedures in these patients with ↑steroid (📖 see Table 7.4).

Clinical features

- Hypotension, shock, coma.
- Vomiting, diarrhoea, most commonly abdominal pain, muscle weakness.
- Hypoglycaemia, hyperkalaemia.
- Adrenal insufficiency most commonly occurs in patients on steroid treatment, particularly if they have been taking high-dose steroids, when steroids abruptly withdrawn.

Investigations

- ACTH stimulation test: give tetracosactide (artificial ACTH) 0.25mg IV, measure cortisol before and 30min after: if 30min cortisol >500nmol/L and increase >200nmol/L above baseline, hypoadrenalism is excluded.
- Concurrent steroids interfere with the results of this test.

Management

- Give hydrocortisone 100mg IV, then hydrocortisone 100mg IV q 6h
- Give NS 1000mL stat, monitor glucose
- Septic screen, empirical antibiotics if infection suspected
- Patients with Addisons disease may also need fludrocortisone

Box 7.2 Side effects of long-term steroid therapy

- ↑susceptibility to, and severity of, infections.
- Impaired wound healing.
- More prone to peptic ulceration, especially if the patient also takes NSAIDs.
- Water and electrolyte imbalance, hyperglycaemia leading to DM.
- Proximal muscle wasting and weakness (take care in moving and positioning these patients).
- Osteoporosis with susceptibility to fractures after relatively minor injury (e.g. moving patient while asleep).
- Skin and blood vessel fragility: bruise easily and dramatically, difficulty getting IV access, pressure sores are more common.

Table 7.4 Guidelines for perioperative steroid therapy

	Steroid therapy	Operation	Perioperative steroid cover
Currently on steroids	<10mg prednisolone per day (or equivalent)	Any	Assume normal HPA response. Additional steroid cover not required (continue maintenance)
	≥10mg prednisolone per day (or equivalent)	Minor surgery	25mg hydrocortisone at induction
		Moderate surgery	Usual preoperative steroids + 25mg hydrocortisone at induction and 100mg/day for 24h
		Major surgery	Usual preoperative steroids + 25mg hydrocortisone at induction and 100mg/day for 48–72h
	High-dose immunosuppression	Any	Usual immunosuppressive doses during perioperative period
Stopped steroids	<3 months	Any	Treat as if on steroids
	>3 months	Any	No perioperative steroid therapy necessary

Thyroid disease

Key facts

- Thyroid surgery may be performed for:
  - Goitre, to relieve respiratory obstruction or for cosmesis.
  - Discrete nodule to exclude or resect malignancy.
  - Recurrent thyrotoxicosis.
- Potentially life-threatening problems after thyroid surgery include:
  - Upper airway obstruction (haemorrhage into the wound, tracheomalacia, laryngeal nerve injury).
  - Hypocalcaemia (📖 see p. 238) due to removal of parathyroid glands.
  - Thyroid crisis.
- Patients undergoing other surgery may present with problems related to their thyroid disease, including hyper- and hypothyroidism.

Hyperthyroidism

Clinical features

- Thyroid crisis: diarrhoea, vomiting, acute abdomen, hyperthermia, tachyarrhythmias, tremor, agitation, hallucinations, psychosis, coma.
- Chronic hyperthyroidism: weight loss, heat intolerance, diarrhoea, tachycardia, AF, tremor, exophthalmus (only in Graves' disease).
- Causes: Graves' disease, toxic multinodular goitre, toxic adenoma, thyroid carcinoma, viral (de Quervain's thyroiditis), drugs (amiodarone, lithium, interferon-α, IL-2).

Investigations

- TSH, T_3 (TSH suppressed, high T_3 and T_4).
- U&E, LFT/Ca^{2+} (may be raised), FBC (anaemia).
- US thyroid ± radioisotope (^{123}I, ^{99m}Tc) scan to identify nodules.

Emergency resuscitation of thyroid crisis

- Sit patient up and give O_2 by face mask.
- Active cooling with cooling blankets, topical ice bags.
- IV hydrocortisone 100–300mg IV.
- Propranolol 1mg IV boluses (up to 10mg); digoxin if fast AF.
- Correction of dehydration and electrolyte abnormalities.

Perioperative management

- Defer elective surgery because of ↑cardiovascular risk.
- Treat first with carbimazole 20mg bd or propylthiouracil 200–400mg daily.
- If surgery cannot be postponed, give propranolol (10–40mg qds) or nadolol 80 to 160mg od to reduce the resting heart rate <90/min.

Thyroid enlargement

- A goitre or thyroid nodule in a patient presenting for surgery is a common incidental finding: rarely needs emergency work-up.
- Exclude a large retrosternal goitre causing thoracic outlet obstruction. (CT neck and chest) and consider flow-volume loop and respiratory function tests as attempts at endotracheal intubation may precipitate acute upper airway obstruction.

Hypothyroidism

Clinical features

- Myxoedema coma: hypothermia, hyporeflexia, bradycardia, seizures, coma, recent thyroid surgery.
- Chronic hypothyroidism: fatigue, lethargy, cold intolerance, weight gain, constipation, bradycardia, non-pitting oedema, hyporeflexia, CCF.
- Common, up to 5% of middle-aged ♀ may be hypothyroid.
- Causes: iodine deficiency, autoimmune, treatment of hyperthyroidism (drugs/surgery), infiltration, drugs (amiodarone, lithium).
- May be precipitated by infection, trauma, surgery, MI, CVA.

Investigations

TSH, T_4 (T_4 low, ↑TSH in 2°; ↓TSH in 1°).

Emergency resuscitation of myxoedema coma

- Sit patient up and give high-flow O_2 by face mask.
- Request T_3, T_4, TSH, FBC, U&Es, cultures, cortisol, and ABG.
- Give hydrocortisone 100mg 8-hourly IV.
- Give T_3 5–20mcg IV slow push.
- Start 100mL/h NS IV (through warmer).
- Active warming with warm air blankets.
- Treat suspected CCF, infection, monitor BM, U&E.

Perioperative management

- Correct hypothyroidism *slowly* with T_4 before elective surgery.
- T_4 can precipitate or considerably worsen IHD—seek senior advice. Correction of hypothyroidism usually takes 3 months.
- Hypothyroidism after total thyroidectomy is treated with a replacement dose of 0.1–0.15mg T_4 (levothyroxine).
- Patients on T_4 may safely discontinue therapy for a few days if they are NBM, as the drug has a long half-life.
- Hypothyroid patients are much more sensitive to narcotics and anaesthetic agents, so these must be administered in reduced doses.
- Hypothermia will aggravate circulatory and respiratory depression.

Airway obstruction after thyroid surgery

- Management of airway obstruction due to tracheomalacia and recurrent laryngeal nerve palsy is described on 📖 p. 207.
- Obstruction due to haemorrhage can occur early (poor haemostasis), or late (due to infection) resulting in haematoma causing dyspnoea, pain, neck swelling, stridor, wound bleeding, in severe cases cyanosis.

Resuscitation

- Give high-flow O_2 (8L/min non-rebreathing mask).
- Large calibre IV access, crystalloid 1000mL if tachycardic/hypotensive.
- ⚠ **Consider opening the wound immediately**. If the patient is cyanosed or unconscious cardio-respiratory arrest is imminent.
  - Immediate decompression of expanding haematoma is vital to maintain airway patency.
  - Loss of blood from opening the wound will be trivial in comparison: clip removers are often placed nearby for exactly this purpose.
- Definitive treatment requires return to theatre for formal control.

Obesity

Key facts
- Obesity (BMI >30) is increasingly common.
- It poses multiple potential problems to surgeon, anaesthetist, and nursing staff, as well as predisposing the patient to serious comorbidity (Box 7.3).
- It is a relative contraindication to day-case surgery.

Preoperative management
Pre-assessment clinic
- Morbid obesity (BMI>40) is a contraindication to day-case surgery.
- Discuss advantages of weight loss (reduction in major complications, as well as improvement in quality and length of life) and provide support (dietician, GP may have access to weight loss resources).
- Look for cardiovascular disease: hypertension (see p. 152 and heart failure should be treated (see p. 124).
- Ask about sleep apnoea (day time somnolence, snoring, home CPAP): these patients will need CPAP as inpatients and are at high risk of respiratory and cardiovascular complications.
- Use the appropriate sized BP cuff (2/3^{rds} arm circumference) as smaller cuffs will over-estimate BP.
- Consider omeprazole 20mg od PO if symptoms of gastric reflux present.

Discuss with anaesthetist
Obese patients undergoing abdominal or thoracic surgery may need prolonged intubation and ventilation postoperatively (ICU bed) or CPAP (HDU bed).

Postoperative care
- All obese patients should receive supplemental O_2 therapy postoperatively.
- A pulse oximeter is useful to determine the adequacy of oxygenation. Sitting the patient up will improve ventilation.
- Chest physiotherapy will be helpful, particularly if the patient has undergone abdominal surgery.
- Obese patients occasionally require a period of postoperative ventilation, particularly after prolonged or emergency major surgery.
- Treat postoperative pain adequately, consider PCA.
- Infections are more common, particularly wound and chest, and should be checked for and treated with appropriate antibiotics.
- Thromboembolism is more likely. Prophylactic measures: two or more of SC heparin, compression stockings, pneumatic compression 'boots', and early will reduce the risk of DVT.

Box 7.3 Perioperative problems caused by obesity

Cardiovascular dysfunction
- Increase in blood volume and in cardiac work, commonly with background coronary artery disease and impaired LV function.
- Hypertension and general atherosclerosis are common.
- Diabetes is much more common with ↑BMI.

Respiratory compromise:
- Vital capacity and functional residual capacity are reduced, and closing volume is ↑.
- Pulmonary blood flowing past inadequately ventilated dependent lung regions ('shunting') causes hypoxia in supine and head-down positions.
- Postoperative atelectasis increases shunt further. It is crucial to achieve early mobilization: sitting out or, at least, sitting up.
- Hiatus hernia: common, and increases risk of pulmonary aspiration.

Transport and positioning
- May be difficult to position: trolleys, operating tables and scanner tables have maximum loads.
- Moving anaesthetized obese patient carries risk to patient/staff.

Anaesthetic problems
- Maintenance of an airway and tracheal intubation can be difficult.
- Venous access may be a problem.
- BP cuffs need to be wider.
- Regional anaesthesia (e.g. epidurals, nerve blocks) are more difficult.

Surgical problems
- Surgery is technically more difficult.
- There is an ↑incidence of wound infection, dehiscence, and pressure ulceration over heels, occiput, and sacrum.

Rare endocrine disorders

Cushing's syndrome

Key facts

- A syndrome of clinical features due to excess levels of plasma cortisol.
- Commonest cause: glucocorticoid steroid therapy (📖 see p. 280).
- 1° adrenal disease (adenoma, carcinoma) Cushing's disease (ACTH-secreting pituitary adenoma), ectopic ACTH secretion (from small-cell lung cancer, carcinoid tumour) make up remainder.

Clinical features

- Truncal obesity, buffalo hump, moon face, acne bruising, striae, thin skin, hirsutism, muscle weakness, menstrual irregularities.
- Lethargy/depression, psychosis, hallucinations.
- Hypertension, osteoporosis, and impaired glucose tolerance/diabetes.
- Impaired wound healing and ↑infection risk.

Diagnosis and investigations

- Tests to prove cortisol excess and establish the cause:
  - Screening: elevated 24h urine cortisol (> 280 nmol/24h) or overnight dexamethasone suppression test (📖 see p. 24).
  - Diagnosis: high-dose dexamethasone test (📖 see p. 24) if screening tests +ve.
  - *ACTH levels:* ↑in Cushing's disease and ectopic ACTH production, ↓in other causes of Cushing's syndrome.
- *CT/MRI:* distinguish adrenal tumour from bilateral adrenal enlargement.
- Pituitary MRI usually shows tumours >1cm in Cushing's disease.

Perioperative management

- Metyrapone decreases cortisol synthesis, get specialist advice.
- Cortisol replacement after unilateral or bilateral adrenalectomy is vital.
  - Patients with solitary adrenal tumours may have an atrophied contralateral adrenal gland; it can take a year for a return to normal function.
  - Start on 50–100mg IV tds hydrocortisone postoperatively. Maintenance dose is usually 20–30mg PO long-term.
  - Patients must be informed about the possibility of an Addisonian crisis triggered by any illness (📖 see p. 278).
- Mineralocorticoid replacement (fludrocortisone 0.1mg) is also necessary after bilateral adrenalectomy.
- Replace cortisol as above after any major surgery in patients with Cushing's syndrome due to exogenous steroids.

Conn's syndrome

Key facts

- Syndrome of hypertension, severe hypokalaemia due to aldosterone hypersecretion with suppression of plasma renin activity.
- Aldosterone-producing adenomas are usually solitary tumours involving adrenal gland: other causes are idiopathic bilateral adrenal hyperplasia (25–30% of cases) and familial hyperaldosteronism.

Clinical features
- Often asymptomatic.
- Weakness, cramps, parasthesiae, intermittent paralysis, headaches, polydipsia, polyuria and nocturia, hypertension, hypokalaemia.

Diagnosis and investigations
- Stop all diuretics and antihypertensives 2 weeks prior to testing.
- Serum K^+ <3mmol/L and urinary K^+ excretion >40mmol/L per day.
- Aldosterone: renin ratio (high as renin suppressed), aldosterone suppression test (fludricortisone suppresses aldosterone production unless aldosterone autonomous), posture test (changing from supine to standing ↑renin leading to ↑ aldosterone, no change in aldosterone in Conn's).
- Abdominal CT to image adrenals.
- If solitary unilateral macroadenoma is identified no other localization studies are necessary: treatment is unilateral adrenalectomy.
- Patients in whom localization is not achieved may have bilateral adrenal hyperplasia and should be treated medically.

Perioperative management
- Correct hypokalaemia preoperatively: spironolactone, oral K^+ or both:
  - Sando $K^®$ 2–3 tablets bd or tds.
  - 20–40mmol K^+ in 1L NS IV over 6–8h by peripheral line.
  - 20–40mmol KCl in 100mL NS over 1h by central line.
- Spironolactone can control hypertension and correct K^+ levels in preparation for surgical treatment.
- Laparoscopic adrenalectomy: for aldosterone-secreting adenomas.

Hormone secreting tumours

Phaeochromocytoma

Key facts

- Rare: incidence of 2–8 cases per million population/year.
- Most common presentation on surgical ward is for elective removal.
- Roughly follows the '10% rule': 10% are bilateral, 10% are extradrenal, and 10% are malignant.
- Produces catecholamines (adrenaline, dopamine, and noradrenaline) leading to episodes of:
  - Headache, sweating, palpitations, a feeling of 'impending doom', hypertension, tachyarrhythmias.
  - Occasionally MI, CVA, seizures occur and are life-threatening complications.
  - Posterior Reversible Encephalopathy Syndrome (PRES) is rare.
- Attacks can be triggered by activities causing mechanical pressure on the tumour (e.g. physical exercise, defaecation, intercourse), by ingestion of alcohol, labour, GA, and surgical procedures.

Diagnosis and investigations

- 24h urine collection and assessment for VMA and noradrenaline is most accurate for diagnosis (both raised).
- Clonidine suppression test (failure of urine levels to fall after clonidine) confirms diagnosis where urine levels are borderline.
- Thoraco-abdominal CT or MRI: first-line imaging especially for adrenal and sympathetic chain tumours.
- MIBG (meta-iodo-benzyl-guanidine) scanning can localize extra-adrenal sites not seen on CT or MRI in the majority of cases.

Perioperative management

- Discuss with anaesthetist: management is complex.
- Key principle is effective BP control:
  - α-blockade (phenoxybenzamine 10mg bd/tds up to maximum dose tolerated) until hypertension controlled and nasal stuffiness occurs.
  - β-blockade (e.g. propranolol) can be added *after* hypertension controlled to combat the β-adrenergic effects (tachycardia). **Never** start with β-blockade.
  - Alternative treatments: doxazosin, labetalol (α/β blocker), Ca^{2+} channel blockers, ACE inhibitors, and GTN/sodium nitroprusside infusions have been required in resistant cases, but are not widely used.
- The principle of surgery is complete resection of the tumour (with negative margins if suspected malignancy).
- Laparoscopic adrenalectomy is the treatment of choice for smaller adrenal tumours (<8cm), open adrenalectomy for larger tumours.

Emergency management

- Hypertensive crisis is an emergency, get help.
- Can occur in patient awaiting definitive surgery, triggers are as described, above
- Treat BP with IV labetolol until stabilized, then use phenoxybenzamine.

Neuroendocrine tumours

Key facts
- Tumours of neural crest origin, secrete serotonin, sometimes insulin, glucagon, bradykinin, thyroid hormones, ACTH, somatostatin.
- Commonest sites are appendix, ileum, rectum, adrenals, but may occur in lung, ovaries and testes, and metastasize to liver.

Clinical features
- Often asymptomatic, occasionally appendicitis, intussusception, obstruction, pain from metastasis (liver, bone).
- *Carcinoid syndrome* (suggests liver or extra-intestinal metastases as secreted vasoactive substances are metabolized in liver): paroxysmal flushing, bronchoconstriction, diarrhoea, valvular fibrosis (usually right-sided) leading to heart failure, fatigue, nausea.
- *Carcinoid crisis* can be triggered by handling tumour during surgery, or administration of exogenous catecholamines (inotropes): life threatening vasodilatation, hypotension, tachycardia, bronchoconstriction.

Diagnosis and investigations
- 24h urinary 5-HIAA (a metabolite of serotonin) makes diagnosis; chromogranin A and B give estimate of disease bulk.
- CT thorax, abdomen, pelvis for staging, dedicated imaging directed at symptomatic sites, or as required to assess for surgery.
- Radiolabelled octreotide or MIBG scan to show extent of disease and determine if radioactive octreotide/MIBG can be used for therapy.

Perioperative management
- Liaise with anaesthetist early as management may be complex.
- Avoid catecholamines.
- Octreotide is a somatostatin analogue which blocks release of serotonin: it may be given as IV infusion or SC injections.
  - If taking long-acting somatostatin analogue (e.g. lanreotide every 28 days) and well controlled, further cover may not be needed.
  - If not on long acting analogue e.g. because of minimal symptoms, consider covering perioperative period with short-acting analogue.
- Treat diarrhoea with loperamide 2mg after each loose motion.

Neurology

Drowsiness and coma

Key facts
- Coma is immediately life threatening, if not protecting airway start ALS.
- Unexplained drowsiness is just one step away from coma.
- Although drowsiness *per se* is not life threatening, many causes of drowsiness *are* medical emergencies (📖 see Box 8.1)
- Being called to assess a drowsy or comatose patient postoperatively is one of the most taxing tasks for a junior doctor.
- Such patients have an ↑ risk of cardiac arrest and death. Rapid assessment and correction of underlying causes is essential in this critical situation. **Call for an anaesthetist or senior help early.**
- Use Glasgow Coma scale (GCS) to assess/monitor change.

Glasgow Coma Scale
- 15 maximum, 3 minimum.
- Below 8, airway is at risk, take measures to secure.

Eyes
- Open spontaneously   4
- Open to command/verbal stimulus   3
- Open to pain (e.g. sternal rub)   2
- No eye opening at all   1

Voice
- Talking appropriately and oriented   5
- Confused conversation   4
- Inappropriate exclamations only   3
- Incomprehensible sounds   2
- No vocalization at all   1

Motor (Score the best response)
- Obeys commands (not just grasp reflex)   6
- Localizes to source of pain (e.g. supraorbital pressure) 5
- Withdraws from source of pain (e.g. nailbed pressure)   4
- Abnormal flexion to pain (e.g. sternal rub)   3
- Abnormal extension to pain (e.g. sternal rub)   2
- No movement at all   1

Box 8.1 Look for causes of drowsiness and coma

Immediately life threatening: hypoxia/hypercapnia (📖 p.180), shock/hypotension (📖 p.116), metabolic (hypoglycaemia (📖 p.278), hyperglycaemia (📖 p.278), acidosis (📖 p.173), hypo/hypernatraemia (📖 p.228 and p.230), drug toxicity, sepsis (📖 p.90), CVA (📖 p.298), status epilepticus (📖 p.306)

After surgery look for: sepsis (📖 p.90) bleeding (📖 p.98), MI (📖 p.122), CVA (bp.298), opioid overdose (📖 p.80), hypoxia and hypercapnia (📖 p.180).

Box 8.2 Emergency resuscitation of comatose patients

1 minute
- AIRWAY: if compromised, relieve obstruction, *call arrest team.*
- BREATHING: if absent/poor respiratory effort, *call arrest team*
- CIRCULATION: if no palpable pulse, *call arrest team.*
- DISABILITY: if GCS <8, put in recovery position, *call anaesthetist.*
- If in any doubt, or patient deteriorating call for senior help.
- If any history of associated fall, stabilize C-spine.

2–5 minutes
- Jaw thrust ± chin lift, oro- or nasopharyngeal airway if tolerated.
- 15L/min O_2 by face mask.
- Continuous monitoring of BP, pulse oximetry, ECG (use defibrillator ECG leads if necessary).
- Identify and treat obvious arrhythmias (📖 p.130–139).
- Check bedside blood glucose: treat hypo- and hyperglycaemia immediately (📖 p.278).
- Identify and treat opioid overdose (📖 p.80).
- Identify and treat seizures (📖 306).
- Venous access: send blood cultures, FBC, clotting, U&Es, glucose, troponin, LFTs; consider drug levels including alcohol.
- After blood cultures, start broad spectrum antibiotics if sepsis suspected.
- Start IV fluids if BP <120/70 (Hartmann's 500mL bolus IV).

5–10 minutes
- Get a brief history from nursing staff or check notes quickly.
- Do rapid clinical examination of CVS, RS, abdo, neuro, surgical sites.
- Do ABG (📖 p.172) and request portable CXR (📖 p.412).

Respiratory failure
- ↓respiratory drive is easily missed, patient may not appear breathless.
- Pulse oximetry will not detect respiratory depression until the minute ventilation is extremely low; then SaO_2 will fall precipitously.
- Check ABGs for a rising $PaCO_2$ (📖 p. 172).
- Hypercapnia/↓pH worsens cerebral oedema; hypoxia and ↓BP also worsen cerebral ischaemia: rapid correction reduces permanent neurological damage.

Anaesthesia and analgesia
- If patient wakes up communicating, and then becomes unrousable, 'the anaesthetic' is not likely to be the cause.
- Opioids given intra- or post-op can cause drowsiness/respiratory depression, more if IV/in epidural, or in hepatic/renal impairment.
- Start resuscitation, discontinue opioid.
- Give naloxone (0.4mg increments to 1mg IV) if necessary.
- Opioid in a spinal/epidural infusion has *extremely* prolonged action. Giving opioids via *second* route is very hazardous—ask for help from an anaesthetist.

Confusion

Key facts

- Confusion is common postoperatively, due to many causes (Box 8.3).
- It may be obvious: a disoriented, uncooperative, or hallucinating patient; or manifest as inactivity, quietness, slow thinking, and labile mood.
- *Actively assess if the patient is oriented in time, person and place.*
- Perform Mini Mental State Examination (MMSE) (📖 Box 8.4, p. 297) if you are still unsure.
- Distinguish from anxiety and psychosis (persecutory ideation).

Emergency management

- Before sedation, try talking to the patient calmly, in a quiet room: involving nurses and relatives may avoid need for sedation.
- Check recent U&Es, FBC: correct metabolic abnormalities and anaemia.
- Perform a neurological examination to look for focal neurological deficit (including pupils) and consider head CT to exclude stroke.
- Assess and treat hypoxia (📖 p. 180) (if face masks are poorly tolerated try nasal cannulae or oxygen tents) and hypotension (📖 p. 116).
- If the patient's behaviour poses physical danger to themselves or others, it may be necessary to sedate as first-line management: haloperidol 0.5–1.5mg up to a total of 10mg in 24h PO/IM/IV, but if patient remains disturbed 1–5mg of midazolam can be given IV, and the patient placed under close observation.
- Beware of sedating the hypoxic or hypotensive patient.
- Reassure patient and relatives: confusion is common, usually reversible, and it is not a sign that the patient is 'going mad'.

Diagnosis and management of perioperative confusion

📖 Stroke, dementia, and epilepsy are dealt with on pp. 296–300, and p. 306.

Hypoxia and hypercapnia

ABG must be checked in any unconscious patient (📖 p. 172).

- Hypoxia produces agitation, confusion, aggression before drowsiness.
- Hypoventilation causes hypercapnia, can result in unconsciousness when the $PaCO_2$ reaches very high levels (>10kPa).
- Can occur solely from accumulation of opioid, may also be seen in pre-existing hypercapnic respiratory failure when precipitated by opioids, pain, chest infection, loss of hypoxic drive after O_2 therapy.
- Hypoventilation is difficult to detect: measure ABGs if any doubt.

Metabolic and endocrine disturbances

- Metabolic conditions causing confusion, drowsiness, or coma include hypo- and hypernatraemia (📖 p. 288), hypo- and hyperglycaemia (📖 p. 278), hypercalcaemia (📖 p. 236), liver (📖 p. 264) and renal failure (📖 p. 212).
- Check blood glucose, U&Es, Ca^{2+}, LFT, TFT, FBC on all patients with altered post-op mental state. Abnormal TFT (📖 p. 220) and steroids may cause delirium.

Box 8.3 Common causes of confusion

- Drugs—benzodiazepines, opioids, anticonvulsants, antipsychotics.
- CVA, encephalitis, meningitis, space occupying lesion, postictal state.
- Hypoxia, hypercapnia.
- Shock.
- Sepsis.
- Alcohol withdrawal, thiamine/vitamin B_{12} deficiency.
- Metabolic disturbances ($\downarrow\uparrow$glucose, $\downarrow\uparrow Na^+$, $\downarrow$pH, $\downarrow\uparrow Ca^{++}$, $\uparrow$creatinine, $\uparrow$urea, $\uparrow$bilirubin).
- Preoperative dementia (may also be unmasked by combination of unfamiliar environment, sleep interruption, medication).
- Surgery is associated with cognitive deficit in some elderly patients.

Sepsis
- Sepsis can cause anything from mild confusion to deep coma.
- Look for other signs of sepsis and its source (🕮 p. 90).
- Sepsis as a cause of delirium is unlikely without fever, but may be seen in overwhelming infection/the elderly/immunosuppressed.
- Combination of fever with acute confusion may herald septic shock. Manage as if septic shock had already developed (🕮 p. 90).

Alcohol withdrawal
- Alcohol withdrawal suggested by history of high pre-op alcohol consumption ± raised γGT, and psychomotor agitation postoperatively.
- Treat with diazepam 2.5mg tds PO/PR or lorazepam e.g. 2mg PO/IV.
- Haloperidol may lower seizure threshold and is best avoided.
- Rarely, letting the patient drink alcohol is safer than the alternatives.
- Remember multivitamins to prevent encephalopathy/psychosis.

Pre-existing dementia
- Patients may retain superficial social skills despite dementia, which is consequently missed if not actively assessed (🕮 p. 296).
- Disruption of a normal routine, sleep deprivation, pain, opioids may unmask dementia leading to confused patient.
- A quiet side-room and patient nurse or relative can help greatly.
- Haloperidol beginning with 0.5–1mg PO alternatively IV/IM.
- Continue usual medication; avoid atropine and hyoscine.

Stroke or space-occupying lesion
- Perioperative CVA commonly embolic, also from hypotension or uncontrolled hypertension: elderly and arteriopaths are at risk.
- Rarely, intra-cranial space-occupying lesion may present post-op due to increased peritumour oedema, with signs of $\uparrow$ICP.
- Stroke is a complication of carotid endarterectomy (~1%), after which permanent neurological damage may be prevented by re-exploration.
- Deteriorating conscious level after craniotomy may be due to intracranial bleeding or cerebral oedema, requiring urgent medical or surgical intervention. Inform neurosurgeon urgently, consider steroids (🕮 p. 307) and/or mannitol.

Dementia

Key facts

- Senile dementia is a hidden disability because of its insidious onset and a deceptive preservation of social skills until relatively late.
- May affect 10% of those >65 years; 20% of those >80 years.
- Commonest causes are Alzheimer's disease, multi-infarct dementia, Lewy body dementia, alcohol abuse, Parkinson's disease.
- Patients with dementia may present for palliative surgery (e.g. ORIF hip fractures, stoma), or for management of problems associated with dementia e.g. faecal impaction, bed sores.
- These patients often are poor historians, difficult to examine, may be poorly compliant with therapy, and may have multiple comorbidities.

Clinical features

- All elderly patients should be screened for dementia by a brief mental state examination and corroborating history from relatives.
- Dementia is characterized by increasing global disturbance of higher mental functions in a patient with normal alertness: increasing forgetfulness, slow repetitive speech, personality change, incontinence.
- Unfamiliar surroundings, sleep deprivation, medication, pain, hypoxia, hypercapnia, sepsis, constipation may cause cognitive crises (📖 p. 294).

Investigations

- MMSE (Box 8.4)
- Consider Na^+, Ca^{2+}, creatinine, glucose, thyroid function, vitamin B_{12}, thiamine to exclude a treatable cause of cognitive impairment (📖 p. 295).

Parkinson's disease

Key facts

- Syndrome of bradykinesia, rigidity, tremor; diagnosis is mostly clinical.
- The 2nd commonest cause of neurological disability after stroke with insidious onset: may go undiagnosed in community for years.
- Associated with depression, dementia and reduced ventilation.

Clinical features and diagnosis

- Coarse tremor, more marked at rest ('pill-rolling').
- Rigidity: resistance to passive movement, with tremor (cog-wheeling).
- Bradykinesia: slowness of movement (initiation and repetition), expressionless face, dribbling, short shuffling steps, slower gut peristalsis.

Perioperative management

- Do not delay surgery for newly diagnosed Parkinson's disease.
- Continue established therapy, via NGT if necessary to avoid post-op akinesia.
- Avoid centrally acting dopamine receptor antagonists (metoclopramide, prochlorperazine, haloperidol). Domperidone does not cross the blood–brain barrier and can be used, as may ondansetron.

Box 8.4 MMSE (maximum score 30 points)

What day of the week is it?	**1 point**
What is the date today?	**1 point**
What is the month?	**1 point**
What is the year?	**1 point**
What season of the year is it?	**1 point**
What country are we in?	**1 point**
What city are we in?	**1 point**
What are two nearby main streets?	**1 point**
What floor of the building are we on?	**1 point**
What is the name of this place?	**1 point**

'I am going to give you a piece of paper. Take it in your right hand, fold it in half, and place it on the table.'   **1 point for each action**

Show a pencil and ask what it is called	**1 point**
Show a watch and ask what it is called	**1 point**

'Repeat after me: "no ifs, ands, or buts"'	**1 point**
'Read what is written at the bottom of this page and do what it says.' (Close your eyes)	**1 point**
'Write a complete sentence on this paper.'	**1 point**
'Here is a drawing please copy it.' (Below)	**1 point**

'I am going to name three objects. Please repeat them back to me and remember them as I will ask you to repeat them in a few minutes: apple, penny, table.'   **1 point for each object**

'Take 7 away from 100. Keep going until I say stop.' (100,93,86,79,72,65)
     1 point for each digit (max 5 points)

'What were the 3 objects I asked you to remember?'
     1 point for each object

CLOSE YOUR EYES

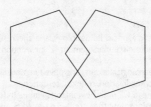

Stroke

Key facts

- Patients at high risk of perioperative stroke: AF, age >70years, arterio-paths, history of CVA/TIA, carotid or cardiac surgery.
- Cerebrovascular disease is very common but may be clinically silent.
- 90% of CVAs are ischaemic and survival is more likely than after intracer-ebral haemorrhage, but distinction can only be made by early CT.
- Early diagnosis and management can dramatically improve functional outcome and prevent potentially life-threatening complications.

Clinical features

- Hemiplegia (middle cerebral artery or total carotid artery occlusion).
- Confusion, altered affect.
- Initial areflexia becoming hyperreflexia and rigidity after a few days.
- Aphasia, dysarthria, ataxia (gait or truncal), inadequate gag reflex.
- Visual deficits, unilateral neglect.
- Persistent, marked hypertension.
- ↓level of consciousness is a poor prognostic sign.

Initial resuscitation

- Assess the airway, breathing, and circulation.
- If the patient is unable to maintain airway insert a Guedel airway, bag and mask ventilate with 100% O_2, call an anaesthetist.
- Otherwise sit the patient up and give high-flow O_2 by face mask.
- Monitor BP, but do not attempt to correct high pressures as these may be critical for adequate cerebral perfusion.
- Monitor SaO_2.
- Secure IV access and give 500mL Hartmann's if systolic BP <100mmHg.
- If the patient is able to maintain their own airway, and is not haemody-namically compromised, explain what is happening and reassure them.
- Perform a neurological exam—it is vital to identify and document the deficits, otherwise recognition of deterioration may be delayed.
- Put the patient NBM if there is any suspicion that gag reflex is compro-mised and request speech and language assessment.
- Send blood cultures if there is any history of endocarditis, pyrexia.
- Send FBC, U&Es, glucose, APTT, and PT.
- Get an ECG.

Establish a diagnosis

Aim to establish the diagnosis, its aetiology, and the resulting functional deficits; these all guide initial management, 2° prevention, and rehabilita-tion plans.

- Carry out a full neurological exam (cognitive function, cranial nerves, and tone, power, co-ordination, reflexes, sensation in all four limbs).
- Modern contrast head CT will show infarcts within 2h (older scanners may not pick up lesions until they are 2–3 days old). Both show haemor-rhage early). You must distinguish between haemorrhagic and ischaemic CVAs (1 in 10 are haemorrhagic).
- MRI is necessary to image brainstem lesions.

Haemorrhagic stroke

- Suspect haemorrhagic CVA (including subarachnoid/subdural haemorrhage, intracranial bleeds) if headache, head injury, or coagulopathy.
- Obtain urgent CT: early neurosurgical intervention may be required.
- If patient anticoagulated, risk of embolic event by reversing anticoagulation must be balanced against risk of further cerebral haemorrhage.

Further management

Perioperative management of chronic CVA is described on 📖 p. 300.

Medical treatment

- Surgical patients are generally not candidates for thrombolysis:
  - Recent major surgery is one of the exclusion criteria.
  - Only effective if given within 3h of onset, consult neurology urgently if new stroke and **no** major surgery.
- Aspirin reduces death/dependency by 13 patients per 1000 treated. Give 300mg/day within 48h (no benefit from heparin/warfarin).

Secondary prevention

- Aspirin, dipyridamole, and clopidogrel reduce recurrence (relative risk reduction >10%).
- Warfarin and heparin reduce recurrence in AF. Restoring sinus rhythm, if possible, also reduces the risk of further stroke.

Ventilation

- In severe stroke, particularly if involving basilar artery territory mechanical ventilation may be needed for respiratory failure due to:
  - Abnormal respiration patterns: apnoeas, Cheyne–Stokes breathing.
  - Loss of protective airway reflexes leading to aspiration.
  - Failure to clear secretions.
- Intubation for apnoea complicating stroke is poor prognostic sign. Most deteriorate neurologically, and few of these patients are successfully weaned from ventilation.
- Intubation for airway protection is more successful; most patients can be weaned, but aspiration pneumonitis may complicate recovery.

Feeding

Protective pharyngeal reflexes may be impaired in stroke. The decision to recommence oral feeding is based on standardized swallow assessments, usually carried out by a speech and language therapist (SALT). Early NG feeding is mandatory until these tests are passed.

- Swallow assessment consists of giving a patient who is alert and able to sit upright, consecutive teaspoons of water followed by a glass of water: the patient fails if at any stage they fail to actively swallow, or if swallowing results in coughing, spluttering, or gurgly voice quality.
- Videofluoroscopy (modified barium swallow) is the gold standard.

Mobilizing

- Structured neurophysiotherapy and intensive nursing is vitally important in preventing complications such as pressure sores, contractures, constipation, and aspiration pneumonitis
- Maximizes early return of function and confidence and reduces respiratory complications eg. atelectasis, pneumonia.

Managing dementia and stroke

Special perioperative considerations

Communication and supportive measures

- Adequate documentation on admission is crucial: assess functional state using the tools on ☐ p. 297.
- Ensure adequate nursing levels and a safe ward environment.
- Anticipate ↑ confusion at night; consider a well-lit side room.
- Return patient to more familiar environment as soon as possible: day case surgery may minimize disruption.
- The carers may need extra support at home: involve social worker.
- *Think* about the effect of your appearance and behaviour on the confused patient.
  - Always explain who you are and why you have come to see them.
  - Smiling, looking at patient directly, speaking in a kind tone all impart reassurance, even in quite severe confusional states when the patient's higher language skills may have been lost. How you speak can be much more influential than what you say.

Medication

- Antihypertensives and aspirin are the mainstay of 2° prevention. Continue unless contraindicated by type of surgery.
- Review medication, some drugs may cause confusion and should be stopped (☐ p. 295).
- Pre-existing cerebral damage causes ↑ sensitivity to all centrally acting drugs, especially hypnotics and other sedatives including opioids. *Reduce dosage of these drugs accordingly, and avoid if you can.*
- A sedative drug may be required for disruptive behaviour, but this may depress respiration, cause hypoxia and worsen confusion.
  - Haloperidol (0.5–1.5mg) or chlorpromazine (12.5–50mg) have wide therapeutic index and are relatively safe (not in Parkinson's).
  - Alternatively, use benzodiazepines, e.g. lorazepam 1–2mg daily, reverse with flumazenil (0.2mg IV, followed by 0.1mg up to 1mg if necessary).
  - Drugs that lower seizure threshold (e.g. tricyclics, major tranquillizers) should be used cautiously.

Respiratory function

- *Exercise tolerance* may be unavailable as a guide to fitness as immobile patients can't exercise to capacity. Weakness may affect the respiratory muscles insidiously, especially the diaphragm. This is most significant when sleeping supine, because of reduced respiratory drive and mechanical disadvantage.
- *Lung function tests* before surgery may demonstrate unexpectedly restricted vital capacity, particularly if done both lying and standing.
- *Oxygenation:* special attention should be paid to adequate oxygenation, chest physiotherapy, and early mobilization.
- If respiratory function is impaired, supplemental O_2 should be given postoperatively. Pulse oximetry is essential. However, significant hypoventilation may coexist with a normal saturation so ABG analysis may be necessary to determine adequacy of ventilation.

Nutrition
- Support fluid intake and nutrition. Assess nutritional state (☐ see p. 246).
- Patients with bulbar weakness may already be both poorly nourished and at high risk of aspiration postoperatively. It may be advisable to keep them NBM if in doubt after surgery.
- A malnourished patient will tolerate the catabolic stress of surgery badly and should *not* be starved postoperatively if possible.
- If normal feeding will be delayed, enteral feeding can be given (NGT, jejunostomy, PEG), or TPN considered. Involve the speech therapist and dietician at an early stage.

Mobilizing
- All patients should get out of bed and mobilize as soon as possible after surgery. This is even more important for postoperative cases with chronic disabilities. These patients should be referred for assessment to physio- and occupational therapists.
- Immobile, undernourished patients are at high risk of pressure sores, (motor neurone disease, more so if spinal cord injury, multiple sclerosis, diabetes mellitus from impaired cutaneous sensation *and* microangiopathy).
- Scrupulous attention must be paid to careful handling, seating, skin traction, plaster casting, and positioning on the operating table.
- Low pressure beds, mattresses, and cushions are vital.
- Incontinence or diarrhoea greatly increases the risk of pressure sores and soft tissue infections.
- Any patient with a paralysed lower limb is at high risk of DVT (40–80%) and PE (1–10%). They should always have graduated antiembolism stockings, intraoperative pneumatic compression and, unless contraindicated, LMWH (enoxaparin 20–40 mg SC od).

Voiding
- Subacute intestinal obstruction 2° to constipation may develop. Remember that both reduced mobility and opioid medication accompanying major surgery will ↑constipation. Patients should be well hydrated and receive early prophylactic suppositories and/or laxatives if necessary (☐ p. 255).
- Neuropathic bladders require careful management. Patients may have significant chronic retention and, if long-standing, reflux nephropathy or stones, increasing the risks of infection.
  - Intermittent self-catheterization (ISC) is increasingly recognized as preferable to a long-term in-dwelling catheter.
  - ISC should be continued in hospital wherever possible, if necessary with the assistance of nursing staff.
  - Resist the temptation to insert a catheter just for convenience.
- Consider UTI if patient becomes confused.

Syncope and blackouts

Key facts

- Syncope: transient loss of consciousness without persistent neurology.
- Careful history is key to accurate diagnosis.
- Majority of syncopal episodes are due to benign causes (vasovagal syncope, postural hypotension) but occasionally underlying diagnosis is important (aortic stenosis, complete heart block and other bradycardias, vertebro-basilar insufficiency). See Box 8.5.

Box 8.5 Causes of syncope

Potentially life-threatening

- Pulmonary embolism.
- Shock: hypovolaemia, sepsis, cardiogenic.
- Cardiac: severe aortic stenosis, HOCM (exertional syncope, AS associated with chest pain/dyspnoea), arrhythmias (e.g. Stokes–Adams attacks in complete heart block).
- Hypoglycaemia.

Benign causes

- Vasovagal (reflex bradycardia and vasodilation) due to pain, fear, standing still too long.
- Postural hypotension: syncope on standing upright, often worse with antihypertensives, especially β-blockers.
- Situational syncope: cough, micturition (♂ at night).
- Carotid sinus hypersensitivity (on turning head).
- Non-syncopal episodes: epilepsy, drop attacks, anxiety, hysteria.

Clinical features

- Try to differentiate between true syncope and non-syncopal events:
  - Loss of consciousness (not syncope without).
  - Falls or collapse without loss of consciousness? (Drop attacks)
  - Neurological deficit ± loss of consciousness? (TIA/CVA)
  - Involuntary movements? (Epilepsy, myoclonic jerks in Stokes–Adams attack; NB not every involuntary movement is epilepsy)
  - Tongue biting, incontinence.
- Ask about associated symptoms or precipitants:
  - Occur while sitting or lying down—usually arrhythmias.
  - Particular stimuli: standing up suddenly, micturition, cough, sneezing, turning head, looking up, exercise.
- Look at medications: antihypertensives (especially β-blockers), anti-arrhythmics, hypoglycaemics.
- Feel pulse, standing and lying BP, auscultate heart (for ejection systolic murmur) and carotids (bruits).
- Quick neurological assessment to exclude focal neurology/CVA.

Diagnosis
- Blood glucose.
- ECG (arrhythmia, heart block), consider 24h monitor
- Consider carotid duplex, TTE.
- Consider tilt-testing if history suggestive of postural hypotension.

Preoperative management
Elective surgery should be postponed if syncope is unexplained or due to newly diagnosed aortic stenosis, HOCM, or TIA.

Postoperative management
- Think about *shock* from any cause (📖 p. 116): this is a potential emergency.
- If there is no clinical evidence of shock look for postural hypotension:
  - Lying and sitting BP: systolic difference should be <10mm Hg.
  - History of syncope or dizziness on standing/sitting up.
  - Reassess (and reduce if indicated) anti-hypertensive medication.
  - Assess volume status (📖 p. 65): if hypovolaemic give 500mL Hartmann's IV bolus, check FBC and transfuse if Hb<9.0g/dL.
  - Give advice on standing slowly, and with assistance.
- Consider PE particularly in the elderly patient (📖 p. 168).
- Look for and treat hypoglycaemia (📖 p. 278), hyponatraemia (📖 p. 288).
- Request 12-lead ECG and discuss with cardiologist if there is evidence of arrhythmias, heart block, or sinus arrest.

Headache

Key facts
- Headache is common on surgical wards. Usually benign and self-limiting, it may occasionally be a serious symptom.
- The history and exam should exclude serious underlying pathology.
- Headaches with altered neurology require urgent investigation.
- See Table 8.1 for clinical features.

Table 8.1 Clinical features of post-op headache in order of frequency

Cause	Features
Tension headache	Feeling of pressure over head or ache around the neck and shoulders. History of similar headaches.
Migraine	Sufferers can often anticipate episode (prodrome—flashing lights/blind spots/mood change/paraesthesiae). May be unilateral facial pain, nausea, vomiting, even focal neurological deficits. History of similar headaches.
Temporal arteritis	Headache lasts days/weeks, no pulse in temporal artery tender to palpation. Temporal headache, >50 years, ESR >50 is temporal arteritis until proven otherwise.
Cluster headaches	Previous history, headaches nightly 4–12 weeks, then pain free for months to years.
$\downarrow PaO_2/\uparrow PaCO_2$	Hypoxia ± hypercapnia can cause arterial dilatation and headache: look for evidence hypo/hyperventilation.
Caffeine withdrawal	Non-specific headache in patients who normally drink a lot of tea or coffee.
Vasodilators	Nitrates, Ca^{2+} channel blockers and other antihypertensives.
Hypertension	Severe hypertension (>180/>100) may cause headaches.
Sepsis	Systemic infection is often associated with headache. Neck stiffness suggests meningism.
Dehydration	Hypovolaemia leads to traction on venous sinuses.
Post-dural puncture	Presents as a severe throbbing pain over the occiput. Worse on sitting or standing upright.
Referred pain	Headache may be only clinical sign of facial/skull fracture after trauma, maxillofacial surgery, otitis media.
Raised ICP	Pain worse on lying flat, coughing, straining, vomiting; drowsiness ± papilloedema. Look for ↓Na, history of head trauma, cranial surgery, coagulopathy, new neurological deficits. Urgent CT head.
Subarachnoid	Sudden onset severe ('thunderclap') occipital headache ± altered neurology: request CT scan urgently.
Meningitis	Patients at risk: recent ENT, maxillofacial, neurosurgical procedures. Photophobia, neck pain/stiffness, seizures, rash or petechiae, sepsis, ↓consciousness /confusion, ↑WCC. LP/blood for culture, antibiotics.

Perioperative management

Tension headache: muscle spasm
- The perioperative period is stressful. Tension headaches account for most cases in surgical patients, are benign but cause undue stress.
- Pain often continuous, with no obvious exacerbating/relieving factors.
- If simple analgesics (📖 p. 78) are ineffective, reassurance/education about relaxation techniques may help. Occasionally, organic causes of muscle spasm (e.g. temporomandibular joint occlusion/arthritis of cervical spine) give rise to tension headaches.

Migraine
- Try simple analgesics (📖 p. 78) and antiemetic (e.g. metoclopramide 10mg) first if not sure about diagnosis.
- In typical attack, give $5HT_1$ agonists (e.g. sumatriptan 50mg PO, up to 300mg/24h, *or* sumatriptan 6mg IV up to 12mg/24h).
- Sumatriptan contraindicated in IHD, may cause drowsiness and low BP.

Post-dural puncture headache (PDPH)
- Loss of CSF after spinal anaesthetic or inadvertent puncture of the dura during epidural anaesthetic may result in post dural puncture headache. Less CSF for cushioning brain and traction on venous sinuses.
- Made worse by sitting up or standing, characteristically patient refuses to get out of bed.
- Post-dural puncture headaches usually resolve within a few days.
- *Inform the consultant anaesthetist* involved in the patient's care: they should be happy to take over management of this problem.
- Bed rest, regular simple analgesics, active hydration (oral or IV). Caffeine tablets (↑CSF production) or coffee may be useful for pain.
- Persistent or worsening symptoms: may require 'blood patch'. (This involves slow injection of ~30mL of the patient's blood into epidural space adjacent to suspected dural puncture. Fibrin plug will stop CSF leak with rapid resolution of symptoms in ~90% cases).

Raised intracranial pressure
- Urgent CT head, and neurosurgical opinion if bleed or trauma.
- Also see sections on hyponatraemia (📖 p. 288), intracranial bleed (📖 p. 298).

Meningitis
- Typical surgery (ENT, maxillofacial, neurosurgical) or from community.
- Mennigococcal septicaemia is an emergency:
  - Petechial rash, septic patient, meningism often absent.
  - Urgent cultures, *then* antibiotics ((cefotaxine 1g IV bd, change on sensitivities).

Temporal arteritis (giant cell arteritis)
- Age >50, ESR >50 ± painful, pulseless thickened artery, treat as GCA.
- Prednisolone 40–60mg/day, biopsy to confirm diagnosis can be next day
- Main threat is blindness. Longer term: side effects from steroid therapy

Investigations
- U&E, FBC, CRP, ESR, blood/urine cultures if evidence of sepsis.
- If there is an associated neurological element, request a CT scan.
- LP in suspected meningitis, but only if no suspicion of raised ICP.

Epilepsy and seizures

Key facts

- Tendency to seizures due to intermittent abnormal brain activity.
- Common: has a prevalence of about 1%; frequency of seizures varies.
- Well-controlled epilepsy does not confer increased perioperative risk, and several general anaesthetic agents are anticonvulsant. Most importantly, ensure that patient receives anticonvulsants as usual.
- Most chronic seizure disorders are idiopathic (without structural abnormality on cranial imaging), but known causes include head injury, CVA, neurosurgery, intracranial tumour, alcohol or benzodiazepine withdrawal (haloperidol can lower seizure threshold, avoid).
- Other seizure triggers include $\downarrow PaO_2$, $\downarrow Na^+$, $\downarrow Ca^{2+}$, $\downarrow$glucose, local anaesthetic toxicity.

Clinical features

- Patients commonly suffer from either *generalized* or *partial seizures*.
  - Tonic-clonic: classical grand mal. Loss of consciousness, limbs stiffen (tonic) and jerk (clonic). Usually drowsy afterwards (post-ictal).
  - Petit mal or absences are loss of awareness <10sec.
  - Focal seizures affect one or more of senses ± $\downarrow$consciousness.
  - Complex partial seizures are transient ± abnormal behaviour.
- *Nature of fits:* review seizure type(s), current frequency, and adequacy of control: for a new diagnosis a clear witness account is vital.
- *Drugs:* establish exact drug regimen, including any controlled-release formulations. Verify compliance if doses are high: toxicity may develop.
- *Shunts?* If neurosurgical shunt in situ consider prophylactic antibiotic cover for procedures likely to cause bacteraemia (📖 p. 60).

Investigations

- *Pharmacology:* almost all anti-epileptic drugs (AEDs) induce liver enzymes and hence their own metabolism. Phenytoin and Phenobarbital may cause elevation of alkaline phosphatase and γGT and may interact with other drugs metabolized by the liver such as warfarin. Sodium valproate is an inhibitor of liver enzymes.
- Check levels of phenytoin or carbamazepine if seizure control is poor. This may guide management if seizures occur postoperatively.

Box 8.6 New seizures

Ask about: witnesses for exact description of fit, headache, previous fits, diabetes, alcoholism, pregnancy, drug/social history including last drink, recreational drugs, family history epilepsy.
Look for: head injury, tongue biting, neck stiffness, incontinence, pregnancy, infection, limb fracture/dislocation, cuts and bruises.
Life-threatening causes: $\downarrow PaO_2$, hypoglycaemia, $\downarrow Ca^{2+}$, $\downarrow\uparrow Na^+$, head trauma, CVA, meningitis, malaria, $\uparrow ICP$, drugs (withdrawal—alcohol, anticonvulsants; toxicity—alcohol, local anaesthetics, tricyclics, amphetamines), eclampsia (pregnancy).

Perioperative management

Emergency resuscitation (Box 8.7)

- Status epilepticus is any seizure lasting >30min, or repeated seizures without intervening clear consciousness. Most seizures are self-limiting.

Continued seizures (>20min) need senior anaesthetic help for sedation ± intubation.

- Status epilepticus usually occurs in known epileptics: if it is first presentation then >50% chance of structural brain lesion. (Box 8.6)
- In pregnant patients contact obstetrics urgently: eclampsia requiring emergency delivery is a possibility.

Maintenance management

- Continue usual medication if possible including when NBM pre-operatively receive morning doses unless specific instructions from anaesthetist.
- Carbamazepine is available as a rectal preparation, but other drugs can be given via NGT if necessary.
- IV preparations available for several antiepileptic drugs: consult *BNF*.
- Maintain IV access until fully recovered from anaesthesia.
- Avoid hyponatraemia, or missing doses of antiepileptics, both lower seizure threshold.

Box 8.7 Emergency resuscitation of seizures

0–5 minutes

- Securing airway (nasopharyngeal/Guedel), give O_2 by facemask, suction if required.
- Place patient in recovery position.
- Pulse oximetry, BP, temperature, *bedside blood glucose test*.
- IV access and bloods: blood cultures, U&Es, LFTs, Ca^{2+}, glucose, anticonvulsant levels, FBC.
- βHCG and external pelvic exam in ♀ of childbearing age.
- Remove objects that are potential causes of trauma.

5–20 minutes

- Call for senior help and telemetry leads to monitor ECG.
- Diazepam 10mg IV (or PR) over 2min, and 5mg/min until seizures stop or respiratory depression occurs, *or* lorazepam 4mg IV over 2min, repeat at 10min.
- ABGs: check hypoxia, acidosis is usually severe but is best treated by terminating the seizures.
- If alcoholism suspected e.g. Pabrinex 7mL (dangers of encephalopathy far outweigh potential for anaphylaxis).
- Dexamethasone 8mg IV if cerebral oedema suspected.

20–40 minutes

- Call for an anaesthetist, for definitive airway management.
- Phenytoin 15mg/kg IV up to 50mg/min.
- If no previous seizures, start to look for an underlying cause.

>40 minutes

- Request urgent transfer to ICU bed for sedation, ventilation, and further IV anticonvulsants. EEG monitoring and brain CT follow.

Dizziness and vertigo

Vertigo

Key facts

- Vertigo is a sensation of rotation, dizziness of feeling faint.
  - *Benign positional vertigo*: sudden onset vertigo following head movement, lasts a few seconds only: refer to physiotherapy for Epley manoeuvre (trying to move debris from inner ear canals).
  - *Meniere's disease*: severe vertigo with tinnitus, nausea and vomiting lasting hours. Cyclizine/metoclopramide, referral to ENT.
  - *Labyrinthitis*: sudden onset vertigo following URTI or fever. Vertigo often severe, lasting days resolving over 2–3 weeks.
- Antiemetics usually effectively treat vertigo from above causes: e.g. cyclizine 50mg PO/IV/IM tds, or metoclopramide 10mg PO/IV/IM tds.
- Pre-syncopal episodes: 📖 see Syncope and blackouts, p. 302.

Table 8.2 Clinical features and causes of dizziness

Symptom	History	Underlying problem
Dizziness	Non-specific symptom that may reflect pre-syncopal episode, vertigo or ataxia	Any of pre-syncope, vertigo, ataxia
Pre-syncope	Light headed, palpitations, sweating, pallor, altered vision/hearing immediately prior to loss of consciousness, no 'spinning' sensation.	Life threatening: shock, hypoglycaemia, CVA Common causes: postural hypotension, anxiety, pain
Vertigo	Sensation of rotational movement, better when still, nausea, occasionally hearing loss/tinnitus, no loss of consciousness.	Benign positional vertigo, labyrinthitis, Ménière's, motion sickness, CVA
Ataxia	Inability to stand, sit, or walk straight, sensation of movement.	Alcohol, ketamine, anti-convulsants, cerebellar lesion, peripheral neuropathy

Ataxia

Cerebellar lesions

- Gross incoordination, wide-based gait, unable to sit or stand upright (truncal ataxia), worse when eyes shut (Romberg's +ve).
- Nystagmus, dysarthria, hypotonia, intention tremor, past pointing, dys-diadochokinesis caused by CVA, MS, infection, anticonvulsants, alcohol, and recreational drugs including ketamine and PCP.

Sensory ataxia
- Damage to spinal dorsal tracts (tabes dorsalis, tumours, skeletal) or peripheral sensory nerves (vitamin B_{12} deficiency, diabetes, alcohol, platin based chemotherapy) leads to loss of proprioception.
- Narrow based (stepping) gait, gross incoordination with eyes shut or in dark, pseudoathetosis, Romberg's +ve, ↓vibration sense.

Perioperative management
- No specific management required for symptom, only for underlying condition

Neuromuscular diseases

Key facts

- Diverse group of conditions: myasthenia gravis (MG), Eaton–Lambert syndrome (ELS), Guillain–Barré syndrome (GBS), muscular dystrophy, motor neurone disease (MND)
- They can all cause problems with perioperative respiratory function, and pose problems linked to the specific pathology.
- For each, careful assessment of respiratory function with spirometry and regular chest physiotherapy to avoid infection are mandatory.
- If respiratory function impaired, likely to require post-op ventilation.
- Patients with well-controlled (MG) or mild disease (ELS, GBS, dystrophy, NMD) undergoing minor or moderate surgery tend to do well.
- Recovery from major surgery may be complicated (postpone in GBS).

Perioperative plan

- Discuss with anaesthetist well before surgery with recent spirometry.
- Decide whether admission to ICU is advisable postoperatively.
- Alert the physiotherapy team—with major surgery intensive chest physiotherapy will be required pre and post-operatively.
- Measuring vital capacity/PEFR, assessing strength of the cough, are good for monitoring function, FEV_1 very useful for GBS.
- Check the SaO_2, blood gases, and CXR.

Myasthenia gravis

Key facts

- An autoimmune condition affecting skeletal muscle acetylcholine receptors associated with thymoma or other autoimmune illnesses.
- Characterized by muscle fatiguability which may be mild, or may be severe enough to cause aspiration and respiratory failure.
- May present for any surgery, (Box 8.8) or undergo therapeutic thymectomy.

Clinical features

- Muscular fatiguability resulting in ptosis, diplopia, facial weakness, and bulbar problems, characteristically worse at the end of the day. Often progresses to involve upper limb and respiratory function.
- *Myasthenic crises:* acute exacerbations with flaccid paralysis/respiratory failure if insufficient anticholinesterases/↓absorption/↑stress.
  - Treat with dose increase. *Call anaesthetist.*
  - Plasma exchange improves muscular function by removing anticholinergic receptor antibodies.
- *Cholinergic crisis:* excess anticholinergics impair neuromuscular transmission (repolarization block), very similar to myasthenic crisis (if bronchospasm, diarrhoea, ↓pulse, miosis, salivation more likely cholinergic). Treat with atropine (📖 p. 139). *Call anaesthetist.*
- Treat with anticholinesterases (pyridostigmine, neostigmine), may be combined with anticholinergics (atropine, propantheline) to reduce muscarinic side-effects such as bradycardia and abdominal cramps.
- *Immunosuppression* is commonly used (prednisolone, azathioprine, ciclosporin). Thymoma may require surgery.

Box 8.8 Perioperative problems due to MG

- Surgical stress can precipitate myasthenic crisis.
- Bulbar palsy may result in ineffective cough and aspiration.
- Muscular weakness may result in respiratory complications including sputum retention, infection, and ventilatory failure.
- Steroid cover may require supplementation.
- $\downarrow K^+$, $\downarrow Ca^{2+}$, $\uparrow Mg^{2+}$, aminoglycosides may worsen weakness.
- Cardiomyopathy is a rare complication.
- Absorption of anticholinesterases may be unpredictable postoperatively.

Additional perioperative considerations for MG

- Plan periop anticholinesterase regimen with anaesthetist/neurology.
- Patients on pyridostigmine PO will need IV neostigmine while unable to absorb from the gut.
  - Pyridostigmine 60mg PO about equivalent to 1mg neostigmine SC/IM.
  - Parenteral neostigmine given in divided doses q4h or more often: patient stable on pyridostigmine 120mg qds needs 8mg neostigmine total daily dose, so prescribe 1.5mg q4h SC.
  - Neostigmine SC/IM may need cover with atropine/glycopyrrolate. Increase steroid dose if indicated (📖 p. 281).
- Myasthenic patients may develop respiratory failure with minimal signs.

Eaton–Lambert syndrome (myasthenic syndrome)

- Pre-junctional reduction in acetylcholine release. Unlike MG, weakness generally improves with repeated or sustained muscular exertion, and anticholinesterases have little or no effect.
- May be associated with malignancy (e.g. small cell carcinoma of lung).

Guillain–Barré syndrome

- Auto-immune condition affecting motor neurones, often triggered by URT or GI infection, occasionally by surgery.
- Progressive weakness, maximal at 3 weeks, with slow recovery over weeks/months. Plasmapheresis, immunoglobulins aid recovery, ventilation if respiratory failure.

Muscular dystrophy

- Group >30 genetic diseases: degeneration of skeletal muscle leads to progressive weakness. Symptoms vary from mild to disabling.
- Duchenne most common and severe form, affects primarily boys.
- No specific therapy available.

Motor neurone disease

- Group of inherited and acquired diseases with degeneration of motor neurones. Age of onset depends on variant of MND.
- Amyotrophic lateral sclerosis is most common.
- No symptomatic treatment, riluzole may improve survival by 2–3 months.

Musculoskeletal

Swollen leg

Key facts

- The development of a swollen leg in a surgical, orthopaedic, or gynae-cology ward is common. The main concern is whether a deep venous thrombosis (DVT) is the underlying cause (📖 see Table 9.1).
- The greatest risk of DVT is after orthopaedic and pelvic surgery and in cancer patients leg trauma.
- These patients are also most likely to develop leg swelling simply because of surgery or trauma itself.
- Any new leg swelling in a surgical patient must be taken seriously.

Assessment of the swollen leg

- *Think about:* DVT, cellulitis, heart failure, surgical site, trauma, compart-ment syndrome, haematoma, renal failure, lymphoedema.
- *Ask about:* usual leg size, better in morning, pain, warmth, fevers, trauma, previous DVT and prophylaxis, mobility, breathlessness, chest pain, post-op weight gain, normal and current diuretic therapy, urine output, serum albumin, Na^+.
- *Look for:* pyrexia, ↓BP, ↑HR, crepitations, ascites, erythema, pitting oedema (truncal, elbows, sacral, and both legs), opposite leg, pus, hae-matoma, varicose eczema, ulcers, pulses, pain on passive foot dorsiflexion?
- *Investigations:*
  - FBC, CRP, U&E, LFTs, BCs: sepsis, ↓ Na^+, ARF, ↓ albumin, ↑urate.
  - D-dimers (normal D-dimers with low clinical suspicion virtually excludes significant DVT).
  - CXR: heart failure, pulmonary oedema.
  - Doppler DP and PT pulses: compartment syndrome.
  - Duplex leg: DVT, venous insufficiency.
  - XR hip and long bones: unidentified fracture.
- See Table 9.1 for causes.

Table 9.1 Common or important causes of postoperative leg swelling

Diagnosis	Clinical features
Common or important causes in post-op patients	
DVT: limited to calf veins	Unilateral calf oedema, calf pain/tenderness, warmth, and redness. Often low grade (<38°C) fever. ↑pain on foot dorsiflexion (Homan's sign) has no differential diagnostic power
DVT: above knee	Oedema of the entire lower limb, cyanosis, superficial venous engorgement, tenderness of the iliofemoral vein itself (in Hunter's canal and the groin). Often low grade (<38°C) fever. The signs of proximal DVT may be the same as calf vein thrombosis
Surgical or post-traumatic oedema	Leg swelling is universal after hip and knee surgery, and common after ankle and even foot procedures. The oedema develops painlessly, without fever, in the first day or two after orthopaedic surgery, and then slowly regresses. A degree of gravitational oedema may persist for a year or more after orthopaedic surgery.

Table 9.1 Common or important causes of postoperative leg swelling (*continued*)

Diagnosis	Clinical features
Cellulitis	Rapidly spreading intense redness and warmth of the skin, fever (less common in elderly), pain, blisters. May be no history of skin trauma. Need iv antibiotics (Table 2.14)
Compartment syndrome	Occurs after trauma/ischaemia to limb. Features are increasing **severe** pain, worse on passive flexion of extremities, tense (almost woody) swelling, paraesthesiae. Needs urgent assessment. Compartment pressures should be measured using a transducer and fasciotomies performed if these are raised
Heart failure or fluid overload with unilateral venous insufficiency	Relatively common (📖 p. 127). Fluid resuscitation of shocked patients often leads to peripheral oedema in the recovery phase. In other patients, excess fluid therapy may precipitate heart failure. If these patients have underlying venous insufficiency (look for telltale signs of varicose eczema, healed ulcers, lipodermatosclerosis), the oedema may appear to be unilateral, but will be seen to be bilateral if the apparently normal leg is examined carefully
Acute gout	Exquisite joint tenderness with redness spreading around the joint. Often triggered by dehydration, sepsis, and catabolism after surgery in a patient with a Hx of gout. The joint most commonly affected is 1st metatarsal phalangial joint. Large joint involvement raises possibility of pseudogout.
Conditions more rarely seen in surgical practice	
Haematoma	Usually history of direct trauma (📖 p. 99). May be spontaneous in overanticoagulated patients. Relatively more common postoperatively after total knee or hip replacement
Thrombophlebitis	Tenderness directly over the course of palpable, lumpy superficial veins. Not often seen perioperatively
Ruptured popliteal cyst	Tenderness in popliteal fossa extending into posterior calf. Uncommon but may occur after trauma
Muscle tear	Only after obvious trauma
Post-phlebitic leg	Gravitational oedema in a patient with previous venous thrombosis and/or varicose veins. Venous insufficiency is improved by bed-rest, so this is an unlikely cause of a newly swollen leg in surgical practice

Rheumatic diseases

Key facts

- The rheumatic diseases affect the bones, joints, and connective tissue.
- Skeletal abnormalities may themselves complicate the management of anaesthesia in particular with relation to the airway.
- Deformities may make the use of regional anaesthesia, including spinals and epidurals, difficult or impossible.
- Some disorders are associated with relevant systemic features including anaemia and inflammatory response (↑WCC, ↑CRP, ↑ESR)
- Long term use of NSAIDs and steroids is common and side effects are potentially serious.
- All these conditions may be associated with reduced mobility and consequent poor aerobic fitness: functional assessment of cardio-respiratory status is often difficult. Also ↓mobility may predispose to thromboembolic disease so DVT prophylaxis is important. Keep the period of immobility associated with surgery to a minimum.

Liaise with anaesthetisst and rheumatology in perioperatve period.

Rheumatoid arthritis

Symmetrical deforming polyarthropathy with systemic features, 📖 see p. 318.

Other connective tissue disorders

- These include systemic lupus erythematosus (SLE), progressive systemic sclerosis (PSS), and other rare conditions.
- Autoimmune multisystem disorders with a chronic course are commonly treated with steroids or other immunosuppressants.

Spondyloarthropathies

- These mainly affect the spine and insertions of tendons and ligaments.
- Systemic features are commonly present, in ankylosing spondylitis:
  - This condition may cause fixed flexion neck deformity making tracheal intubation impossible.
  - Reduced chest expansion and associated restrictive ventilatory defect are common.
  - Aortic regurgitation may also occur.

Scoliosis

- In this condition, there is progressive lateral curvature of the spine associated with progressive ankylosis and an associated restrictive ventilatory defect.
- Congenital scoliosis may be associated with hypoplasia of the odontoid process resulting in atlantoaxial instability.
- This may make tracheal intubation hazardous. (Asymptomatic atlantoaxial instability can also occur in Down syndrome.)

Osteoarthritis

- There are no systemic features, but this is a disease of the elderly and intercurrent disease is common.
- Severe OA in needs may make intubation more different.

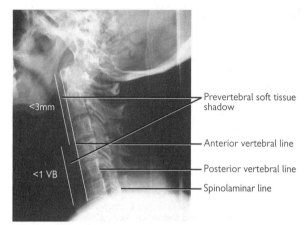

Fig. 9.1 Landmarks in neck imaging. Lateral cervical spine X-ray must visualize all 7 cervical vertebrae from upper border of T1 to skull base. All three lines on the diagram above should have a smooth curve with no steps or discontinuities. The prevertebral soft tissue shadow is less than 50% the width of a vertebral body above ch4. Reproduced with permission from Collier M and Brinsden M (2006). *Oxford Handbook of Clinical Specialties*, 7e. Oxford University Press, Oxford.

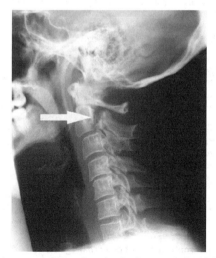

Fig. 9.2 Spinous process fracture. Reproduced with permission from Collier M and Brinsden M (2006). *Oxford Handbook of Clinical Specialties*, 7e. Oxford University Press, Oxford.

Rheumatoid arthritis

Key facts
- Affects 1% of the population, ♀ > ♂.
- Associated with specific anaesthetic problems in relation to the airway and relevant systemic features.

Clinical features

Articular disease
- Joint deformities may make IV access and positioning for other procedures difficult. Bone density is often very low due to a combination of female sex, advanced age and chronic steroid use.
- Previous joint replacements, particularly THR, at risk of dislocation when moving unconscious patient (transfer with pillow between legs to reduce risk of flexion + adduction which can dislocate prosthesis).
- Effects of the disease on the airway are most important.
  - *Cervical spine:* ask about headaches, neck pain, and possible neurological symptoms. The really worrying symptoms are radicular ones, i.e. nerve root pains or paraesthesiae going down the limb(s). Neck pain is noteworthy; radicular pain is really serious. Carefully assess the neck. Note any deformity and range of movement. Assess the angle between maximum flexion and extension achieved. Radiological changes occur in up to 86% patients with rheumatoid arthritis but may be asymptomatic particularly when the patient is on steroids. Atlantoaxial subluxation may make tracheal intubation and patient transfer hazardous as the cervical cord may be compromised with extremes of flexion or extension. Subaxial subluxation can also occur and may be exacerbated by flexion or extension. Fixed flexion deformities occur later in disease again making tracheal intubation difficult.
  - *Temporomandibular joints:* assess mouth opening as arthritis of these joints may limit mouth opening and make intubation difficult.
  - *Cricoarytenoid joints:* laryngeal involvement is common. Rarely stridor and upper airway obstruction may occur.

Systemic disease
- *Cardiovascular system:* ask about exercise tolerance and chest pain: pericarditis, valvular involvement.
- *Respiratory system:* ask about breathlessness, wheeze, and look at CXR—pulmonary fibrosis, rheumatoid nodules and pleural effusions.
- *Haemopoietic system:* check FBC—normochromic normocytic anaemia is associated with active disease. Drugs may cause BM suppression, azathioprine (AZA), methotrexate with bleeding tendency, particularly if on NSAIDs.
- *Renal system:* Interstitial nephritis and amyloid may occur. The toxic effects of treatment (especially NSAIDs) are potentially serious.
- *Nervous system:* peripheral neuropathy can occur. Symptoms and signs in arms and or legs may be 2° to cervical spinal cord compression.

Common complications of drug management
- *NSAIDs:* GORD, renal impairment including a ARF.
- *Disease-modifying drugs (e.g. gold, penicillamine):* proteinuria, bone marrow suppression.

- *Immunosuppressants (AZA, methotrexate):* marrow suppression.
- *Steroids:* hypokalaemia, hypertension, impaired glucose tolerance.

Perioperative prescribing

- *Continue disease-modifying drugs* (except azathioprine) up to the time of surgery. Azathioprine has been associated with major wound complications and should be discontinued 3 weeks before surgery.
- NSAID use is associated with an ↑risk of bleeding complications after major joint surgery. It may be appropriate to stop aspirin pre-op (📖 p. 58) or to continue NSAIDs up until surgery using agents with a short half-life, e.g. diclofenac. Continue NSAIDs post-op unless contraindicated using rectal or IV routes if oral route unavailable.
- Stop NSAIDs immediately if the patient is volume depleted or if there is significant deterioration of renal function.
- Start DVT prophylaxis: 📖 p. 61 and GERD prophylaxis (📖 p. 82)
- Plan postoperative pain control and counsel patient in conjunction with relevant staff. PCA may be difficult to use if the hands are affected.
- Increased steroid cover for intermediate or major surgery. (📖 see p. 281.)
- Resume rheumatoid medication as soon as practicable.

Perioperative management

- Pre-op blood transfusion not usually necessary.
- Maintain adequate fluid intake and monitor renal function.
- Maintenance of mobility associated with good pain control is important. If the patient is immobilized, chest physiotherapy and passive exercises may be required.

Table 9.2 Preoperative investigations in rheumatoid arthritis

All patients	To exclude
FBC	GI loss, drug effects
U&E	Renal involvement, drug toxicity
ECG	Ventricular hypertrophy. Low voltages might suggest pericardial effusion ESR, CRP assess disease activity
CXR	Pulmonary fibrosis, pleural effusion, pericardial effusion, rheumatoid nodules, steroid-induced osteoporosis
Selected patients	Indications
Cervical spine radiographs	Anaesthetist requests
PFTs	Unexplained dyspnoea
Indirect laryngoscopy	Hoarseness, stridor
Echocardiography	Pericardial/valvular involvement

Trauma

The ATLS protocol is on the inside cover of this book.

Key facts

- Trauma is the leading cause of death in the first four decades of life but three people are permanently disabled for every one killed.
- Death from injury occurs in one of three time periods (trimodal).
  - First peak—within seconds to minutes from severe injury.
  - Second peak—within minutes to several hours from major injury.
  - Third peak—days to weeks from sepsis and multiple organ failure.
- The 'golden hour' refers to the period when medical care can make the maximum impact on death and disability.
- These patients most commonly end up on surgical wards for observation—even if they do not require an operation.

The Advanced Trauma Life Support (ATLS) System

- Standard for trauma care in 'golden hour', focuses on '2nd peak'.
- Emphasizes that injury kills in certain reproducible time frames in a common sequence: loss of airway, inability to breathe, loss of circulating blood volume, expanding intracranial mass.
- The 1° survey aims to identify and treat life-threatening conditions according to priority following these areas (ABCDEs) Simultaneous resuscitation is emphasized (Box 9.1).

Pre-hospital care and the Trauma Team

- Effort is made to minimize scene time, emphasis on immediate transport to the closest appropriate facility (scoop and run).
- Information from paramedics includes **M**echanism of injury, **I**njuries identified, vital **S**igns at scene, **T**reatment administered (MIST).

Management of trauma patients on the ward

- *Do not assume the primary or secondary survey was 100% correct or complete, or that things have not changed since then.*
- Repeat a careful history and examination once patient stabilized, review all lines and investigations, and previous hospital records:
  - Change in cognition suggesting neurological injury.
  - PMHx, full Dx, allergies, last meal/drink.
  - HR, BP (note trend—may reveal slow clinical deterioration), peripheral perfusion, wounds.
  - Always repeat full thoracic examination: cardiac tamponade, tension pneumothorax, pulmonary contusion, haemothorax may be insidious in onset, but life threatening within hours.
  - Review the CXR again, check position of NGT, CVP line.
  - Review the spinal films again: if they appear ok but were not cleared in A&E contact a radiologist as nursing medical care and rehabilitation is much easier if the patient allowed to sit up and move.
  - Review the echo report: *any* fluid in the pericardium in the setting of tachycardia + chest trauma is suspicious.
  - Chase laboratory tests including toxicology screens.
  - Antibiotics (📖 p. 86), DVT prophylaxis (📖 p. 61), fluids (📖 p. 64), analgesia (📖 p. 78) anti-tetanus, antiemetics (📖 p. 252), usual medication.

Falls on the ward

Key facts
- Risks: unfamiliar environment, post-op confusion, sedatives, postural hypotension, encumbered by Foley catheter, drains, drip stands.
- Fractures common even with low energy impact in elderly patients.

Emergency management: resuscitation
- See patient immediately to assess and treat loss of consciousness (📖 p. 302), confusion (📖 p. 294), stroke (📖 p. 298), seizures (📖 p. 306), shock (📖 p. 116).
- Transfer patient to bed or trolley.
- Assess airway, breathing, circulation, GCS.
- Careful history for loss of consciousness, dizziness, collapse vs. straight-forward trip over object.
- Ask about previous falls, site of impact, any pain (limbs, head, back, neck, drain sites, Foley site, wound), inability to weight bear, reduced range of movement.
- Ask about amnesia, check orientation time, person, place, ask about visual disturbance, headache.
- Examine scalp, clavicles, spine, wrists, hip and ankles for tenderness, swelling or obvious deformity.
- Pay particular attention to sites of any bony surgery (sternal wound, athroplasty/ORIF) and recent wounds.
- Ask the patient to stand and check that they can weight bear.

Investigations
- In younger patients usually no investigation required.
- Investigation of underlying cause, especially in older patients: Box 9.1.
- CT head in patient with history of head trauma and loss of consciousness, or subsequent neurological deficit to identify ICH.
- C-spine if history suggests likely trauma e.g. fall onto head.
- AP and lateral hip if local tenderness, inability to weight bear, rotational deformity and shortening to lower limb to identify fracture with fracture.
- AP and lateral wrist if local tenderness, swelling, reduced range of movement, deformity to identify fracture with fracture remember to palpate the scaphoid too.

Box 9.1 Important causes of post-op falls

- Trips: drips, Foley, drains, dark, unfamiliar environment.
- CNS: stroke, seizure, dementia, Parkinson's, visual defect.
- Cardiac: postural hypotension, shock, bleeding, arrhythmias, syncope (AS, vasovagal).
- Respiratory: PE, hypoxia, hypercapnia.
- Endocrine: Hypoglycaemia.
- Drugs: alcohol, opioids, benzodiazepines.

Oncology and palliative care

Basic concepts

Surgery in patients without known malignancy

- Cancer is on the differential diagnosis of virtually all surgical problems, with the work-up of the patient according to the presenting complaint.
- If malignancy is confirmed, refer to oncology for consideration of adjuvant/palliative management. This requires a tissue diagnosis.
- A management plan should then be formulated by the cancer multi-disciplinary team before definitive intervention.
- Cancer surgery is specialized, and should be performed in the non-emergency setting by appropriately trained surgeons where possible.
- Surgical management of specific malignancies is beyond the scope of this book.

Surgery in patients with known malignancy

- When asked to see an oncology patient, do not automatically assume symptoms are due to cancer, even if this is often the case.
- Surgery for non-oncological problems is appropriate in many cases; factors to consider are life expectancy, patient wishes, likely success of surgery.
- Some 'surgical' problems may be best treated with non-surgical methods (e.g. (sub-) acute bowel obstruction in peritoneal dissemination).

📖 See Tables 10.1 and 10.2 for staging tumours and grading patients' performance status.

Table 10.1 General principles for staging of solid tumours

Stage	Description	Therapy
1	Localized tumour, minimal invasion, very good prognosis	Local therapy only
2	Localized tumour, more extensive invasion, no metastasis, good prognosis	Often only local therapy required, systemic adjuvant therapy if poor prognostic features
3	Tumour with loco-regional metastasis (usually lymph nodes), reasonable prognosis	Local therapy and systemic adjuvant therapy
4	Disseminated malignancy, often incurable (NB but not always!)	Systemic therapy

*Local therapy: either surgery or radiotherapy, or both.

Table 10.2 Grading of performance status (PS)

Performance status	Description
0	No symptoms from malignancy
1	Some symptoms, able to do light work
2	Sedentary for <50% of waking hours
3	Sedentary for >50% of waking hours
4	Bed bound

Oncological emergencies

Basic principles
- Consider these possibilities in any patients with known malignancy.
- Rapidly assess tumour staging, response to treatment, prognosis, and the wishes of patient (±relatives): they have bearing on management.
- You should never have to make treatment decisions without back-up by the oncology team: know primary stage, PS (🕮 see p. 325), current and previous treatment, when discussing a patient.

Neutropaenic sepsis
Key facts
- A true emergency: untreated Gram −ve septicaemia has 80% mortality.
- Neutropaenia can complicate most chemotherapy, including for non-malignant disease.
- Where organism identified, Gram +ve causes 60%, Gram −ve causes 20%, fungal sepsis in prolonged/severe myelosuppression or antibiotic therapy.
- Most important intervention is prompt empiric broad-spectrum antibiotics. If in doubt, treat! And do it quickly.

Clinical features
- High index of suspicion: in absence of neutrophils usual focal and systemic signs of sepsis may be absent—many patients never have a positively identified source for their sepsis.
- Look for common sites of sepsis (🕮 p. 90), perform full septic screen *prior* to antibiotics.
- Diagnosis: neutrophils ≤0.5 plus 1 of: temperature (≥38°C on a single occasion, or 37–38°C for >24h), evidence of local or systemic sepsis (hypotension, hypoxia, DIC, ARDS, multi-organ failure).

Treatment
- Check local guidelines; otherwise gentamicin 5mg/kg IV od + piperacillin 4.5g IV q6h (ceftazidime 2g IV q8h if penicillin allergy).
- Do not use G-CSF routinely.

Acute tumour lysis syndrome
Key facts
- Results from rapid release of cellular contents, due to massive cell death after anti-cancer therapy in very sensitive tumours.
- Can lead to multi-organ failure and death.

Clinical features
- Signs develop within 1–5 days of therapy.
- Weakness, myalgia, nausea and vomiting, acute renal failure.
- Characterized by $\uparrow K^+$, $\uparrow\uparrow$urate, $\uparrow PO_4$, $\downarrow Ca^{2+}$.

Treatment
- Prevention: hydration, allopurinol 300mg od PO.
- Aggressive IV fluids (u/o 2mL/kg/h), correct $\uparrow K^+$ (🕮 p. 218) and $\downarrow Ca^{2+}$.
- Alkalinize urine with oral $NaHCO_3$ (aim for urinary pH>7).
- May need dialysis, liaise with renal team/ITU early (🕮 p. 212).

Spinal cord compression

Key facts
- Complicates course of up to 10% of all cancer patients.
- True emergency: delayed treatment may result in paraplegia.
- Caused by extradural metastasis, vertebral collapse, bony metastases from: breast, prostate, lung, kidney, thyroid, myeloma, bone tumours.

Clinical features
- New onset back pain and tenderness, not improving with analgesics.
- May be worse on coughing/sneezing/straining/overnight/lying flat.
- Motor and sensory deficits, urinary retention and constipation are late signs with poor prognosis, if >24h recovery unlikely.

Treatment
- Exclude fracture as cause of pain with XR (if no neurology), confirm compression with urgent (same day) whole spine MRI.
- Dexamethasone 8mg bd PO (first dose stat), lansoprazole 30mg od.
- Radiotherapy for sensitive tumours; consider surgical decompression if paralysis <24h and life expectancy >3 months; may give tissue diagnosis.

SVC obstruction

Key facts
- Compression/thrombosis/fibrosis of SVC preventing venous return from head and neck and upper extremities.
- Up to 20% of cases due to non malignant disease.
- Not usually immediately life threatening, although sudden obstruction causes cerebral oedema as venous collaterals are not well developed.

Clinical features
- High index of suspicion, especially if lymphoma, small cell lung cancer, mediastinal cancer.
- Neck, face, and arm swelling, dyspnoea, cough, epistaxis, haemoptysis.
- Worse on bending forwards, stooping, lying down.
- Signs include: distended neck (↑↑JVP) and chest veins, facial oedema and plethora, occasionally stridor.
- CT reveals source of obstruction, collaterals, guides fine needle biopsy.

Treatment
- Supportive: O_2, diuretics, head elevation, dexamethasone 8mg bd PO (first dose stat) may help, lansoprazole 30mg od.
- Therapy targeted to histological diagnosis, unless impending airway obstruction/↑ICP when emergency radiotherapy may help.

Upper airway obstruction
In malignancy this may be due to extraluminal compression or intraluminal tumour. Diagnosis and management is detailed on 📖 p. 207.

Raised intracranial pressure
This is dealt with on 📖 p. 295.

Hypercalcaemia
This is described on 📖 p. 236.

Urgent referral

Urgent referral for work-up to the appropriate specialist/cancer network should be carried out for patients with the problems listed, with no current diagnosis of cancer. In some countries (e.g. UK), oncologists will generally accept patients only with histologically confirmed malignancy.

Lung
- Emergency: signs of SVC obstruction or stridor.
- Urgent: persistent haemoptysis in smoker/non-smokers >40 years.
- Suspicious CXR (mass, pleural effusion, chronic consolidation).
- Normal CXR but high index of suspicion (COPD/smokers).
- Chest pain or dyspnoea with history of asbestos exposure.

Upper gastrointestinal
- Urgent referral for dyspepsia plus any one of: dysphagia/chronic GI bleeding/persistent vomiting/chronic unintentional weight loss/epigastric mass/Fe deficiency anaemia/suspicious barium study/supraclavicular node.
- Urgent referral for isolated dysphagia.
- Unexplained abdominal pain and weight loss.
- Obstructive jaundice, especially without pain.
- New onset of upper GI symptoms in patients with Barrett's, dysplasia, atrophic gastritis, or peptic ulcer surgery >20 years previously.

Lower gastrointestinal
- >40 years with PR bleeding *and* bowel habit change >6 weeks.
- >60 years with PR bleeding or bowel habit change >6 weeks.
- Any age with right lower abdominal mass/rectal mass.
- ♀ or ♂ with ↓Fe anaemia and Hb <10 or 11g/dL respectively.

Breast
- >30 years with discrete lump persisting after a period/menopause.
- <30 years with a lump that is enlarging/fixed hard and family Hx.
- Previous breast cancer with new lump or suspicious symptoms.
- Unilateral eczematous skin or nipple change unresponsive to topical treatment.
- Recent nipple distortion.
- Spontaneous bloody unilateral nipple discharge.
- ♂ >50 years with unilateral firm, subareolar mass.

Gyynaecological
- Examination or pap smear suggestive of cervical cancer.
- Postmenopausal bleeding in non-HRT patients/after 6 weeks off HRT.
- Vulval lump or bleeding.
- Persistent inter-menstrual bleeding.
- Any abdominal or pelvic mass not GI/urological in origin.

Urological
- Hard, irregular prostate (refer with PSA).
- Raised PSA even with normal prostate (>4.0 if <40 years).
- Painless macroscopic haematuria.
- >50 years with microscopic haematuria.
- Any abdominal mass arising from the urological tract.
- Mass within the body of the testis/penis.

Central nervous system
- Progressive neurological deficit, new onset seizures, headaches, mental changes, cranial nerve palsy, unilateral sensori-neural deafness.
- Recent onset headaches with symptoms of ↑ICP e.g. vomiting, drowsiness, posture-related headache, pulse-synchronous tinnitus.
- New onset Horner's syndrome—partial ptosis, miosis, anhydrosis, enophthalmos.

Skin
- Any changing pre-existing or suspicious mole: check ABCDE (Asymmetry, irregular Border, Colour change, Diameter >6mm, Evolving lesion).
- Hard-firm nodules or chronic skin ulcers in sun-damaged skin areas (especially head, shoulders, arms).
- Associated enlarged LN or satellite lesions.

Head and neck
- Hard irregular lumps or ulcers on oro-pharyngeal mucosa, especially in smokers or heavy drinkers.
- Oral erythro- or leukoplakia.
- Palpable, firm neck LN.
- Persistent hoarse voice.

Bone
- Bone pain and swelling in young adults without Hx of trauma.
- Suspicious/diagnostic XR: bone destruction, new matrix formation, periosteal reaction (onion skin).

Soft tissue
- Suspicious lumps in soft tissues: >5cm, firm, deep seated, no history of trauma.
- Avoid needle biopsy as sarcomas can seed along biopsy tract, if malignant tumour is suspected, aim for excision biopsy by specialist surgeon (sarcomas can infiltrate a long way and complete excision may be difficult even for clinically relatively small lamps).

Neutropaenic surgical patients

Key facts

These patients may present with unique surgical problems including:

- Oncological emergencies, 📖 see p. 326.
- Unusual causes of acute abdominal symptoms.
- Perioperative management of neutropaenia, immunocompromise, DIC, and elevated WCC.

Abdominal pain in the neutropaenic patient

Neutropaenic enterocolitis

- Most common cause of abdominal pain in neutropaenic patient.
- Mortality >50%.
- Chemotherapy- or radiotherapy-induced destruction of normal mucosa.
- Intramural haemorrhage due to thrombocytopaenia.
- Leads to colitis which may progress to necrotic bowel.
- Treatment medical and surgical individualized to patient:
  - NGT decompression (may need platelet transfusion first if ↓↓ platelets) to avoid life-threatening epistaxis.
  - IV fluids and parenteral nutrition.
  - Broad spectrum antibiotics to cover aerobes and anaerobes.
  - Surgery for perforation, haemorrhage, abscess, obstruction.

Disseminated abdominal infections

- Fungal organisms 2nd commonest after bacteria in neutropaenia.
- *Candida* and *Aspergillus* in 90% of fungal infections.
- Occasionally HSV or CMV may necessitate surgery.
- Can involve liver or spleen and occasionally kidneys.
- Upper quadrant abdo pain, anorexia, nausea and vomiting.
- Surgery for perforation, haemorrhage, abscess, obstruction.

Bone marrow patients

- Up to 50% of bone marrow transplant patients present with acute abdominal pain within 100 days of transplant, with about 10% requiring laparotomy.
- Causes include graft-versus-host disease (GVHD) involving GI tract and liver, infectious colitis, cholecystitis, and gastroduodenal ulceration.
- Hepatic thrombosis is a common non surgical cause of RUQ pain

Acute tumour lysis syndrome

📖 See p. 326.

Anorectal infection in acute leukaemia

- Mortality rate >50%, complicates almost 10% of cases.
- Neutropaenia, febrile, rectal pain, with perianal cellulitis/fluctuance.
- Do not perform digital rectal exam – may cause infection/bleeding.
- Commonest organisms *Enterobacter,* anaerobes, *Pseudomonas*.
- Treatment is broad spectrum antibiotics, sitz baths, warm compresses.
- Surgical drainage and debridement if abscesses don't spontaneously drain.

Perioperative care of the neutropaenic patient

Management of sepsis
- Start empiric antibiotic therapy even if afebrile.
  - Follow local guidelines or sepsis algorithm.
  - Consider antifungal agent if fever persists for 72h on antibiotics.
  - Differential diagnosis much broader in immunocompromised patient.
- Wait for granulocyte cell count to recover before surgery unless life-threatening condition.

Management of blood products
- If unsure, ask for advice from a Haematologist.
- For any transfusion in leukaemia/BMT patients use irradiated products to prevent potentially lethal transfusion-associated GVHD.
  - Occurs when donor competent T-cells attack recipient cells.
  - No effective therapy and mortality is 90%.
- Use leukocyte-depleted blood products to decrease risk of refractoriness to platelet transfusion in patients needing long-term platelet Tx (i.e. BMT, leukaemia, and lymphoma patients)
- Use CMV –ve products in patients with unknown or documented CMV –ve status.
- In patients sensitized by repeated transfusion of blood products use HLA-matched/platelet cross-matched single donor transfusion.
- Transfuse blood to maintain Hb >8.0g/dL.
- Maintain platelets >50,000/µL,preoperatively.
- Avoid aspirin, clopidogrel, and other NSAIDS preoperatively.
- Do not use G-CSF/erythropoietin without specialist advice.

Management of disseminated intravascular coagulation
- All leukaemias can be associated with DIC (📖 p. 101).
- Treat underlying illness.
- Aggressive platelet transfusion in bleeding patients until platelets >50,000/µL.
- Transfuse FFP if INR >1.5 and cryoprecipitate if fibrinogen <1.2g/L.
- Antifibrinolytic agents e.g. tranexamic acid may be beneficial in bleeding.

Management of immunocompromised patients
- Immunocompromise in patients with advanced or haematological malignancy/after chemotherapy/bone marrow irradiation is caused by ↓serum Ig, ↓CD4 helper T cells, ↑CD8 suppressor cells, ↓↓antigen response which may persist for years after treatment.
- Discuss prophylactic antimicrobial therapy with microbiologist (📖 p. 60).

Radiotherapy and chemotherapy

Key facts: radiotherapy

- Ionizing radiation causes direct and indirect (via free radicals) damage to DNA. Depth of tissue penetration depends on type of radiation.
- Malignant cells are more vulnerable than normal cells due to their higher rate of division.
- The total dose is fractionated (divided into small parts and given over time) to magnify this effect. Most fractionation schedule is 1.2–3.0Gy per day, 5–7 days a week, for 3–8 weeks.
  - 2 or 3 fractions a day may be used to treat certain tumours which regenerate more quickly e.g. CHART—continuous hyperfractionated accelerated radiotherapy used for lung cancer.
- Three methods of delivery:
  - *External beam:* usually applied to tumour, + margin of normal tissue (to allow for motion and error) ± draining lymph nodes.
  - *Brachytherapy:* 'Seeds' can be implanted to deliver radiation locally, e.g. ^{125}I in prostate cancer.
  - *Unsealed source:* ingestion/injection of soluble radioactive substances e.g. ^{131}I for thyroid cancer.
- Radiation may be:
  - *Radical:* used with intent to cure cancer: given in 15–40 daily fractions, may be combined with chemotherapy to improve response.
  - *Adjuvant:* used after surgery to treat micrometastases.
  - *Neoadjuvant:* used before surgery to down-stage /debulk cancer.
  - *Palliative:* used to treat symptoms e.g. bone pain, haemoptysis, cough, dyspnoea: given in 1–10 daily fractions (e.g. 20Gy in 5 fractions).

Early side effects of radiotherapy

- Skin reactions: erythema, dry or wet desquamation, ulceration.
- Mucositis: oral ulceration, pharyngitis, oesophagitis, dysphagia, diarrhoea, nausea and vomiting, cystitis, urinary frequency.
- Oedema: soft tissue swelling, including cerebral → raised ICP.
- Bone marrow suppression if large areas treated.
- Infertility: treatment designed to avoid direct exposure to gonads.
- Generalized fatigue or somnolence (in cranial irradiation).

Late side effects of radiotherapy

- Fibrosis: loss of elasticity in tissues, may result in strictures of oesophagus or bowel needing dilatation, bladder fibrosis, vaginal stenosis, dyspareunia, xerostomia.
- Atherosclerosis and calcification: accelerated changes in vessels and cardiac valves years after mediastinal irradiation.
- Pneumonitis: dry cough and dyspnoea.
- Hypothyroidism.
- Somnolence, spinal cord myelopathy, brachial plexopathy.
- Cancer: 2° malignancies due to radiotherapy seen in small minority of patients many years after radiotherapy (e.g. breast cancer after mediastinal RT for lymphoma).

Perioperative care

No indication to change preoperative management. However, be aware that wound healing may be compromised, and skin and epithelial surfaces are broken much more easily, e.g. pressure sores.

Key facts: chemotherapy

- Anti-neoplastic drugs used to treat cancer in standardized regimen.
- May be given as 1° (sole) therapy e.g. haematological malignancies.
- More often combined modality chemotherapy- with radiation/surgery:
  - *Neoadjuvant:* preoperative treatment to downstage tumour to improve survival or operability.
  - *Adjuvant:* postoperative treatment for potential micrometastic disease.
- Palliative: to decrease tumour load—aim to control symptoms and increase life expectancy without curative intent.
- Generally even IV as out-patient, occasionally by PICC or Hickman line for continous infusions, or orally. High-dose reqimes requires admission.

Side effects of chemotherapy

- Nausea and vomiting—usually after administration, may be delayed.
- Diarrhoea—may coincide with neutropaenia, if in doubt, treat as infectious.
- Alopecia—think of wigs, self-esteem is very important for patients!
- Fatigue.
- Neutropaenia—within 5–14 days, 📖 see p. 326.

Box 10.1 Lymphoedema after axillary clearance

- Lymphoedema (swollen arm) is a debilitating and disfiguring condition which is difficult to treat, affecting up to 40% of patients after axillary clearance, particularly if radiotherapy is also given.
- Patients who have undergone axillary clearance (usually for breast cancer, but also upper limb melanoma) are advised *not* to let anyone take blood, cannulate veins, use BP cuffs or phlebotomy tourniquets in that arm, to try to avoid lymphoedema developing or making existing lymphoedema worse.
- This is based on the following premises:
  - Removal of deep lymphatics particularly with level 2 and 3 clearance means patients depend on superficial lymphatics.
  - Subdermal lymphatics may be damaged by pressure cuffs.
  - Superficial lymphatics more easily overwhelmed by minor infection or venous congestion.
  - Cannulation is likely to be difficult in lymphoedematous arm.
- Although there is only anecdotal evidence that routine careful phlebotomy/BP measurements predispose to lymphoedema, it is appropriate to explore all alternative avenues (including re-examining need for cannulation/phlebotomy) first.
- If a patient subsequently develops lymphoedema after your uneventful cannulation, the latter is very likely to be recalled by the patient as the triggering event; particularly when they asked you not to do it.

Palliative care

Key facts
- Care is focused on improving quality of life rather than length of life.
- Applies to any patient in the last stages of any major illness.
- Competent palliative care is based on four basic principles:
  - *Symptom control:* physical and psychological.
  - *Communication:* open and sensitive communication should extend to patients, informal carers, and professional colleagues. Your duty is to the patient, although those most in need may be the relatives.
  - *Autonomy:* respect the patient's autonomy and choice (e.g. over place of care, treatment options, communication with family).
  - *Support for relatives and friends.*
- Complex problems benefit from specialist palliative care: refer early.
- Surgery may occasionally have a role in palliative care, e.g. unstable, pathological fracture of a long bone may cause pain which is resistant to medical management, justifying surgical fixation for pain control.
- Review the benefit/burden balance for every drug and intervention. For instance, antihypertensive or lipid-lowering drugs are usually not necessary; anticoagulants or metformin may even be dangerous.
- Minimize observations, blood tests, medication, and imaging.
- Discuss resuscitation status; and document it clearly, see 📖 p. 110.

Pain (Table 10.3 and Box 10.2)
- Terminal patients are often on opioids preoperatively: continue these peri- and postoperatively unless the surgical management will immediately relieve the pain for which the opioids were prescribed.
- Be aware that, due to tolerance, the doses will often be much higher than the 'usual' doses of opioids used for other surgical patients (📖 Box 10.2).
- The predicted daily dose of SC morphine postoperatively will be approximately $1/3^{rd}$ of the previous oral dose (📖 see also Table 10.3).
- If PCA is not used, prescribe SC bolus opioids for break-through or postoperative pain in doses of approximately $1/6^{th}$ of the preoperative 24h oral dose.
- Review opioid prescribing *frequently* (at least bd) if surgery is likely to have removed or reduced the source of pain.

Table 10.3

Drug	Dose	Strength*	Class
Oral (tablet/suspension/solution)			
Morphine	5–40mg/4h	1 ×	Opioid
Morphine m/r tablets	15–120mg/12h	1 ×	Opioid
Oxycodone	5mg/4h	2 ×	Opioid
Paracetamol	1g/6h		Non-opioid
Ibuprofen	200–400mg/6–8h		NSAID
Diclofenac	50mg/8h		NSAID

Table 10.3 (*Continued*)

Drug	Dose	Strength*	Class
IV/SC			
Morphine	5–40mg/4h	2 ×	Opioid
Diamorphine	2.5–20mg/4h	3 ×	Opioid
Oxycodone	5mg/4h	3 ×	Opioid
Diclofenac	75mg/12h (max 2 days)		NSAID
Paracetamol	1g/6h		Non-opioid
PCA			
50mg morphine in 50mL NS with 10mg metoclopramide: 1mL bolus, with 5min lock-out. Titrate bolus size to achieve symptom control			
Transdermal (patch)			
Fentanyl	25/50/75/100mcg per hour patches (change patch every 72h)	150 ×	Opioid
Suppository			
Paracetamol	1g/6h		Non-opioid
Diclofenac	75mg/12h		NSAID
Topical/nerve block			
May help with wound or bone pain: discuss with anaesthesia/pain service			
Some patients report feeling better using NSAID in gel form			
Non-pharmacological methods (e.g. massage, gentle heat) may also help			

*Strength relative to oral morphine
NB some patients may already be on doses much higher than those indicated above, if in doubt, involve local palliative care team.

Box 10.2 Tips for prescribing opioids

- Patients often worry that opioids are addictive: reassure that this is not a problem in the acute pain or palliative care setting.
- Tolerance is *normal* so increases in regular doses are to be expected. Higher doses do not mean that the patient is deteriorating.
- Patients may also worry a morphine pump is tantamount to euthanasia: reassure that overdosing with pump or PCA is impossible if correctly used, and opioids have no impact on life expectancy.
- Include total quantity in figures *and* words when prescribing.
- Include the formulation (liquid/tablet/suspension).
- Rewrite in full if dose changes.
- Give amount in milligrams for liquids.
- Always think about prescribing adjuncts to reduce opioid requirement and side effects: anxiolytics, antiemetics and laxatives.
- If patient intolerant of one opioid, try another.

Common problems

Fluid management
- Resuscitative perioperative fluids may not be appropriate in advanced disease where there is no expectation of recovery.
- In irreversible intestinal obstruction, NGT and IV infusion can give relief, **or** great distress. Review benefits and burdens carefully.
- Bed-bound and cachectic patients may require and wish for very little fluid: ↓insensible fluid loss and catabolism produces much endogenous water. Fluid requirements may be only a few hundred mL per day.
- In patients with end-stage terminal cancer, SC or IV fluids are unnecessary unless the patient is thirsty. If fluids are needed, SC is preferable to repeatedly resiting IV cannulae.
- Spironolocatone 100–400mg/24h PO in divided doses may help ascites, minimizing the need for invasive procedures such as paracentesis.

Breathlessness
- Careful history and examination, pulse oximetry (± ABGs) and CXR to identify pleural/pericardial effusion, pneumonitis, lobar collapse.
- Give supplementary (humidified) O_2. Nasal cannulae may be better tolerated than mask, but even this can create claustrophobia.
- Pleural effusion can be treated with diuretics, therapy to underlying malignancy, pleurocentesis, pleurodesis.
- Treat pericardial effusion with pericardiocentesis or pericardial window (📖 p. 128) which may be performed percutaneously.
- Remember that ascites may splint diaphragm and cause breathlessness.
- Benzodiazepines or (dia)morphine provide symptomatic relief; this is especially important when the underlying cause cannot be reversed.
- Consider other causes of breathlessness, especially PE.

Bowel obstruction
- Obstructive symptoms may be functional rather than mechanical, so in a significant minority of cases spontaneous resolution occurs.
- If abdominal pain due to colic, pro-kinetic drugs (metoclopramide, domperidone) and bulking/stimulant laxatives should be stopped.
- Treat persistent colic with SC hyoscine butylbromide (Buscopan®) infusion 20–60mg/24 h (sometimes more).
- Treat continuous abdominal pain with SC diamorphine. Add 20–400mg diamorphine to 5mL water and infuse at 0.2mL/h.
- Treat persistent nausea with an antiemetic (Table 10.4).
- Dexamethasone has 2nd line antiemetic activity and is used in some centres in intestinal obstruction, but evidence for benefit is poor.
- Octreotide has antisecretory and bowel relaxant effects, but is expensive and is best used by specialists when conventional therapy fails.

Constipation
- Careful history and examination to exclude bowel obstruction.
- Common with opioids.
- Bisacodyl 5mg at night.
- Co-danthramer 5–10mL at night with glycerine suppository in morning.
- Movicol sachet 2–4/12h ± phosphate enema for resistant cases.

Table 10.4 Choice of antiemetic in palliative care

Antiemetic	Dose	Comment
All of these can be given as part of PCA or NCA		
Metoclopramide	10mg/8h IV/IM/PO	Prokinetic—good for gastric stasis
Domperidone	10–20mg/8h PO or 60mg 12h PR	Fewer extrapyramidal side effects than metoeloppramide
Ondansetron	4–8mg IV/IM/PO	Good for opioid/chemotherapy-induced nausea
Haloperidol	1–1.5mg/12h IV	Antipsychotic—good for drug related nausea
Levomepromazine	3–12.5mg/12h	Sedative effect—can be desired

Nausea and vomiting

Choice of antiemetics in general surgery is discussed on, p. 252.
Hyoscine 0.4–0.6mg/8h SC helps in setting of upper GI obstruction.
- Possible causes include chemotherapy, constipation/bowel obstruction, drugs e.g. opioids, antibiotics, severe pain, cough, oral thrush, gastritis, sepsis, renal failure, raised ICP, anticipatory, liver disease.
- Take a careful Hx, including a detailed DHx, and full exam.
- Treat reversible causes with laxatives, antibiotics, PPI, reviewing medication (with a view to avoiding polypharmacy—consider changing, stopping, or reducing drugs wherever possible).

Dry mouth or dry cough

- Use humidified O_2 (nebulized NaCl 5mL PRN).
- Treat candida with nystatin suspension 5mL q6h.
- Promote good oral hygiene with chlorhexidine mouth washes and saliva substitutes.
- Ice chips to suck, or chewing gum, often help.

Pruritus

- Causes include allergy, drug reactions (including morphine), diabetes, anaemia, malignancy, jaundice, uraemia, contact dermatitis (including from adhesive dressings, tape, ECG electrodes, etc.).
- Take careful Hx and exam; request FBC, LFTs, U&Es, TFTs.
- Treat 1° cause.
- Try emollients e.g. E45® cream or Diprobase® or calamine lotion.
- Antihistamine: chlorpheniramine 4mg/8h PO (10mg/8h IV).
- Cholestyramine 4-8g/24h PO 1h after other drugs helps in jaundice
- In obstructive jaundice, consider ursodeoxycholic acid (400mg tds PO).

Psychological

- Allow the patient to express anger, fear, sorrow.
- Specialist counselling can help, particularly if done in advance: e.g. meeting preoperatively with stoma nurse or mastectomy nurse.
- Biofeedback or relaxation techniques may help reduce treatment side effects.
- Consider whether transfer to a dedicated palliative care facility, or even home, is feasible for the last days of life.

Communication

Key facts

- Sensitive, effective communication with patients and those close to them is often the key factor in maintaining a sense of control and meaning towards the end of life.
- The starting point is always active, unhurried listening to the patient's story. Only in this way can important misunderstandings be avoided, and assumptions minimized.
- If you do not feel able to handle communication with dying patients, ask for someone to help you or rehearse the strategy of your interview with the nursing staff beforehand.

Preparation

- *Be absolutely sure of your facts: right patient, right diagnosis, understand the plan and prognosis.*
- If possible warn patient: "I'm going to come back in half an hour to go through your test result". and try to time discussion so partners or other support can also be present.
- Ask the patient if they wish anyone who happens to be with them to stay while you talk. And never assume that the person of similar age and opposite sex sitting by the bed is the patient's partner—ask them how they are related.
- Switch off your mobile and pager, or give them to someone else.
- Ask a nurse to be with you when you talk to the patient to help continuity of communication and support when you leave.
- Try to create a sense of quiet and privacy: if a private room is not appropriate at least draw curtains around the bed.
- Introduce yourself by name and by role.
- Whenever possible, sit down. This brings you to a similar level to the patient and indicates that you are not imminently going to walk away.
- If the set-up is not right, change it, even during the discussion.

Diagnosis

- Ask the patient what they have already been told, and try to understand what their expectations are, how much they want to know and how much they will understand.
- Indicate in outline what information you already have, and its source, e.g. from family doctor, previous hospital notes.
- Be prepared to explain the patient's problem in layman's terms, e.g. 'a blockage in the bowel causing pain and sickness'.
- If it is cancer, use the word 'cancer' and be prepared to give a realistic assessment of what may be achieved, e.g. 'we expect to be able to control your pain and vomiting, but although we can slow this down this is not an illness that we can cure', or 'we can cure most people with this problem, and we would expect you to be one of those'. *Avoid giving percentages or survival figures in months/years.*
- If the patient asks directly if they have cancer, share their anxiety if the diagnosis is likely, but not proven.
- Be honest but gentle if the diagnosis is confirmed.
- Be sensitive: if the patient is too distressed, do not plough on.

Management options

- Recognize that some people will want full explanations and options for treatment; others will find these details burdensome. Sometimes it will be right to be explicit, but let the patient guide you as to how much to say: 'Would you like to know more now, or would it help to have some time to think over what I've just said?'
- Give a realistic assessment of the consequences of each option. Avoid coercing patients into a particular decision by exaggerating the risks or benefits of different approaches. It is the patient who will have to bear the consequences, not you.
- Take care not to offer options that are clearly against the patient's best interests, or that the team is not prepared to undertake.
- Be clear what a successful outcome to a proposed operation might be; and put it in the context of progressive, incurable disease. For instance, 'success' might be reducing symptoms, even without prolonging life.
- If their choice is 'wrong', remember it is *their* decision not yours.

Prognosis

- Even those who do not ask will have the question 'how long have I got' in their minds. Even if we as doctors cannot know the answer, patients should not be made to feel this is a silly question.
- Never leave a patient without hope, nor with the suggestion that 'there is nothing more that can be done for you'.
- Any mention of a specific time, even if heavily qualified, is likely to be remembered as 'the doctor gave me 6 months to live': try to give a general idea 'years rather than months', or 'probably days not weeks'.
- Explore what particular reasons there may be for wanting an estimated survival time: then try to address those personal or business needs.
- The question 'how long have I got' can actually mean 'how will I die'?
- If the disease is incurable, say so; do not be so evasive over prognosis as to fail to acknowledge the tragedy of a significantly shortened life.

Family and other informal carers

- Only the patient, or their legal guardian, can make health-care decisions for the patient (but *not* relatives, or even the next-of-kin).
- Information about the patient should be shared only with those whom the patient wants to know.
- Never lie to the patient, and do not tell relatives information before the patient as this risks harmful collusion.
- Your primary duty is to the patient, but bear in mind that relatives and friends will survive the patient; also manage their grief.

Reaction to terminal diagnosis

- The classic Kübler model consists of 5 stages: denial, anger, bargaining, depression, and acceptance.
- Patients may also experience numbness, resignation, shock, or panic.
- Denial and anger are only problems if jeopardizing coping mechanisms.
- Patients and close ones may direct anger at medical staff. Don't take it personally, get angry or become defensive in return: it's not an accusation of failure, it is part of the grieving process.

Procedures

How to change a vacuum dressing

Key facts

- Vacuum dressing is the choice for large open wounds, often associated with sepsis where 1° closure is not possible or desirable.
- The creation of a hostile environment to most organisms, combined with immediate removal of effluent from the wound, creates optimal conditions for wound healing.
- The dressings consist of a micropore sponge placed directly onto a wound, sealed with a clear, occlusive, adhesive membrane through which an intermittent or continuous vacuum can be applied at 75–150kPa.
- Although it is possible to use wall suction, normal vacuum dressings are supplied with an individual unit to generate the vacuum containing a canister to collect wound exudate; portable canister are available.
- Vacuum dressings should be changed every 48–96h, more frequently if suction is occluded by wound debris, or the vacuum seal is broken.
- Aseptic technique is preferable but not mandatory, except where internal viscera or prostheses are at risk of exposure.

Equipment

- Sterile gown, gloves, and drapes.
- Vacuum dressing pack (comes in 10 × 15cm, 30 × 15cm, 40 × 30cm).
- Vacuum pump and canister: wall suction if these are not available.
- Sterile disposable scalpel or scissors.
- Betadine or chloroprep.
- Duoderm if skin excoriated around the dressing.
- Forceps and gauze.
- Microbiology swabs.

Preparation

- Explain to the patient what you are going to do.
- Ask nurse to give 2.5–5mg morphine IV.
- Switch off the vacuum pump: the sponge should decompress and become soft to touch.
- Remove the occlusive dressing completely from the skin around the wound, and gently lift the sponge out of the wound without touching the wound.
- Prep the skin around the wound with betadine or chloroprep.
- Gown and glove.
- Take a microbiology swab, and use the gauze and forceps to de-slough.
- Make a note of exposed prosthesis, sutures, bone, or viscera.
- Dry the skin thoroughly: if the edges are raw, cut Duoderm® to size and place around the wound.
- Cut the adhesive dressing to size so that it overlaps the wound by 5–10cm all the way round, particularly where there are deep skin folds.
- Cut the sponge so that it is about 1cm larger than the wound all the way round (it's easier to do this with a scalpel than the scissors), and place the sponge in the wound.
- Peel the backing labelled '1' off the adhesive and place it over the sponge, making sure it sticks to the skin all the way around the wound.

- Peel off the backing labelled '2' (usually striped).
- Stab the adhesive dressing and sponge once with the scalpel in the middle of the sponge, and place the sticky pad end of the suction tubing over the stab hole.
- Connect to the vacuum pump or wall suction.
- Check the suction tubing is unclamped, switch on the suction, and you should see the sponge compress down into the wound, and become almost hard, as well as a small amount of wound exudate or blood in the suction tubing.
- See Box 11.1 for troubleshooting.

Box 11.1 Troubleshooting vacuum dressings

The vacuum pump says there's a leak, and the sponge doesn't deflate
- Check the connections along the suction tubing.
- Check the dressing for obvious areas where the adhesive isn't sticking to the skin, especially skin creases: the sponge should deflate if you press on the area where the leak is, and it's sometimes possible to correct these by sticking a tegaderm, or more adhesive dressing on top once you've dried the skin.
- Change the dressing, and make sure the skin is dry, and the adhesive is placed deep into skin folds and creases.

The vacuum pump registers a vacuum, but the sponge won't deflate
- Check the connection tubing isn't clamped.
- If there is debris or blood clots in the suction tubing change it.
- Change the canister.
- Look at the dressing: if it is full of clot, change it.

The canister is full of blood
- It may be blood-stained pus or transudate, which is common.
- If blood appears to be actively draining from the wound think what may be below the wound (vascular anastomosis, ventricle, vascular graft?) treat as for surgical bleeding (📖 p. 98).
- If drainage is limited but constant, it will reduce the efficiency of the vacuum dressing: correct coagulopathy, take down the dressing, and apply direct pressure to bleeding areas for 5–10min (Surgicel® is very effective).

Endotracheal intubation

Box 11.2 Caution

⚠ Effective bag and mask ventilation is better than multiple attempts at endotracheal intubation in the arrest setting. Except in a dire emergency this procedure should not be performed without expert supervision.

- Patients not in cardiac arrest or who maintain a gag reflex will usually need to be anaesthetized and paralysed prior to oropharyngeal intubation, i.e. administration of a hypnotic agent plus muscle relaxant which should only be done by an anaesthetist or practitioner with formal training.
- *The best setting to learn intubation is preoperatively in the anaesthetic room of a theatre with good supervision in controlled conditions.*

Equipment
- 10mL syringe.
- ET; size 7–9 for ♀; 8–10 for ♂.
- Laryngoscope.
- Ribbon to secure tube, lubricating jelly.
- Suction
- Stethoscope

Preparation
- Preoxygenate the patient by bag and mask ventilation with 100% O_2.
- Ensure that the laryngoscope and ET tube cuff are functioning.
- Remove any dentures and suction excess saliva and secretions.
- Flex the neck, extend the head (unless C-spine injury suspected) (pillows adjust under head, chin lift).

Technique
- Insert laryngoscope with your left hand pushing the tongue to the left.
- Advance the scope anterior to the epiglottis and lift gently but firmly upwards to expose the vocal cords. *Take care not to lever on the upper teeth with the 'heel' of the scope.*
- Insert the lubricated ET tube between the cords into the trachea.
- Confirm correct positioning of the tube by observing chest movements, and listening over lung bases and stomach. If you have a colorimetric device to confirm CO_2 in exhaled air, use it.
- Progressively inflate the cuff and attach ventilation equipment, while holding ET tube in position, prior to securing it with tape.
- Confirm correct cuff inflation by listening for whistling or bubbling in the larynx suggesting air leak and secure the tube in place with ribbon.
- Reconfirm that both sides of the chest are moving. If the tip of the tube is too far in, it will go past the carina and only ventilate one lung (usually the right). Withdraw the tube 3cm and reassess.
- Secure tube in position with tape ribbon.

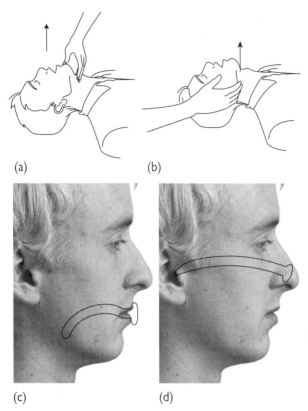

(a)   (b)

(c)   (d)

Fig. 11.1 Safe alternative methods of temporarily maintaining airway until anaesthetic expertise is available, used in conjunction with bag and mask ventilation. (a) Performing a chin-lift. (b) Performing a jaw-thrust. (c) Choose the size of the oropharyngeal airway by measuring from the patient's teeth to the angle of the mandible. (d) Choose the size of the nasophayngeal airway by measuring the patient's nostril to the tragus. Reproduced with permission from Thomas J and Monaghan T (2007). *Oxford Handbook of Clinical Examination and Practical Skills*, Oxford University Press, Oxford.

Venepuncture

This is a mandatory skill to learn for all doctors but many patients will have 'difficult' veins and regular practice is needed.

Indications

Obtaining venous blood samples for laboratory analysis, venesection.

Equipment

- Tourniquet.
- 23G or 21G needle (blue or green).
- Syringe (appropriate size: 10–20mL).
- Alcohol swabs.
- Appropriate laboratory sample tubes.
- Cotton-wool ball and tape.

Most hospitals now have vacuum tube systems as an alternative to the 'needle and syringe' approach for obtaining blood samples.

Preparation

Apply tourniquet above the elbow and inspect the arm for suitable engorged veins.

Method

- Confirm the patient's identity (including against their ID bracelet) and explain what you are about to do.
- Clean the skin thoroughly at the site of access and allow to dry completely.
- Pull the skin over the site under tension with your left hand.
- Pass the needle obliquely through the skin at a point approximately 1–2mm distal to the point of planned entry to the vein.
- Advance the needle until a 'give' is felt as the vein is entered and a 'flash-back' is seen in the syringe hub.
- Aspirate the desired amount of blood while holding the barrel of the syringe firmly.
- If you're using self-vaccing tubes, keep the needle in place with your right hand, and with your left hand place the sample tubes in turn on the other end of the needle.
- Release the tourniquet *before* gently withdrawing needle and syringe.
- Apply pressure to the site to arrest any bleeding. Do not assume the patient can help with this, e.g. stroke patients.

Tips and problems

- *Poor veins:* if the patient is cold and the samples non-urgent, place the arm in warm water—this may aid venodilation. Veins on the dorsum of the hand may be the only ones readily available—try using a smaller or butterfly needle to obtain samples.
- *Obese patients:* try the dorsum of the hand or the radial aspect of the wrist, access may be easier here.
- *Failed attempts:* repeated failed attempts will distress the patient and demoralize the doctor! Ask someone to help. If the samples are extremely urgent, a femoral stab may be the best option for obtaining blood samples, e.g. during cardiac arrest.
- *IV cannulae:* if blood samples and IV access are needed, a sample can be taken immediately after inserting the cannula. However, do not use a

peripheral cannula for routine samples; they can be haemolysed, contaminated by IV fluids and unreliable.
- *Sample bottles and request forms:* ensure these are labelled correctly and the appropriate tests are ordered. If in doubt about a particular investigation, seek advice from a senior or the laboratory.
- *Blood cultures:* ensure that the skin is cleaned thoroughly. Do not touch the skin again. Once the sample is taken, change the needle before transferring the sample to the appropriate culture bottle. Document whether the patient was on antibiotics at the time of the sample and ensure the sample is not placed in the fridge during transfer to the lab.

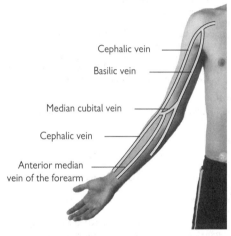

Cephalic vein

Basilic vein

Median cubital vein

Cephalic vein

Anterior median vein of the forearm

Fig. 11.2 Representation of peripheral veins of the upper limb. Reproduced with permission from Thomas J and Monaghan T (2007). *Oxford Handbook of Clinical Examination and Practical Skills*, Oxford University Press, Oxford.

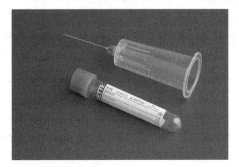

Fig. 11.3 Vacutainer® blood collection system, ready for use. Reproduced with permission from Thomas J and Monaghan T (2007). *Oxford Handbook of Clinical Examination and Practical Skills*, Oxford University Press, Oxford.

Intravenous cannulation

A similar skill to that of simple venepuncture but needs plenty of practice to become competent. If having difficulty, observe a few experts in action—an ideal setting is in the anaesthetic room of theatres.

Indications
Venous access for administration of IV fluids, blood, or IV drugs.

Equipment
- Tourniquet.
- Cannula: 20G or 18G (pink or green).
- Adhesive dressing/tape.
- Skin cleaning solution.
- 5mL syringe containing 0.9% saline or heparinized saline.
- IV fluid bag with giving set, if necessary.
- 1% lidocaine in a 2mL syringe, with an orange needle

△ *In the emergency setting, use at least 18G (green) cannula, preferably 16G (grey) or 14G (brown) to facilitate fluid resuscitation.*

Preparation
Apply tourniquet above or below the elbow and inspect the arm for suitable engorged veins.

Method
- Clean the skin thoroughly at the site of access.
- Identify a suitable vein. Inject a 'bleb' of lidocaine into the skin to raise a small bump at the site of proposed insertion. Do this for 18G cannulae and larger unless it is an emergency.
- Pull the skin over the proposed puncture site under tension with your left thumb.
- Pass the cannula obliquely through the skin at a point approximately 1–2mm mm distal to the point you wish to enter the vein.
- Advance the cannula smoothly until the vein is entered: a 'give' will be felt and a 'flashback' seen in the hub of the cannula.
- Hold the hub of the needle with one hand and advance the cannula into the vein either with your index finger or the other hand, while maintaining skin fixation until the cannula is well into the vein.
- Remove the tourniquet and press on the vein proximal to the cannula as the needle is removed to prevent back-bleeding. Place the needle straight into a sharps container, or a separate receiver.
- Apply the screw cap to the end of the cannula.
- Secure the cannula in place with a transparent dressing. Write the time and date on the dressing.
- If the cannula is not going to be used immediately, flush with 5mL heparinized saline: if a swelling appears in the skin, the cannula is not properly in the vein—remove it and try again elsewhere.
- If the needles and syringes you have used are not already safely disposed of, do this now.

Tips and problems

- *Poor veins, obese patients, and failed attempts*: ☐ see Venepuncture p. 346.
- *Agitated or fitting patients*: try not to place the cannula over a joint, as these tend to become easily dislodged or 'tissued'. Consider bandaging the arm where cannulated to a padded board.
- *Secure the cannula*: cannulae are all too easily dislodged because of poor fixation to the skin. Use of two cannula dressings (one placed above and one below) is often needed. Use tape to secure any attached tubing so it does not pull the cannula out by accident.
- *Hairy arm*: shaving the skin at the planned cannula site seems tedious but will allow the cannula to be secured adequately.
- *Non-dominant hand*: placing the cannula in the non-dominant hand or arm, if possible, will allow the patient a little bit more freedom and may prevent the cannula becoming dislodged accidentally.
- *Fragile veins*: this tends to a problem in elderly or debilitated patients. Try using a smaller cannula: the dorsum of the hand is often a good site.
- *Poor peripheral access*: in some patients with multiple collapsed or damaged veins, alternative cannula sites may have to be considered, e.g. feet. If peripheral cannulation becomes impossible, a central line will have to be considered.
- *Blood transfusion*: it is a myth that blood cannot be given through a pink 20G cannula (or even blue 22G), but beware that often blood transfusions are given to those requiring volume as much as Hb, and fast transfusion through 16G (grey) or 14G (brown) cannula is preferred.

Complete failure to cannulate

- Is a cannula necessary?
  - Can IV medication or fluids be omitted until elective central/long line insertion is possible?
  - Can medication or fluids be given orally, via SC, or via NGT?
  - Discuss with microbiology if antibiotics are involved: changing route of administration often requires appropriate changes in antibiotic.
  - Fluid and insulin regimens can be modified to be given subcutaneously if desperate.
  - Many painkillers and antiemetics can be given PR or IM.
- Ask another member of your team to try: sometimes a 'fresh' pair of hands is all that is needed.
- If no-one in your team can site the cannula, ask the on-call anaesthetist if they can help, but remember they are **not** a cannulation service!
- If peripheral access is impossible, or required for a long time (e.g. IV antibiotic regimens for infected prostheses) consider:
  - Elective PICC line insertion (long-term line inserted electively by specialist nurse into basilic vein).
  - Elective central line insertion: this should be done in an anaesthetic room rather than on the ward, and during daytime hours (☐ p. 352).
  - Femoral line insertion (less ideal as this site is more prone to line sepsis).

Arterial cannula insertion

Key facts
- Used for continuous monitoring of arterial BP in unstable patients or those on inotropic support in an HDU or ICU.
- Allows frequent ABG sampling.

Equipment
- Two 20G arterial cannulas with guidewire.
- Connectors and 3-way tap.
- 2mL 1% lidocaine injection.
- 5mL syringe and blue needle.
- 10mL saline injection.
- Skin prep.
- Gauze swabs.

Preparation
- Make sure the appropriate monitoring set-up is available: a nurse should have a flushed and zero'd pressure transducing line, with a 3-way tap connecting it to a short extension ready.
- Explain the procedure to the patient if appropriate.
- It is good practice to perform Allen's test (📖 see Box 11.3) to demonstrate that the ulnar arterial supply to the hand arcades is intact.
- For radial artery cannula insertion place the forearm on a pillow so that the wrist is dorsiflexed; for femoral artery insertion abduct and flex the hip slightly.

Landmarks
Radial artery
Lies between tendon of flexor carpi radialis and head of radius.

Femoral artery
Lies midway between the anterior superior iliac spine and the symphysis pubis.

Technique
- Prepare and check equipment and prep skin.
- Infiltrate 1–2mL LA in the skin but avoid distorting the anatomy.
- Palpate pulse between two fingers 2–3cm apart.
- Pass cannula at 45° into skin using either of the techniques described next.
- Once the cannula is in situ, aspirate, connect to the pressure line extension and flush about 5mL slowly either using a syringe via the 3-way tap, or at the level of the transducer.

Transfixion technique
The cannula is passed through both artery walls, the needle completely withdrawn, and the cannula then withdrawn slowly until flashback occurs at which point it is advanced into the artery.

Partial transfixion technique
The cannula is advanced until flashback stops, and the needle with-drawn while holding the cannula steady, which is then advanced into the artery.

Artery not transfixed
The cannula is advanced carefully in 0.5mm increments until flashback is seen, at which point the catheter is carefully slid off the needle in the artery.

Troubleshooting

No or poor arterial trace
- Confirm that the patient has a pulse: if no detectable pulse start ALS protocol and call arrest team
- Check the BP with cuff measurement: ⌨ Management of shock and hypotension are described on p. 116.
- If pulse detectable:
  - Cannula may not be in the artery: check that you can aspirate arterial (not venous) blood.
  - Check that the BP cuff is not inflated more proximally.
  - There may be a problem with the monitor: check that the scale is appropriate (0–200mmHg), and if you shake the connection tubing that an irregular trace appears on the monitor: if it doesn't ask the nurse to recheck the transducer connections and set-up.
  - The cannula or connection tubing may be blocked or kinked: check that the 3-way stopcocks are all open, that the cannula and tubing are not kinked (this may vary with the position of the patient).
  - Try flushing the cannula with 5mL NS.
  - Try rewiring the cannula: put the guidewire down the cannula, remove the old cannula and thread a new one over the guidewire.

Guidewire
A guidewire is useful where it is possible to get flashback, but difficult to advance the catheter up the artery.

Complications

Ischaemia, thrombosis, bleeding, damage to radial and median nerve. Inadvertent intra-arterial injection of drugs.

Box 11.3 Allen's test

Used to demonstrate a patent palmar collateral circulation: the patient clenches their fist to exclude blood from palm, and the doctor firmly compresses both ulnar and radial pulses while patient opens their palm which should be blanched. The doctor releases the ulnar compression whilst still occluding the radial pulse: the palm becomes pink in <5sec if there is good collateral supply from the ulnar artery. About 3% of people do not have a collateral palmar supply: hand ischaemia is a real risk if the radial artery is cannulated and pressure readings are more accurate from proximal arteries: brachial, axillary, and femoral.

Central venous catheter insertion

Key facts
- Used for monitoring CVP to provide information to guide fluid balance and inotropic support in an HDU or ICU setting.
- Used for administration of inotropes, pressors, and TPN.
- Catheters can be single or multi lumen, sheaths (for insertion of PA catheters and pacing wires), tunnelled, or long lines.

Equipment
- Appropriate central venous catheter.
- US probe if this is to be utilized.
- Enough 3-way taps for all individual lumens.
- 10mL 1% lidocaine injection.
- 10mL syringe.
- Blue needle and a green needle.
- 20mL saline injection.
- 2 or 3/0 silk on a large handheld needle.
- 11 blade scalpel.
- Skin prep, sterile drape, sterile gloves and gown.
- Gauze swabs.

Preparation
- Explain the procedure to the patient if appropriate.
- Ask a nurse to be present.
- Patient's ECG and pulse oximetry should be continually monitored.
- Ensure that there is adequate light, a space behind the bed which you can work in, and that it is possible to place the bed in Trendelenberg.

Landmarks
Internal jugular vein
- *Central approach:* apex of triangle formed by clavicular and sternal heads of sternocleidomastoid muscle, aiming the needle towards the ipsilateral nipple.
- *Posterior approach:* point where line drawn horizontally from the cricoid cartilage to the lateral border of the clavicular head of sterno-cleidomastoid, aiming the needle towards the sternal notch.
- *Anterior:* medial border of the sternal head of sternocleidomastoid, aiming needle towards ipsilateral nipple.

Subclavian vein
Advance the needle at 45° to the junction of the outer and middle 1/3rd of the clavicle 1–2cm, then direct needle towards sternal groove.

Technique
There are numerous techniques only one technique is described here:
- Prep the patient.
- Drape so that all landmarks are exposed.
- Palpate the carotid pulse.
- Infiltrate LA around the planned puncture site.
- Spend 2–3min laying out the equipment in the order of use, secure 3-way taps to central line and turn to closed position.
  Ask the nurse to place the bed in 10–20° of Trendelenberg (head-down).

- Ballot the internal jugular vein.
- Using aseptic technique and a green needle on a 10mL syringe enter the skin at 45° as described in 📖 Landmarks on p. 352.
- On aspirating venous blood remove the syringe but leave the green needle in situ as an exact marker of position, depth, and direction.
- Take the large-bore hollow needle attached to the 10mL syringe and using the green needle as a guide cannulate the internal jugular vein.
- Aspirate 3–5mL of blood when there is flashback and then remove the syringe leaving the wide-bore needle in situ. The blood should look dark and nonpulsatile rather than bright and pulsatile.
- Pass the guidewire down the wide bore needle and keeping hold of it at all times.
- Once an adequate length of wire is in place, remove the needle over the wire, and apply pressure to the vein.
- Make a 3mm nick in the skin over the wire with a scalpel.
- Pass the dilators over the wire through the skin but not into the vein making sure you hold the wire *AT ALL TIMES*.
- Remove the dilators, apply pressure, and pass the central venous catheter over the wire into the vein until it reaches the skin. Before advancing the catheter into the vein, make sure you are holding the top of the wire where it protrudes out of the lumen's hub. Only then can you slide the catheter.
- The wire normally protrudes through the brown distal lumen of a triple lumen line which should therefore be left open.
- Aspirate, flush, and close all lumens and suture the catheter to the skin.
- Check that there is a satisfactory pressure trace in a transducer is used.
- Chest XR to identify pneumothorax.

Complications

Immediate

Damage to nearby structures (carotid artery puncture, pneumothorax, haemothorax, chylothorax, brachial plexus injury, arrythmias) air embolism, loss of guidewire into right side of heart.

Late

Sepsis, thromboembolism, AV fistula formation.

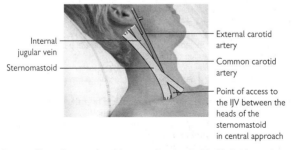

Internal jugular vein

Sternomastoid

External carotid artery

Common carotid artery

Point of access to the IJV between the heads of the sternomastoid in central approach

Fig. 11.4 The surface anatomy of the internal jugular vein. Modified with permission from Thomas J and Monaghan T (2007). *Oxford Handbook of Clinical Examination and Practical Skills*, Oxford University Press, Oxford.

Intercostal drain insertion

Indications (British Thoracic Society guidelines)

- Pneumothorax:
  - In any ventilated patient.
  - Tension pneumothorax after initial needle decompression.
  - Persistent or recurrent pneumothorax after simple aspiration.
  - Large 2° spontaneous pneumothorax in patients >50 years.
- Malignant pleural effusion.
- Empyema and complicated parapneumonic pleural effusion.
- Traumatic haemopneumothorax.
- Postoperative for example, thoracotomy, oesophagectomy, cardiac surgery.

Equipment

- 28G intercostal drain.
- Underwater seal containing water to up to mark.
- Connection tubing.
- Line clamp.
- Roberts or other instrument for blunt dissection.
- 20mL 1% lidocaine injection.
- 10mL syringe.
- Blue needle and a green needle.
- 20mL saline injection.
- 2 or 3/0 silk on a large handheld needle.
- 11 blade scalpel.
- Skin prep.
- Sterile drape.
- Sterile gloves and gown.
- Gauze swabs.

Preparation

- Explain the procedure to the patient if appropriate.
- Ensure continual monitoring of pulse oximetry.
- Position the patient at 45° with the arm abducted (📖 see Fig. 11.5).

Technique

- Usual insertion site is the 5th intercostal space in the mid axillary line. (It may extend anteriorly to the anterior axillary line.)
- Prep and drape the skin.
- Infiltrate site for tube insertion with LA ensuring anaesthesia at all layers down to and including parietal pleura, and the periosteum of the ribs posterior to the line of the incision.
- A 2cm transverse skin incision is made and the intercostal space is dissected bluntly staying perpendicular to the skin to avoid creating a false track between muscle and fat layers.
- Firmly and carefully pass a blunt-ended clamp over the lower rib through the pleura, and spread to widen the hole.
- Place a finger into the pleural space to ensure there are no adhesions.
- Pass a chest tube **without a trocar** into the pleural space, guiding it superiorly for a pneumothorax and basally for a haemothorax.
- Secure drain with at least one strong suture, and connect immediately to an underwater seal.

Complications

- Misplacement: SC, intraparenchymal.
- Trauma to other structures: diaphragm, **spleen, liver, heart, aorta, lung parenchyma, intercostal arteries** (entry sites too low, posterior or trocar used instead of blunt dissection).
- Surgical emphysema.
- Wound infection, empyema.

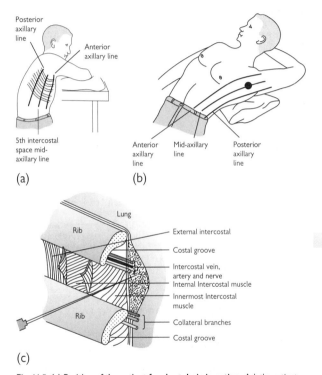

Fig. 11.5 (a) Position of the patient for chest drain insertion. Ask the patient to lean forwards over a table or the back of a chair, since this opens up the rib spaces and prevents them from moving too much. **(b) Alternative position of the patient for chest drain insertion.** Position the patient at about 45° with their arm above and behind the head, exposing the axilla. **(c) Safe pleural aspiration approach to avoid neurovascular bundles.** The main bundle sits just beneath the inferior rib edge, though collateral branches are located adjacent to the superior border. The safe approach is to advance the needle above a rib, but not right against its superior edge. Reproduced with permission from Sanders S, Dawson J, Datta S, and Eccles S (2005). *Oxford Handbook for the Foundation Programme*, Oxford University Press, Oxford.

Intercostal aspiration/pleurocentesis

Indication
- Simple pneumothorax in patient.
- Diagnostic fluid aspiration.
- Drainage of pleural effusion.

Equipment
- Cannula: 18G.
- Skin preparation fluid.
- 10mL syringe and blue needle.
- 5mL 1% lidocaine injection.
- Adhesive dressing/tape.
- 3-way tap
- 50mL syringe
- Drainage bag with Luer lock.
- Sterile container for fluid specimen for cytology, MC&S.

Preparation
- Explain procedure to patient if appropriate.
- Check CXR for fluid or air, percuss level of fluid if present.
- Position patient sitting leaning forward (fluid) or (semi) supine for air.

Technique

Simple aspiration of fluid
- Clean area of insertion: 1 intercostal space caudal to fluid level, posterior mid-clavicular linne.
- Entering above the rib, infiltrate site with LA ensuring anaesthesia at all layers down to and including parietal pleura, and the periostium of rib (💷 see Fig 11.5)
- During infiltration, aspirate at regular intervals, and once in pleural space, draw sufficient sample for tests required.
- Seal puncture wound with airtight plaster.

Pleurocentesis/thoracocentesis
- Check all required equipment is present.
- Clean area of insertion.
  - *Air*. 2nd intercostal space, mid-clavicular line.
  - *Fluid*: 1 intercostal space caudal to fluid level, posterior mid-clavicular line.
- Entering above the rib, infiltrate site with LA ensuring anaesthesia at all layers down to and including parietal pleura, and the periostium of rib (💷 see Fig 11.5).
- Insert 18G cannula into pleural space, withdraw needle and attach closed 3-way tap to cannula.
- Attach 50mL syringe to 2nd port of 3-way tap, and if aspirating fluid, sealed bag too 3rd port.
- Withdraw repeated volumes of 50mL, expel into bag (if present), until resistance felt, no further air aspirated, or 1000mL of fluid withdrawn.
- Cannula can be left in-situ for 24h for further drainage of fluid.
- Seal puncture wound with airtight plaster.

It is also possible to use a Seldinger technique to insert a pigtail drain:

Set-up and patient positioning is as described for intercostal aspiration.

After insertion of local anaesthetic insert the large blue needle into the pleural space, aspirating until fluid is obtained.

Remove the syringe, and insert the wire down the needle, then remove the needle.

Make a small nick in the skin where the wire enters with a scalpel and insert the dilators over the wire, just deep enough to enter the pleural cavity.

Remove the dilators.

Next thread the pigtail up to its hilt. Remove the wire, suture the pigtail securely in place and connect to drainage.

Nasogastric tube insertion

Indications
- Intestinal obstruction.
- Paralytic ileus.
- Perioperative gastric decompression.
- Enteral feeding adjunct (fine bore tube).

Equipment
- NGT; sizes 10–12 French.
- Gloves.
- Lubricating gel.
- Lidocaine throat spray.
- NG collection bag.
- Litmus paper.
- Stethoscope.
- Tape.

Preparation
- Chill NGT in fridge prior to passing. This stiffens the tube and makes it easier to pass.
- Position the patient, preferably in a sitting position, with the head tilted slightly forward.

Method
- Lubricate the tip of the NGT with gel.
- Pass the tube horizontally along the floor of the nasal cavity aiming towards the occiput.
- As the tube engages in the pharynx ask the patient to swallow and the tube should pass into the oesophagus.
- Advance the tube approximately 60cm.
- Check the position of the tube by:
  - Aspirating gastric contents, which will turn blue litmus red.
  - Blowing air down the tube will produce bubbling which can be heard on auscultation over the stomach.
  - Feeding tubes must be x-rayed prior to use to exclude inadvertent bronchial intubation.

Tips and problems
- *Patient has problems swallowing:* ask the patient to swallow sips of water as the tube is passed.
- *Constant coiling in the mouth:* your tube may be too soft—cool in the fridge.
- *Resistance to passing:* there may be an anatomical reason for this, e.g. oesophageal stricture. The tube may need to be passed under XR control.

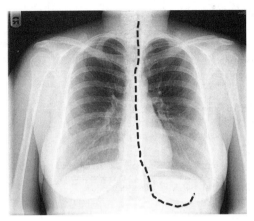

Fig. 11.6 Correct positioning of NGT, visible in stomach below the level of the left hemidiaphragm: if you cannot see the NGT and its tip, do not use it; check it isn't coiled up in the nasopharynx, and ask for repeat CXR with greater penetration.

Urethral catheterization

Catheterization of ♀ patients is usually performed by nursing staff but it is useful to learn the technique as the doctor will be asked to try if they fail!

Indications
- Perioperative monitoring of urinary output.
- Acute urinary retention.
- Chronic urinary retention.
- Aid to abdominal or pelvic surgery.
- Incontinence.

Male catheterization

Equipment
- Foley catheter (size 16–20G: always use the **largest** available to avoid creating a false tract/inflating balloon in prostate).
- Dressing/catheter pack containing drapes.
- Cleansing solution.
- Sterile gloves.
- Lidocaine gel.
- Gauze swabs.
- Drainage bag.
- 50mL bladder syringe.
- A universal specimen pot for MSU.

Preparation
- Ensure the area is screened off from public view and lay patient supine.
- Expose the genital area and cover with a sterile drape with a hole in it.

Method
- Clean hands and put on sterile gloves.
- Pick up the glans penis with your non-dominant 'dirty' hand, through the hole in the drape: the other hand will be your 'clean' hand.
- Retract the foreskin with your 'dirty' hand and, holding a swab soaked in sterile saline with your clean hand, use it to clean the urethral orifice and glans thoroughly, so that your clean fingers only touch the swab not the glans penis.
- Without letting go of the penis, discard the swab and pick up the sterile lidocaine gel with your clean hand and inject into the urethra. Warn the patient. It stings.
- Still holding the penis in a vertical position introduce the catheter with the clean hand and advance gently for approximately 10cm.
- Lower the penis to lie horizontally and advance the catheter fully (through the prostatic urethra) up to the hilt.
- Inflate the balloon now in the bladder via the smaller catheter channel with the 10mL sterile water: some catheters have an integral bulb of air which when squeezed inflates the balloon.
- ⚠ **Never** *inflate the balloon until the catheter is fully inserted as this risks inflating the balloon within the prostatic urethra, causing urethral rupture: ideally you should see urine before inflating the balloon.*
- Attach a catheter bag firmly to the catheter.
- *Replace the foreskin to avoid paraphimosis.*

Tips and problems
- *No urine immediately*:
  - The bladder has just been emptied: insert a 2mL syringe into the end of the catheter and aspirate any residual urine.
  - The catheter tip may be blocked with lidocaine gel—try gently instilling 15–20mL of sterile water and gently aspirating.
- *Still no urine:* the patient may be anuric or a false passage may have been created—palpate to see if the bladder is empty or if you can feel the catheter balloon (which should not normally be palpable).
  - Treat anuria appropriately: 📖 see p. 212.
  - Consult a senior colleague if a false passage may have been created.
- *Inability to insert:* try a smaller catheter or a silastic (firmer). If unsuccessful, ask a senior for help; suprapubic catheterization may be needed.
- *Decompression of grossly distended bladder:* rapid decompression of a distended bladder (from chronic retention, for example) may result in mucosal haemorrhage. Empty the bladder by 250–500mL every 30min until empty. Then monitor urine output closely, as a brisk diuresis and dehydration may follow.
- *Bypassing catheter:* usually due to catheter blockage. Check urine output, flush the catheter, and observe. If urine is flowing down the catheter and bypassing it, the catheter may be too small—try a slightly larger size.
- *Catheter stops draining.* The catheter may be blocked. Flush as described; if unsuccessful, try inserting a new catheter. Is the patient oliguric or anuric? Treat appropriately.

Female catheterization

⚠ *In many hospitals ♂ are not allowed to catheterize* **awake** *♀. Check before doing do and request a ♀ chaperone.*

Equipment
📖 As for ♂, see Male catheterization p. 360.

Preparation
Ensure privacy. Lie patient on back with knees bent. Ask the patient to place heels together and allow knees to fall apart as far as possible.

Method
A similar technique is employed here to ♂ catheterization, but note:
- Separate the labia minora with the left hand and ensure the whole genital area is adequately cleaned using the right hand
- Identify the external urethral orifice. If this proves difficult in obese patients, an assistant may help by retracting the dependant fat from the pubic area.
- Lubricate the tip of the catheter with sterile water or lidocaine gel and pass gently into the urethra.

Tips and problems
Difficulty identifying urethral orifice: after warning the patient, place an index finger in the vagina to elevate the anterior vulva. Guide the catheter along the finger into the urethra (📖 see Fig. 11.7, p. 363).

Suprapubic catheterization

Indications

Urinary retention with failed or contraindicated urethral catheterization.

Cautions

- Do not perform suprapubic catheterization on a patient with known bladder tumour or previous bladder surgery—seek expert advice.
- Ensure by clinical examination (and, if available, US bladder scanning) that the bladder is full and distended.
- Check clotting: if INR >2.0, platelets <50 or APTT >50 get senior advice before proceeding.

Equipment

- Dressing pack.
- Gloves.
- Cleansing solution.
- Two 10mL syringes.
- 25G and 21G needle.
- 10mL 1% lidocaine injection.
- Prepacked suprapubic catheter set (usually containing catheter, trocar, and scalpel).
- 1/0 silk suture.
- Catheter bag.

Preparation

- Ensure privacy. Lie patient supine and expose abdomen.
- Confirm clinically an enlarged, tense bladder.
- Identify catheterization site, 3–4cm (two finger breadths) above the symphysis pubis.

Method

- Clean the skin thoroughly around the site and apply drapes.
- Inject lidocaine into skin and SC tissues, injecting and aspirating in turn *until urine is withdrawn.*
- Two systems for introducing a suprapubic catheter are available.

'Nottingham' introducer (uses trocar)

- Make a 1cm incision at the identified site.
- Advance the catheter, with trocar in place, through the incision and SC tissues. A 'give' will be felt as the bladder is entered.
- Withdraw the trocar and ensure that there is free flow of urine from the catheter.
- Inflate the catheter balloon and suture the flange of the catheter to the skin.
- Attach a catheter bag.

Bonanno (based on the Seldinger technique)

- Make a 5mm nick in the skin.
- Take the introducer needle and advance it aspirating until urine is withdrawn.

- Remove the syringe and pass the guidewire down the needle into the bladder, then remove the needle, holding the guidewire in place.
- Pass the dilator firmly over the wire, into the bladder.
- Remove the dilator and pass the catheter into the bladder, securing it as above.

Tips and problems

- *Bypassing urine:* with some types of catheter and trocar, urine may initially bypass the catheter. This will cease with full advancement of the catheter and decompression of the bladder.
- *No urine, or faeculent matter in catheter:* obtain help—you may have entered the peritoneum or bowel.

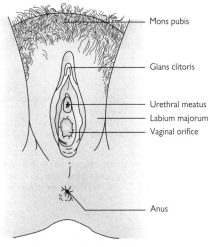

Fig. 11.7 Diagrammatic representation of the ♀ external genitalia showing position of the urethral meatus. ♀ urethral catheterization. Reproduced with permission from Thomas J and Monaghan T (2007). *Oxford Handbook of Clinical Examination and Practical Skills,* Oxford University Press, Oxford.

Paracentesis abdominis

This is a useful technique in some patients for the diagnosis and management of ascites, often in a patient with malignancy.

Indications
- Diagnostic evaluation of ascites.
- Therapeutic drainage of ascites.

Equipment
- Dressing pack.
- Gloves.
- Cleansing solution.
- 10mL syringe and 21G and 25G needles.
- 10mL 1% lidocaine injection.
- 1/0 silk suture.
- Bonano catheter or paracentesis catheter, 3-way tap and collecting bag for therapeutic drainage.
- Specimen container if appropriate.
- Dressing.
- Scalpel

Preparation
- Ensure privacy. Position the patient supine and expose the abdomen.
- Percuss out and identify the position of ascites.
- Identify a suitable tap site: the right lower quadrant is the commonest with the patient turned semilateral to ensure the ascites fills this area.

Method
- Prepare the skin at the appropriate site and place sterile drapes.
- Infiltrate LA into skin and SC tissues down to the peritoneum. Aspirate as the needle is advanced, to avoid accidental vessel puncture.

Diagnostic tap
- While injecting LA, enter peritoneal cavity. A 'give' should be felt and fluid freely aspirated at this point.
- Withdraw 10–20mL of fluid for a diagnostic evaluation.
- Remove the needle carefully and apply an occlusive dressing.

Therapeutic drainage
- Make small incision into abdominal wall and introduce catheter until 'give' felt. Trial aspirate with a syringe if ascites not draining spontaneously.
- Slide catheter into peritoneal cavity while holding needle stationary. Stop if resistance is encountered.
- Secure catheter with stitch and dressing and attach catheter bag.
- Drain up to 3000mL of ascites before clamping. If drainage is too fast, large fluid shifts can cause haemo dynamic compromise, especially if ascites is a transudate.
- Remove catheter once drainage complete.

Tips and problems

- *Unable to aspirate adequate quantity of fluid:* the ascites may be loculated. Drainage under US guidance may be helpful.
- *Blood or faeculent material:* continual staining of the ascitic fluid with fresh blood or any staining with faeculent material may indicate puncture of a vessel or viscus. This is potentially serious—inform a senior colleague.
- Some patients who require repeated ascitic drainage may benefit from daily drainage of ascites for symptomatic relief. There is a risk of peritonitis and only a short period of use is usually recommended, e.g. 2–3 days.
- The volume of ascites drained should be closely monitored along with the patient's serum albumin and overall fluid balance. A maximum drainage of 2L/day is usually advised if ascites a transudate.

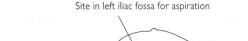

Site in left iliac fossa for aspiration

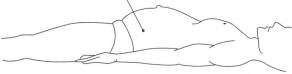

Fig. 11.8 Performing a diagnostic tap. Reproduced with permission from Thomas J and Monaghan T (2007). *Oxford Handbook of Clinical Examination and Practical Skills,* Oxford University Press, Oxford.

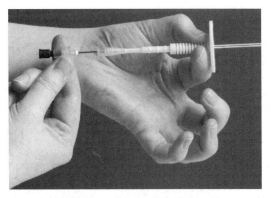

Fig. 11.9 The assembled catheter components. Reproduced with permission from Thomas J and Monaghan T (2007). *Oxford Handbook of Clinical Examination and Practical Skills,* Oxford University Press, Oxford.

Rigid sigmoidoscopy

This is a useful skill to learn. It is usually performed in the outpatient department as part of the investigation of lower GI complaints, but may have to be performed on the ward, e.g. acute admissions with rectal bleeding.

Indications
- Investigation of anorectal symptoms.
- Visualization of the rectum.

Equipment
- Rigid sigmoidoscope with obturator and light source.
- Lubricating jelly.
- Gloves.
- Gauze swabs.

Preparation
- Position the patient in the left lateral position with the hips flexed as fully as possible and knees partially extended.
- Carry out a digital examination of the rectum to identify low-placed lesions or faecal loading, which may prevent safe insertion or obscure a useful view.

Method
- Lubricate the sigmoidoscope with jelly.
- With the obturator in place, introduce the scope gently through the anal sphincter in the direction of the umbilicus for approximately 5cm.
- Remove the obturator, attach light source, insufflator, and eyepiece.
- Introduce small amounts of air to open up the lumen.
- Advance the instrument slowly under direct vision, ensuring that a patent lumen is identified prior to advancing the scope further.
- Note the appearance of the mucosa and the presence of any mucosal lesions. The level of any lesion should also be noted using the marked scale on the outer casing of the sigmoidoscope.
- If the patient experiences significant discomfort do not persist.
- Withdraw the scope slowly, again under direct vision.
- Clean the area around the patient's anus.

Tips and problems
- *Biopsy:* unless experienced in the skill, do not attempt biopsy of lesions. Note and document their position and inform a senior colleague.
- *Unable to see the upper rectum:* remember that the rectum has a sacral curvature often pronounced in ♀, gently use the tip of the scope as a 'lever' to push the anterior wall of the rectum forward to open to lumen. If this isn't easy and painless—don't persist, it may represent pathology.
- *Rectosigmoid junction:* negotiation of the rectosigmoid junction can be difficult. The best view that can be hoped for is to see the last sigmoid fold above the junction. Do not attempt to pass the scope into the distal sigmoid—this is the role of flexible sigmoidoscopy.

Local anaesthesia (LA)

LA is used in a variety of settings and is easy to deliver. It is essential to become familiar with the different agents, their relative merits, and potential dangers.

Indications

- Minor procedures requiring anaesthesia, e.g. insertion of a chest drain, central venous access, suprapubic catheterization, etc.
- Excision of skin or SC lesions.
- Infiltration of surgical wounds postoperatively.

Cautions

- *Allergy:* do not use LA if there is a history of allergy to LA.
- *Infection* at site of infiltration: injection may spread infection. The effect of the LA will be diminished (due to an acidic environment) and injection may be more painful.
- ↑ *risk of toxicity:* heart block, low cardiac output, epilepsy, myasthenia gravis, hepatic impairment, porphyria, β-blocker, or cimetidine therapy.
- *Adrenaline:* causes vasoconstriction reducing bleeding locally and prolonging anaesthetic effect. It should not be used for injections into fingers, toes, ears, or penis (all supplied by end arteries), or where skin flaps are involved, (risks flap necrosis).

Agents

The two most commonly used agents are lidocaine and bupivacaine. Other agents, e.g. prilocaine, are less commonly used.

Lidocaine (previously known as lidocaine)

Used for local infiltration for minor procedures.

- *Concentrations:* 0.5%, 1%, and 2 %. Plain solutions (with no added adrenaline) or solutions containing adrenaline.
- *Duration of action:* rapid onset (2–3min), lasts 30–90min
- *Maximum dose:*
  - Plain solutions: 3mg/kg: 21mL 1 % or 10.5mL 2% for 70kg adult.
  - Solutions with adrenaline: 7mg/kg as systemic absorption is much slower: 49mL 1% or 24.5mL 2% for a 70kg adult.

Bupivacaine

Useful in some prolonged procedures, wound infiltration, and regional blocks as it has a longer duration of action than lidocaine.

- *Concentrations:* 0.25–0.5 % plain solutions or with adrenaline.
- *Duration of action:* slower onset than lidocaine. Effects last 3–8h.
- *Maximum dose:* 2mg/kg (depending upon indication).

Equipment
- Syringe.
- Needles 21G–25G.
- Alcohol swabs.
- Disinfecting solutioon for skin

Preparation
- Identify site of infiltration and check for any sign of infection or obvious SC blood vessels.
- Calculate maximum dose of anaesthetic for each individual patient.
- Draw up anaesthetic and check details of drug and dose.

Method
- Clean skin thoroughly.
- Inject anaesthetic slowly with a fine needle to area required, aspirating before each delivery to prevent accidental IV injection.
- Injecting LA in a fan-shaped area subcutaneously from a single skin entry-point is often more comfortable for the patient.
- Field block. Injecting anaesthetic into the tissues surrounding the area which is to be anaesthetized (e.g. a cutaneous lesion) will often produce a field block, including the area itself.

Tips and problems
- *You are more likely to achieve good anaesthetic block with a large volume of less concentrated LA, than a small volume of more concentrated LA: generally use 1% rather than 2%.*
- *Allow 2–3min for the LA to take effect: spend this time setting up your instruments and draping the patient.*
- *Accidental IV injection:* Stop injection. Place patient on cardiac monitor or rhythm abnormalities. Keep a finger on their pulse and engage them in conversation so that if they become drowsy or arrest, it is very obvious. ALS guidelines apply.
- *Inadequate analgesia:* infiltrate more anaesthetic up to the patient's maximum calculated dose. If the patient is still not tolerating the procedure, alternative anaesthetic methods may have to be considered, e.g. regional anaesthesia (note maximum LA dose), sedation, or GA.
- The smaller the needle, and the more slowly you inject initially, the less painful it is for the patient.
- Use the smallest needle that is long enough for the depth of injection required.
- If a 21G (green) needle is required, short with 25G (orange) at the short and change over once anaesthetised.

Intercostal nerve block

This may be a useful skill to learn, although it is usually performed by anaesthetists.

Indications
- Pain due to fractured ribs.
- Post-thoracotomy pain relief.

Equipment
- Dressing pack.
- Skin antiseptic.
- Gloves.
- 20mL syringe and needle.
- 20mL of LA, e.g. bupivacaine.

Preparation
The patient is positioned as for pleural aspiration (📖 see Pleural aspiration, p. 356) and the site of infiltration is identified:
- *Broken ribs:* medial to the site of fracture on the posterior aspect of the chest wall.
- *Post-thoracotomy:* medial to the posterior edge of the scar on the posterior chest wall.

Method
- Ensure that the skin is prepared thoroughly with antiseptic. Drapes are placed appropriately.
- Insert the needle and syringe containing anaesthetic through the skin, inferior to the rib (unlike pleural aspiration) associated with the nerve to be blocked.
- Aspirate the syringe to ensure that the needle has not entered a blood vessel or the pleural space. If no blood or air is withdrawn, the site is infiltrated with 4–5mL of anaesthetic.
- This is repeated at various sites.
- Obtain a CXR to ensure a pneumothorax has not complicated the procedure.

Note
- *Multiple blocks:* Ensure that the patient does not receive a toxic dose of LA.
- *Air or blood is aspirated:* withdraw the needle slowly, repeat procedure in different place. Compress bleeding vessel if arterial puncture.

A-Z of surgical procedures

Individual procedures are described with an estimate of their impact on the patient (major, intermediate, minor), Indication, preoperative investigations and expected postoperative course are detailed, together cross-references for common complications.

📖 See Box 11.4 for a definition of common surgical terms used to describe surgical procedures.

Box 11.4 Commonly used terms

Most operations are described in the following way:

Organ or area operated:

Lapar-	Abdomen (laparus = flank)
Nephro-	Kidney
Pyelo-	Renal pelvis
Cysto-	Bladder
Chole-	Bile/the biliary system
Col(on)-	Large bowel
Hystero-	Uterus
Thoraco-	Chest
Rhino-	Nose
Mast-/Mammo-	Breast

Other elements involved:

Docho-	Duct
Angio-	Vessel (blood or bile carrying)
Litho-	Stone

Type of procedure:

-otomy	To cut (open)
-ectomy	To remove
-plasty	To change shape or size
-pexy	To change position
-raphy	To sew together
-oscopy	To look into
-ostomy	To create an opening in (stoma =mouth)
-paxy	To crush
-graphy/-gram	Image (of)

Approach:

Percutaneous	Via the skin
Trans-	Across
Per	Through
Antegrade	Forward
Retrograde	Backwards
Scopic	Video assisted through small ports
Peri	Near or around
Hemi	Half

So: laparoscopic cholecystectomy—removal of the gall bladder from the abdomen by video-assisted keyhole surgery.

A–Z of surgical procedures

A

Abdominal aortic aneurysm (AAA) repair (Table 11.1)

- Emergency much higher risk.
- Elective AAA repair also performed using endovascular stent.

Table 11.1 Replace aneurysmal abdominal aorta with Dacron graft via laparotomy (major + cardiovascular)

Preoperative	XM6U, 2UFFP, 10UPlts, CT, US, ?TTE/carotids, book ICU	
Indication	Postoperative course	Specific problems
AAA (elective or emergency)	NBM 48h, passing flatus by 48 h, drains out by 72h, BO and eating and drinking by 72h, H 5–7 days,	Death, CVA (📖 p. 298), MI (📖 p. 122), ARF (📖 p. 212), gut ischaemia (📖 p. 157), limb ischaemia (📖 p. 158), damage to ureters (📖 p. 213), bleeding (📖 p. 98)

Abdominoperineal (AP) resection (Table 11.2)

If it is possible to preserve the anal sphincter, it may be possible to avoid the need for a stoma by creating an ileoanal pouch: this is sometimes done as a 2-stage procedure, with a temporary ileostomy (📖 see p. 94)

Table 11.2 Resection of anus, rectum, sigmoid colon via laparotomy and perineal approach, with formation of end colostomy (major +)

Preoperative	XM2U, histology, imaging, CT, mark stoma, book HDU	
Indication	Postoperative course	Specific problems
Low rectal cancer	NBM 24h, passing flatus by 24h, drains out by 72h, stoma output 24h, remove Foley 72h, eating and drinking by 72h, *histology 5 days*, H 7 days,	Death (1–2%), stoma (📖 p. 94), ileus (📖 p. 256), phantom rectum, anastomotic leak (📖 p. 262), damage to pelvic ureters (📖 p. 213), SBO or LBO (📖 p. 256),

Adhesiolysis (Table 11.3)

Table 11.3 Division of adhesions from previous surgery via laparotomy or laparoscopy ± resection of infarcted small bowel (intermediate)

Preoperative	G&S, contrast study, HDU if emergency presentation	
Indication	Postoperative course	Specific problems
(Small) bowel obstruction	Mobilize and oral fluids day 1, normal diet day 2 on return of normal bowel function, continue IV fluid resuscitation, home day 5–10	Death, 5%, stoma (📖 p. 94), ↓Na⁺ (📖 p. 228), ↓K⁺ (📖 p. 232), ileus (📖 p. 256), anastomotic leak (📖 p. 262)

Adrenalectomy (Table 11.4)

Preoperative alpha and beta-blockade for phaeochromocytomas (📖 p. 288).

Table 11.4 Removal of either/both adrenal glands via laparotomy or subcostal or posterior subcostal or laparoscopy (major)

Preoperative	XM2u, CT or MRI, MIBG scan, mark side, book HDU	
Indication	Postoperative course	Specific problems
Adrenal cancer Phaeodiromocytoma	NPO 24h, passing flatus by 24h, H 7–10 days, (1–2 days if laparoscopic) histology, phaeo pts need haemodynamic monitoring for 72h postop, all pts supplement gluco + mineralocorticoids (p. 286)	Addisonian crisis (📖 p. 286), ileus (p. 256)

Amputation (AKA/BKA/TKA) (Table 11.5)

Table 11.5 Removal leg above/below/ through knee (intermediate)

Preoperative	G&S, mark leg	
Indication	Postoperative course	Specific problems
Limb ischaemia, trauma	Mobilize non weight-bearing 24h, drains out 48h, prosthesis fitting day 4, H 5 days	Stump healing (📖 p. 166), residual ischaemia, phantom limb pain or sensation, psychosocial issues

Anorectal abscesses (Table 11.6)

Table 11.6 Opening anal fistula, draining pus (intermediate)

Indication	Postoperative course	Specific problems
Anorectal abscess	Mobilizing, eating and drinking day 1. H 1–2 days	Bleeding (📖 p. 98)

Anterior resection (Table 11.7)

More acceptable to patients than AP resection which involves a stoma and perineal incision with loss of anus.

Table 11.7 Resection of upper 1/3rd of rectum via laparotomy, and primary anastomosis (major)

Preoperative	XM2U, contrast studies, histology	
Indication	**Postoperative course**	**Specific problems**
High rectal cancer	NPO 48h, passing flatus by 48h, drains out by 72h, BO and eating and drinking by 72h, H 5–7 days, histology 5 days	Ileus (📖 p. 256), anastomotic leak (📖 p. 262),

Aortic valve replacement (AVR) (Table 11.8)

Tissue valves do not normally need warfarinizing.

Table 11.8 Replacement of aortic valve with tissue or mechanical prosthesis via median sternotomy on cardiopulmonary bypass (major+ cardiac)

Preoperative	XM2U, angiogram, TTE, carotids, dentist, book ICU	
Indication	**Postoperative course**	**Specific problems**
Severe AS Severe AI	On ICU 24h, extubated by 6–12h, drains out 24h, off inotropes 24h, remove pacing wires day 3–4, start warfarin (📖 p. 399), eating and drinking 48h, mobilizing 24–48h, ECG day 1–3. Daily weights, postop TTE day 4, H 5–7 days,	Death, CVA (📖 p. 298), MI (📖 p. 122), AF (📖 p. 136), CHB (📖 p. 133), ARF (📖 p. 212), bleeding (📖 p. 98), tamponade (📖 p. 128)

Aortobifemoral (trouser) graft (Table 11.9)

Table 11.9 Replace aneurysmal abdominal aorta + iliacs with Dacron graft via laparotomy (major+ cardiovascular)

Preoperative	XM2U, contrast study, book HDU	
Indication	Postoperative course	Specific problems
AAA (elective or emergency)	NPO 48h, passing flatus by 48h, drains out by 72h, BO and eating and drinking by 72h, H 5–7 days,	Death, CVA (📖 p. 298), MI (📖 p. 122), ARF (📖 p. 212), gut ischaemia (📖 p. 157), limb ischemia (📖 p. 158), damage to pelvic ureters (📖 p. 213), bleeding (📖 p. 98)

Appendicectomy (Table 11.10)

Perforated appendix associated with longer operation, more systemically unwell, prolonged postoperative course.

Table 11.10 Removal of appendix via small laparotomy or laparoscopically (intermediate)

Preoperative	G&S	
Indication	Postoperative course	Specific problems
Appendicitis	NPO 24h, mobilizing and passing flatus by 48h, eating and drinking by 72h, H 3–5 days, histology 5 days	Ileus (📖 p. 256), residual sepsis or stump leak (📖 p. 262),

Austin Moore (📖 see Hemiarthoplasty hip, p. 381)

B

Breast reconstruction (TRAM flap/Lat dorsi flap) (Table 11.11)

Table 11.11 Post-mastectomy creation of new breast using skin and muscle flap, with blood supply either pedicled or re-anastomosed. For rectus abdominus (TRAM) donor incision is long suprapubic, for latissimus dorsi donor incision is long posterior (major)

Preoperative	XM2U, mark side, book HDU if free flap planned, preoperative photo	
Indication	Postoperative course	Specific problems
Post-mastectomy (can be delayed or immediate)	Eat, drink, mobilize day 1, drains out day 2–3, check flap every hour for signs of ischaemia (warm, cap refill, colour), postop photo day 7, H 7–10 days,	Two wound sites: haematoma (📖 p. 99), flap necrosis, seroma, prosthesis infection, lymphoedema (📖 p. 333)

C

Carotid endarterectomy (CEA) (Table 11.12)

Table 11.12 Removal of plaque from internal carotid artery and closure with patch angioplasty (Dacron or saphenous vein) via 10cm longitudinal lateral neck incision (major)

Preoperative	G&S, duplex or angiography	
Indication	Postoperative course	Specific problems
Carotid stenosis ± CVA/TIA	Mobilize, eat and drink 1, 4, day 3–4	CVA (📖 p. 298), need for re-exploration, injury to CN XI, X, XI, bradycardia (📖 p. 138), haematoma (p. 99), cerebral hypoperfusion

Cervical discectomy (Table 11.13)

Table 11.13 Removal of intervertebral disc with curettes via either 8–10cm incisions along sternocleidomastoid, or midline posterior (intermediate)

Preoperative	XM2U, cross-sectional imaging	
Indication	Postoperative course	Specific problems
Herniated disc with root compression	Mobilize, eat and drink day 1, H 1–2 days, postop X-ray day 1 or 2 if bone graft or internal fixation/fusion	Spinal cord or nerve root injury (📖 p. 421), vertebral or carotid artery injury, oesophageal or tracheal injury, RLN injury (📖 p. 207) haematoma (📖 p. 99)

Coronary artery bypass grafting (CABG), offpump CABG (OPCAB) (Table 11.14)

All patients should receive aspirin, statin and beta blocker or ACE-inhibitor.

Table 11.14 Anastomosis of saphenous vein to aorta and coronary arteries, and/or left internal mammary artery to coronary artery via median sternotomy with or without cardiopulmonary bypass (major+ cardiac)

Preoperative	XM2U, angiogram, TTE, carotids, check veins, book ICU	
Indication	Postoperative course	Specific problems
Severe IHD	On ICU 24h, extubated by 6–12h, drains out 24h, off inotropes 24h, start aspirin, statin, eating and drinking 48h, mobilizing 24–48h, daily weights to monitor diuresis, ECG day 1–3, H 5–7 days	Death, CVA (📖 p. 298), MI (📖 p. 122), AF (📖 p. 136), ARF (📖 p. 212), bleeding (📖 p. 98), tamponade (📖 p. 128)

Cholecystectomy (Table 11.15)

Table 11.15 Removal of gall bladder usually laparoscopically, very occasionally via 15cm right subcostal incision ± ERCP (intermediate–major)

Preoperative	G&S, HIDA or US scan, mark side	
Indication	Postoperative course	Specific problems
Cholecystitis	Mobilize, eat and drink day 1 for elective op, emergencies may need to wait 48h until return normal bowel activity, H1–2 days laparoscopic, 3–4 days open	Conversion to open (5%), bile duct injury (📖 p. 266), subhepatic abscess (📖 p. 251)

Cleft palate surgery (Table 11.16)

Table 11.16 Use of mucoperiosteal flaps to lengthen palate and close palatal defect via facial and sub labial incisions (intermediate)

Preoperative	G&S	
Indication	Postoperative course	Specific problems
Cleft palate	Mobilize from day 1. NPO 24h, with IV fluids. Liquid diet 1 day for 1 week. 4 day 1–2	Respiratory compromise (📖 p. 180), dehydration (📖 p. 65), poor nutrition

Common bile duct (CBD) exploration (Table 11.17)

Death rates up to 20% in emergencies, or malignancy.

Table 11.17 Open CBD, insert T tube, close duct round T tube, cholangiogram, via subcostal incision or laparoscopically (intermediate)

Preoperative	G&S (XM2U if stricture not gallstones), ERCP, US	
Indication	Postoperative course	Specific problems
Blocked CBD due to gallstones/ stricture/ cancer	Mobilize, drink clear liquids day 1 for elective op, emergencies may need to wait 48h until return normal bowel activity, T-tube cholangiogram POD 6, clamp if NAD, unclamp if pain, remove 2–3 weeks in OPD, H 5–10 days	Death 1–2%, conversion to open (5%), bile duct injury (📖 p. 266), T tube displaced—bile peritonitis, pancreatitis, retained CBD stone

Craniotomy (Table 11.18)

Table 11.18 Entry skull via 10–15cm scalp skin flap and burr-holes connected by craniotome (major)

Preoperative	XM2U, cross-sectional imaging, book neuro ICU bed	
Indication	Postoperative course	Specific problems
Space occupying lesion, intracranial haematoma, aneurysm	Intubated and ventilated until appropriate conscious level 0–24h, removal spinal CSF drain if present, when ICP normalizes, removal staples 10 days, H 2–5 days	Haemorrhage requiring surgical evacuation (📖 p. 295), infection and cerebritis, cerebral oedema (📖 p. 295), CVA (📖 p. 298), seizures (📖 p. 306), CSF leak

Cystectomy and urinary diversion (Table 11.19)

Table 11.19 Removal of bladder, ± pelvic lymphadenectomy ± construction of either ileal conduit to stoma, or reservoir from small and/or large bowel, connected to skin by small stoma via laparotomy (major)

Preoperative	XM2U, histology, bowel prep, book HDU bed	
Indication	Postoperative course	Specific problems
Bladder cancer, neurogenic bladder	Mobilize day 1, NPO then clear liquids when normal bowel activity resumes day 3–4, contrast neo-cystogram day 5, H histology H day 7–10	Ileus (📖 p. 256), infarcted conduit, anastomotic leak (📖 p. 262), ARF/oliguria, bleeding (📖 p. 98). Obturator nerve injury, UTI (📖 p. 88), mucus occlusion catheter (📖 p. 361)

D

Debridement (Table 11.20)

Table 11.20 Removal dead skin, muscle and bony tissue and contaminants from wound using combination of surgical resection, pulsatile lavage ± antibiotic solution, scrubbing (intermediate-major)

Preoperative	G&S	
Indication	Postoperative course	Specific problems
Contaminated or infected wounds	Mobilize, eat and drink day 1, if vacuum dressing change every 48–72h for 2–10 weeks, aggressive physiotherapy	Haematoma (📖 p. 99), wound infection (📖 p. 96)

Dynamic hip screw (DHS) (Table 11.21)

- Usually elderly, with multiple comorbidity and at high risk of postoperative complications, and sequelae of whatever caused the fall including:
  - Cardiovascular problems: MI, CVA, AF, heart failure.
  - Respiratory problems: chest infection, atelectasis, COPD.
  - Renal and fluid balance: ARF, fluid overload, dehydration.
  - Gastrointestinal problems: peptic ulcers, malnutrition.
  - Pressure sores, urinary retention, confusion.
- Long term residential care may be needed: start planning this early.

Table 11.21 Insertion metal rod through femoral trochanters across fracture, held in place with 3–4 screws into a plate via longitudinal incision over lateral hip (intermediate)

Preoperative	XM2U, mark side, X-rays, start discharge planning	
Indication	Postoperative course	Specific problems
Fracture neck of femur(NOF)	Mobilize weight bearing as tolerated day 1, eat and drink day 1 postop, physio, PA and lateral X-ray day 4–5 to check prosthesis alignment, drains out day 3–4 if present. H day 5–7	Low grade fever, DVT and PE (🕮 p. 194), haematoma (🕮 p. 99), peroneal nerve palsy (🕮 p. 421), stiffness

E

Endoscopic sinus surgery (ESS) (Table 11.22)

Table 11.22 Removal of tumour, repair CSF leak, drain sinus and intraorbital abscesses via endoscopic approach (intermediate)

Preoperative	G&S, MRI head/sinuses, bleeding	
Indication	Postoperative course	Specific problems
Recurrent sinusitis, tumours	Eat, drink, and mobilize from day 1. 4 day 1–2	MRI head/sinuses, bleeding (🕮 p. 98), CSF leak, ophthalmic complications including blindness

F

Femoropopliteal/femorodistal bypass graft (Table 11.23)
Femoral distal graft more prone to failure than femoropopliteal graft

Table 11.23 Anastomosis saphenous vein or Dacron graft to femoral artery and popliteal or more distally via long incision along course of saphenous vein, or two or three smaller incisions (major cardiovascular)

Preoperative	XM2U, arteriography	
Indication	Postoperative course	Specific problems
Chronic limb ischaemia	Mobilize, eat and drink day 1, elevate leg to reduce oedema, SQH, monitor DP and PT pulses, sometimes duplex conduit day 4, H day 4–6	Death, CVA (📖 p. 298), MI (📖 p. 122), bleeding (📖 p. 98), leg oedema (📖 p. 314), graft thrombosis (📖 p. 158), graft infection (📖 p. 90)

Femoral embolectomy (Table 11.24)

Table 11.24 Use balloon tipped flexible catheter (Fogarty) to remove embolus from femoral artery and distally via 4cm groin incision (intermediate)

Preoperative	G&S, arteriography	
Indication	Postoperative course	Specific problems
Acute limb ischaemia	Mobilize, eat and drink day 1, elevate leg to reduce oedema, SQH, monitor DP and PT pulses, look for source of embolus (TTE, CT angio) 4, H day 4–6	Death, CVA (📖 p. 298), MI (📖 p. 122), bleeding (📖 p. 98), leg oedema (📖 p. 314), compartment syndrome (📖 p. 314), leg ischaemia (📖 p. 158), haematoma (📖 p. 99), nerve paresis (📖 p. 421), lymphocele

Femoral intramedullary nail (Table 11.25)

Table 11.25 Insertion large metal rod through femoral shaft across fracture, nailed into place via longitudinal incision over lateral hip (intermediate)

Preoperative	XM2U, mark side, X-rays	
Indication	Postoperative course	Specific problems
Trauma	Mobilize weight bearing as tolerated day 1, eat and drink day 1 postop, physio, PA and lateral X-ray day 4–5 to check prosthesis alignment, drains out day 3–4 if present	Low grade fever, DVT and PE (📖 p. 194), haematoma (📖 p. 99), peroneal nerve palsy (📖 p. 421), stiffness

G

Gastrectomy (Table 11.26)

Table 11.26 Resection of whole stomach (total) or antrum only (subtotal) via laparotomy for the primary treatment of gastric cancer. Lymph node dissection to at least D2 improves outcome and is mandatory (major)

Preoperative	G&S, cross-sectional imaging, staging laparoscopy	
Indication	Postoperative course	Specific problems
Gastric Cancer, peptic ulcer disease (rarely)	NPO until oral contrast study day 3–4, feed via PEG or PEJ ± TPN. Mobilise day 1, drains out day 2–3. Flatus 48h. Epidural out day 2–4. *Histology* day 5. H day 10–14.	Death, anastomotic leak (📖 p. 262) pneumonia (📖 p. 192), ileus (📖 p. 256)

Gastric banding (Table 11.27)

Table 11.27 Intermediate

Preoperative		
Indication	Postoperative course	Specific problems
Morbid obesity	Common post-op complications in these patients are detailed on 📖 p. 284	

H

Hemiarthroplasty hip (Thompson/Austin Moore) (Table 11.28)

These patients are often elderly, with multiple comorbidity and are at high risk of postoperative complications, as well as the sequelae of whatever caused the fall including:

- Cardiovascular problems: MI, CVA, AF, heart failure.
- Respiratory problems: chest infection, atelectasis, COPD.
- Renal and fluid balance: ARF, fluid overload, dehydration.
- GI problems: peptic ulcers, malnutrition.
- Pressure sores, urinary retention, confusion.
- Long term residential care may be needed: start planning this early.

Table 11.28 Replacement head of femur with metal prosthesis either cemented (Thompson) or uncemented (Austin Moore) (intermediate)

Preoperative	XM2U, mark side, X-rays, start discharge planning	
Indication	Postoperative course	Specific problems
Intracapsular fracture NOF	Mobilize weight bearing as tolerated day 1, eat and drink day 1 postop, physio, PA and lateral XR day 4–5 to check prosthesis alignment, drains out day 3–4 if present	Low grade fever, DVT and PE (📖 p. 194), haematoma (📖 p. 99), nerve palsy (📖 p. 421), stiffness

Hemicolectomy (Table 11.29)

Table 11.29 Resection of ascending and transverse colon (right) or transverse and descending (left) and 1° anastomosis ± defunctioning ileostomy via laparotomy (major)

Preoperative	XM2U, contrast studies, histology	
Indication	Postoperative course	Specific problems
Colon cancer	NPO 48h, passing flatus by 48h, drains out by 72h, BO and eating and drinking by 72h, H 5–7 days, *histology* day 5	Ileus (📖 p. 256), anastomotic leak (📖 p. 262)

Hepatic resection (Table 11.30)

Table 11.30 Resection part of liver via large subcostal incision, with vascular inflow occlusion or ligation portal vein and hepatic artery (major+)

Preoperative	XM2U, MRI lives book HDU	
Indication	Postoperative course	Specific problems
Hepatic malignancy Trauma	NPO 24h, start NG feed, oral liquids and mobilize 48h, remove subhepatic drains 5 days, H 7–10 days	Death, hypoglycaemia (📖 p. 278), pleural effusion, pyrexia (📖 p. 90), bleeding (📖 p. 98), hepatic failure (📖 p. 264), perihepatic abscess

Hernia repair (inguinal/incisional/umbilical/femoral/ epigastric) (Table 11.31)

Table 11.31 Identifying and returning herniated abdominal contents to abdominal cavity, closure of defect in abdominal wall ± mesh via 5–6cm incision over hernia, or occasionally endoscopic (intermediate)

Preoperative	G&S, mark hernia	
Indication	Postoperative course	Specific problems
Femoral Hernia	Mobilize, eat and drink day 1, often daycase procedure, H day 1–2	Haematoma (📖 p. 99), mesh infection (📖 p. 90), residual strangulated bowel (📖 p. 256)

Hiatal hernia repair (Nissen, Belsey, Hill) (Table 11.32)
All patients should receive regular chest physio, nebulized saline and bronchodilators, and daily portable CXRs.

Table 11.32 Reposition stomach below diaphragm and restore gastro-oesophageal sphincter competence via laparotomy or laparoscopically (major)

Preoperative	XM2U, contrast study	
Indication	Postoperative course	Specific problems
Hiatus hernia	Mobilize, eat and drink day 1 for elective op, emergencies may need to wait 48h until return normal bowel activity, contrast swallow day 5, H 7–10 open, 2–5 laparoscopic	Left lower lobe atelectasis (📖 p. 76), left subphrenic abscess (📖 p. 90), dysphagia, ulceration, splenic injury

L

Laryngectomy (Table 11.33)

Table 11.33 Removal of larynx, ± part of oropharynx, mandible and tongue ± neck dissection ± reconstruction with muscle flap (major)

Preoperative	XM2U, histology, book ICU or HDU bed	
Indication	Postoperative course	Specific problems
Carcinoma of upper aerodigestive tract	Some patients may be ventilated via tracheostomy, mobilize carefully day 1, NPO and NG or PEG feed until day 10, oral contrast study day 10 to check closure, remove drains when <20mL/24h by day 4–5, H 10 days Histology day 5	Bleeding (📖 p. 98), fistula shoulder pain (CNXI), oesophageal perforation, airway obstruction

Liposuction (Table 11.34)

Table 11.34 Infiltration 1–2L fluid and LA, and removal of 500g–2kg fat through rigid suction tube via 2–4 5mm–1cm incisions usually over abdomen, or upper legs (intermediate)

Preoperative	G&S, contour marking by surgeon, preoperative photo	
Indication	Postoperative course	Specific problems
Non-uniform weight loss, Lipodystrophy	Mobilize, eat and drink day 1, compression garments, H same day or day 2	Pulmonary fat embolus (📖 p. 195), volume depletion (📖 p. 116)

Lobectomy(Table 11.35)

All patients should receive regular chest physio, nebulized saline and bronchodilators, and daily portable CXRs.

Table 11.35 Removal one or more lobes of lung via thoracotomy or occasionally thoracoscopically (major)

Preoperative	XM2U, CXR, CT, PET, histology, PFTs, book HDU	
Indication	Postoperative course	Specific problems
Lung cancer Emphysema	Mobilize day 1, eat and drink day 1 if adequate cough, drains out when no air leak and minimal drainage day 2–4, epidural out when drains out, daily CXR, Foley out when mobile, *histology* day 5, H day 5–7	Death 1%, pneumothorax (📖 p. 202), URTI (📖 p. 192), respiratory failure (📖 p. 180), prolonged air leak, AF (📖 p. 136), bleeding

Lumbar discectomy (Table 11.36)

Table 11.36 Removal of intervertebral disc with curettes via either 8–10cm posterior midline incisions or endoscopically (intermediate)

Preoperative	XM2U, MRI spine	
Indication	Postoperative course	Specific problems
Herniated disc with root compression	Mobilize, eat and drink day 1, H 1–2 days, postop XR day 1 or 2 if bone graft or internal fixation/fusion	Spinal cord or nerve root injury (📖 p. 421), CSF fluid leak, haematoma (📖 p. 99), recurrent herniation

M

Mastectomy/lumpectomy (Table 11.37)

📖 see Lymphoedema p. 333.

Table 11.37 Removal part/all breast tissue ± axillary lymph nodes (clearance) ± reconstruction with TRAM/lat-dorsi flap (intermediate–major)

Preoperative	G&S, histology, mark by surgeon	
Indication	**Postoperative course**	**Specific problems**
Breast cancer	Eat, drink, mobilize day 1, drains out day 2–3, H day 2–3 lumpectomy day 3–4 for mastectomy, longer for flaps, *histology* day 5	Haematoma (📖 p. 99), flap necrosis, seroma, prosthesis infection, lymphoedema (📖 p. 333). Flap donor site wound

Mitral valve surgery (MVR) (Table 11.38)

Tissue valves do not normally need warfarinizing.

Table 11.38 Repair or replacement of mitral valve with tissue or mechanical prosthesis via median sternotomy on cardiopulmonary bypass (major+ cardiac)

Preoperative	XM2U, angiogram, TTE, carotids, dentist, book ICU	
Indication	**Postoperative course**	**Specific problems**
Severe MS Severe MR	On ICU 24h, extubated by 6–12h, drains out 24h, off inotropes 24h, remove pacing wires day 3–4, start warfarin (📖 p. 61, 398), eating and drinking 48h, mobilizing 24–48h, daily weights to monitor fluid balance, post op TTE day 4, H 5–7 days,	Death, CVA (📖 p. 298), MI (📖 p. 122), AF (📖 p. 136), CHB (📖 p. 133), ARF (📖 p. 212), bleeding, (p. 98) tamponade (📖 p. 128)

N

Neck dissection (Table 11.39)

Table 11.39 Removal of cervical lymph nodes via longitudinal incision along sternocleidomastoid (intermediate)

Preoperative	G&S	
Indication	**Postoperative course**	**Specific problems**
Head and neck cancer	Eat, drink, and mobilize from day 1 H day 2–3, occasionally tube feeding required for several days	Bleeding (📖 p. 98), fistula, shoulder pain (CNXI), oesophageal perforation, airway obstruction.

Nephrectomy (Table 11.40)

Table 11.40 Removal of kidney ± adrenal gland and perirenal tissue ± IVC and adjacent organs via laparotomy or subcostal or posterior subcostal or laparoscopic approach, occasionally with cardiopulmonary bypass if extension of tumour up IVC to right atrium (major cardiovascular)

Preoperative	XM2U, CT or MRI, MIBG scan, mark side, book HDU	
Indication	**Postoperative course**	**Specific problems**
Renal cell carcinoma, cystic kidneys	NPO 24h, passing flatus by 24 h, H day 7–10 day, (1–2 if laparoscopic) *histology* day 5, daily U&Es, all pts supplement gluco+ mineralocorticoids	Addisonian crisis (📖 p. 286), ileus (📖 p. 256), pneumothorax (📖 p. 202), DVT and PE (📖 p. 194), bowel injury

Nissen fundoplication (Table 11.41)

Table 11.41 Wrapping cardia of stomach partially around lower oesophagus (intermediate)

Preoperative	G&S	
Indication	**Postoperative course**	**Specific problems**
GORD	Oral fluids day 1, normal diet day 3, remove on day 1 H day 3–4	Left lower lobe atelectasis, left subphrenic abscess, dysphagia, ulceration, splenic injury

O

Oesophagectomy/oesophagogastrectomy (Ivor Lewis) (Table 11.42)

Table 11.42 Resection oesophagus ± proximal stomach ± colonic interposition, via right thoracotomy and laparotomy (Ivor Lewis) or laparotomy and neck incision, or occasionally laparoscopically (major+)

Preoperative	XM2U, cross sectional imaging, histology	
Indication	Postoperative course	Specific problems
Oesophageal cancer, perforation, Banetts, oesophagus	NPO until oral contrast study day 3–4, feed via PEG or PEJ ± TPN. Mobilize day 1, drains out day 2–3. Flatus 48h. Epidural out day 4–5. *Histology* day 5. H day 10–14.	Death 1–2%, anastomotic leak (📖 p. 262), mediastinitis (📖 p. 90), pneumonia (📖 p. 192), ischaemia, ileus (📖 p. 256)

Open reduction and internal fixation (ORIF) (Table 11.43)

Table 11.43 Incision over fracture, soft tissue dissection to visualize bone, manual fracture reduction which is held in place by plate and screws, or nails, or wires (intermediate)

Preoperative	XM2U, cross-sectional imaging AP	
Indication	Postoperative course	Specific problems
Unstable fracture	Mobilize (weight bearing for all except foot and ankle fractures), eat and drink day 1, H day 3–7, postop AP and lateral XR day 1 or 2 to visualize alignment, most patients will have plaster cast	DVT and PE (📖 p. 194), prosthesis infection (📖 p. 90), haematoma (📖 p. 99), regional nerve injury (📖 p. 421)

P

Pneumonectomy (Table 11.44)

CXR should normally show pneumonectomy side gradually filling up with fluid post operatively.

Table 11.44 Removal of entire lung via posterolateral thoracotomy (major)

Preoperative	XM2U, CXR, CT, PET, histology, PFTs, book HDU	
Indication	Postoperative course	Specific problems
Lung cancer, Trauma	Mobilize day 1, eat and drink day 1 if adequate cough, drain normally out day 1, epidural out day 4–5, daily CXR to monitor fluid level which normally increases until ipsilateral hemithorax is whited out, Foley out when mobile, *histology* day 5, H day 5–7	Death 1%, pneumothorax (📖 p. 202), Chest infection (📖 p. 192), respiratory failure (📖 p. 180), prolonged air leak, AF (📖 p. 136), bleeding, bronchopleural fistula, cardiac herniation

Portal shunt (Table 11.45)

All patients should receive regular chest physio, nebulized saline and bronchodilators, and daily portable CXRs.

Table 11.45 Anastomosis between portal vein and IVC via laparotomy major or percutaneous (TIPS, transjugular intrahepatic portosystemic shunt) (minor-intermediate)

Preoperative	XM4U, book ICU bed	
Indication	Postoperative course	Specific problems
Portal hypertension ± bleeding varices	NPO 24–48h, resume oral intake when normal gut activity returns day 3–4, mobilize day 1, daily weights and girth to monitor ascites, US to evaluate shunt day 4–5, H day 7–10 days	GI bleed (📖 p. 260), shunt occlusion, ascites, hepatic encepalopthy (📖 p. 264), hepatorenal syndrome (📖 p. 264)

Prostatectomy (radical) (Table 11.46)

📖 see also TURP, p. 392.

Table 11.46 Resection of prostate, seminal vesicles, vas deferens, and pelvic lymph node dissection via perineal or retropubic approach or occasionally laparoscopic or robot assisted (major)

Preoperative	XM2U, histology	
Indication	Postoperative course	Specific problems
Carcinoma of prostate	Mobilize, eat and drink from day 1 as tolerated, H day 3–4	Ileus (📖 p. 256), urinary incontinence, impotence, retrograde ejaculation

Pyloroplasty ± vagotomy (Table 11.47)

Table 11.47 Division of pyloric sphincter ± denervation via upper laparotomy or laparoscopically (intermediate)

Preoperative	G&S, contrast studies	
Indication	Postoperative course	Specific problems
Gastric outlet obstruction secondary to PUD	NPO 24h, clear fluids when flatus 48h, H day 4–5	Dumping, diarrhoea (📖 p. 254)

S

Small bowel resection (Table 11.48)

Table 11.48 Removal part of small bowel with end stoma or 1° anastomosis ± temporary defunctioning stoma via laparotomy or laparoscopically (intermediate–major)

Preoperative	G&S, histology, contrast studies, mark stoma	
Indication	Postoperative course	Specific problems
Infarction, IBD, neoplasm, AVM, Meckels	Oral fluids day 1, flatus day 1, mobilize day 1, if all small bowel removed need TPN, stoma ouput 48h, BO 72h, normal diet 72h, *histology* day 5, H day 5–7	Death anastomotic leak (📖 p. 262), stoma (📖 p. 94), ileus (📖 p. 256), residual ischaemia (📖 p. 157)

Spinal fusion (Table 11.49)

Table 11.49 Decompression of neural structures, bone grafting, stabilization with metal internal fixation via anterior and/or posterior approaches (major +)

Preoperative	XM2U, cross-sectional imaging	
Indication	Postoperative course	Specific problems
Severe kyphosis or scoliosis	Mobilize, eat and drink day 1 if tolerated, log roll hourly, intensive specialist physiotherapy, H day 5–7 postop XR day 4 or 5 if bone graft or internal fixation/fusion	Spinal cord or nerve root injury (📖 p. 421), respiratory failure (📖 p. 180), DVT and PE (📖 p. 194), urinary retention (📖 p. 216), ileus (📖 p. 256)

Splenectomy (Table 11.50)

Death rate <1% for elective splenectomy, >30% for splenectomy associated with trauma (depending also on other injuries).

Table 11.50 Removal of spleen through laparotomy or occasionally laparoscopically (intermediate)

Preoperative	XM2U	
Indication	Postoperative course	Specific problems
Trauma, ITP and anaemias with hypersplenism	Mobilize, eat and drink day 1 for elective op, emergencies may need to wait 48h until return normal bowel activity, monitor Hb, WCC, Plts, anti *Haemophilus* and *Meningococcus* vaccine, H day 5–10	Bleeding Left lower lobe atelectasis, left suprhenic abscess, ↑↓Plts (📖 p. 100), sepsis (📖 p. 90)

T

Thompson

📖 see Hemiarthoplasty hip p. 381.

Thyroidectomy (Table 11.51)

Table 11.51 Resection either or both lobes of thyroid via 5cm transverse collar incision or endoscopically (intermediate)

Preoperative	G&S, propranolol, histology, imaging	
Indication	Postoperative course	Specific problems
Thyroid tumours, thyroid goitre, thyrotoxicosis	Eat, drink, and mobilize day 1. Daycase/H day 1–2	Bleeding (📖 p. 98), hypoparathyoidism (📖 p. 238), laryngeal nerve injury (📖 p. 207), thyroid storm (📖 p. 282)

Tonsillectomy (Table 11.52)

Day-case procedure in children, but more prolonged postoperative course in adults because of pain and bleeding.

Table 11.52 Removal of tonsillar ± adenoidal lymphoid tissue via oral route (intermediate)

Preoperative	G&S	
Indication	Postoperative course	Specific problems
Recurrent tonsillitis	Eat, drink, and mobilize from day 1. H day 1–2	Bleeding (📖 p. 98), dehydration (📖 p. 64)

Total hip replacement (Table 11.53)

Table 11.53 Replacement hip joint with metal on polyethylene prosthesis cemented to resected heads of femur and acetabulum via longitudinal incision over lateral hip (intermediate)

Preoperative	XM2U, mark side, XRs	
Indication	Postoperative course	Specific problems
OA or RA hip	Mobilize weight bearing as tolerated day 1, eat and drink day physio, PA and lateral XR day 4–5 to check prosthesis alignment, drains out day 3–4 if present Avoid hip adduction and flexion to minimize dislocation	Low grade fever, DVT and PE (📖 p. 194), haematoma (📖 p. 99), peroneal nerve palsy (📖 p. 421), stiffness, dislocation

Total knee replacement (Table 11.54)

Table 11.54 Replacement knee joint with metal prosthesis cemented to resected heads of femur and tibia via intermediate longitudinal anterior incision

Preoperative	XM2U, mark side, XRs	
Indication	Postoperative course	Specific problems
OA or RA knee	Mobilize weight bearing as tolerated day 1, eat and drink day 1 physio, AP and lateral XR day 4–5 to check prosthesis alignment, drains out day 3–4 if present Avoid hip	Low grade fever, DVT and PE (📖 p. 194), haematoma (📖 p. 99), peroneal nerve palsy (📖 p. 421), stiffness

Tracheostomy (Table 11.55)

Table 11.55 Placement hole in trachea for intubation via transverse collar incision or percutaneous Seldinger technique (intermediate)

Preoperative	G&S, stop NG feed and heparin 6h preop	
Indication	Postoperative course	Specific problems
Prolonged intubation, unprotected airway	Resume NG feeds within 6h, may be able to eat and drink, wake patient in 1–2 weeks.	Death Loss of airway (📖 p. 283), trauma to trachea, tracheal stenosis, tracheo-innominate fistula, mediastinitis tracheal ring fracture

Transphenoidal surgery (Table 11.56)

Table 11.56 Resection of pituitary tumours via sublabial, transseptal, or endonasal approach (intermediate)

Indication	Postoperative course	Specific problems
Sellar and suprasellar tumours	Mobilize eat and drink day 1, avoid coughing, sneezing and nose-blowing, use nasal decongestant, corticosteroids, monitor CSF rhinorrhoea, H day 3–4 days	CVA (📖p. 298), visual loss, diabetes insipidus, CSF rhinorrhoea

Transurethral resection of prostate (TURP) (Table 11.57)

Table 11.57 Resection of urethral prostate via cystoscopic approach using radiofrequency metal loop, and copious irrigation with Foley catheter inserted at end to tamponade bleeding (intermediate)

Preoperative	XM2u, cross-sectional imaging	
Indication	**Postoperative course**	**Specific problems**
Benign prostatic hypertrophy	Mobilize, eat, and drink day 1, H day 1–3 once voiding after Foley removal	Gross haematuria (common), urinary retention (📖 p. 216), UTI (📖 p. 88), prostatic capsular perforation with drainage urine into pelvis, TUR syndrome

U

Uvulopalatopharyngoplasty (Table 11.58)

Table 11.58 Removal of posterior soft palate, uvula, pharyngeal mucosa and tonsils via oral approach (intermediate)

Preoperative	XM2U, book HDU if severe obstructive sleep apnoea	
Indication	**Postoperative course**	**Specific problems**
Obstructive sleep apnoea	Eat, drink, and mobilize from day 1. H day 1–2	Bleeding (📖 p. 98), dehydration (📖 p. 64), nasopharyngeal reflux of liquids

V

Varicose veins stripping (high tie/saphenous ligation/avulsion) (Table 11.59)

Table 11.59 Removal of varicose veins via several 5mm incisions over course of vein (avulsion) ± ligation and avulsion of long saphenous vein at level of femoral vein via 4cm groin incision (intermediate +)

Preoperative	G&S, Duplex veins, mark varicosities	
Indication	Postoperative course	Specific problems
Varicose veins	Compression bandages, mobilize, eat, and drink normally day 1, often day-case procedure	Haematoma (p. 99), failure to identify all varicosities,

W

Whipple procedure (pancreatoduodenal resection) (Table 11.60)

Table 11.60 Removal head, neck and body of pancreas, duodenum, distal CBD, and antrum of stomach ± cholecystecomy with anastomosis duodenum to end stomach and remaining pancreas via laparotomy (major +)

Preoperative	XM4U, CT or MRI, PET, histology, HDU or ICU bed	
Indication	Postoperative course	Specific problems
Cancer head of pancreas or distal CBD	Mobilize day1–2, NJ/PEJ feeding from day 1, oral clear liquids and diet with return of normal bowel function day 2–3, erythromycin, remove drains day 5–7, *histology* day 5, H 2–3 weeks	Death 2–5%, delayed gastric emptying, pancreatic fistula, intrabdominal abscess, hyperglycaemia (p. 274)

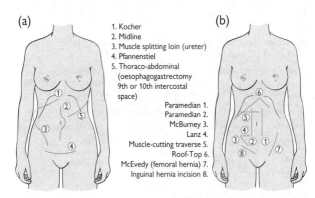

(a)

1. Kocher
2. Midline
3. Muscle splitting loin (ureter)
4. Pfannenstiel
5. Thoraco-abdominal
   (oesophagogastrectomy
   9th or 10th intercostal
   space)

(b)

Paramedian 1.
Paramedian 2.
McBurney 3.
Lanz 4.
Muscle-cutting traverse 5.
Roof-Top 6.
McEvedy (femoral hernia) 7.
Inguinal hernia incision 8.

Fig. 11.10 Surgical incisions in the abdomen. Adapted with permission from Longmore M, Wilkinson, I, Turmezei, T and Cheung, CK (2007). *Oxford Handbook of Clinical Medicine*, 7th edn, Oxford University Press, Oxford.

Useful information

Cardiovascular drugs

There are no large trials evaluating the use of cardiac drugs in reducing surgical risk. Only β-blockers have been shown to be of value in small trials and should be considered in all patients with known coronary disease where there are no specific contraindications such as asthma 206 or heart failure (📖 see p. 124).

Aspirin

Aspirin reduces the risk of arterial thrombosis but increases the risk of bleeding intra- and postoperatively. For some procedures (e.g. neurosurgery), aspirin may need to be stopped 10 days beforehand, but this is unnecessary for most surgery.

Clopidogrel

Clopidogrel reduces the risk of arterial thrombosis but greatly increases bleeding intra- and postoperatively. It is prescribed for patients past MI or with drug-eluting stents which are at high risk of thrombosis in the first year after implantation if clopidogrel is stopped. For many procedures clopidogrel may need to be stopped 10 days beforehand, so this should be discussed with a cardiologist.

β-blockers

β-blockers reduce heart rate, BP, and myocardial contractility. This in turn leads to reduced myocardial O_2 consumption. β-blockers have been shown to confer a survival advantage when given after acute MI. Abrupt withdrawal should be avoided; this may result in a rebound tachycardia and precipitate acute myocardial ischaemia.

Ca^{2+} antagonists

Ca^{2+} antagonists may be used to treat angina or hypertension. There is currently a question mark over the use of dihydropyridine Ca^{2+} channel blockers (nifedipine group), particularly short-acting preparations, which have been implicated in increasing the risk of AMI. Continue nifedipine in haemodynamically stable patients, but stop it if the BP is already controlled. It is better not to change patients from their usual brand/preparation of Ca^{2+} antagonists to another, as a rule. The effects of this class of drugs are notoriously variable between different preparations, even when they contain the same drug, and the same dose.

Nitrates

Nitrates are useful in treating the acute attack of angina when given sublingually and may be given intravenously for perioperative ischaemia. Long-acting preparations (oral or topical) are often taken by angina sufferers, but there needs to be a nitrate-free period to prevent tolerance developing.

ACE inhibitors

ACE inhibitors have been shown to improve survival in patients with LV dysfunction due to ischaemic heart disease or dilated cardiomyopathy. They can cause profound, long-lasting hypotension in critically ill patients. Stop ACE inhibitors in emergency patients at risk of hypotension, but continue them in elective cases after checking with the anaesthetist. Caution may be required when restarting ACE inhibitors in view of the profound hypotensive effect of most of these agents in hypovolaemic patients. Similarly, in patients whose serum urea and creatinine have appreciably deteriorated perioperatively, the serum values should be well on the way back to normal prior to reintroduction of ACE inhibitors—and their renal function requires close monitoring after that.

Angiotensin II inhibitors

Angiotensin II inhibitors have also been shown to improve survival in patients with LV dysfunction due to ischaemic heart disease. They act further down the same pathway as ACE inhibitors, but notably produce less coughing. Patients often are on ATII inhibitors because of this; the perioperative issues are the same as for ACE inhibitors.

Warfarin

Key facts

- Warfarin is commonly used: it inhibits vitamin K synthesis preventing formation of factors II, VII, IX, and X. It therefore takes several days for anticoagulation to peak and wear off.
- Warfarin **must** be monitored: measure INR, the ratio of patient's PT to a laboratory control. Dose needed to achieve same INR varies considerably from patient to patient (due to age, size, liver function, and concurrent medication). INR is only a useful measure of coagulation in patients taking warfarin.
- Once warfarin is stopped it takes on average 4 days for the INR to reach 1.5.
- Many drugs interact with warfarin metabolism, always check *BNF* if prescribing in patients taking warfarin.

Table 12.1 Indications for anticoagulation (BNF recommendations, updated according to the British Society for Haematology) (2005)

Indication	Target INR*	Duration of therapy
Low risk		
Prophylaxis of DVT	2	Until mobile after surgery
Use with Hickman lines**	1mg	While line in situ
Medium risk		
Proximal DVT	2.5	6 months
Pulmonary embolism	2.5	6 months
Calf vein thrombosis: non-surgical	2.5	3 months
Calf vein thrombosis: postsurgical	2.5	6 weeks
Recurrence of thromboembolism	2.5	At least 6 months
Chronic AF (any cause)	2.5	Permanent
MS with embolism	2.5	Permanent
Cardiomyopathy	2.5	Permanent
MI with mural thrombus	2.5	3 months
Symptomatic inherited thrombophilia	2.5	Permanent
Cardioversion	2.5	3 weeks pre to 4 weeks post
High risk		
Recurrent thromboembolism on warfarin	3.5	Permanent
aortic	3.0	
mitral	3.5	
Mechanical prosthetic heart valves**		Permanent
Antiphospholipid syndrome	3.5	Permanent

* Aim is ±0.5 INR units of target

** INR may be 0.5 units lower for tilting disc values

Managing anticoagulation preoperatively

Elective surgery

- Stop anticoagulation or perform surgery with the INR <2.0.
- For minor surgery, oral anticoagulants should be stopped/adjusted to achieve a target INR of approximately 2.0 on the day of surgery.
- For major surgery, stop warfarin at least 3 days before surgery.
- **Short-term** (24h) risk of thromboembolism in patients with mechanical valves is small off anticoagulants (8 per 100 patient-years).
- If medium or high risk (Table 12.1), start unfractionated heparin when INR <2.0.
- If the patient's INR is too high on the day of surgery the options are:
  - Delay surgery (usually most appropriate solution).
  - Talk to surgeon, who may be happy to proceed.
  - Give vitamin K 5–10mg IV and recheck INR in 2h (exposes patient to small risk of anaphylaxis, complicates restarting warfarin).
  - Give 2U of FFP not more than 1h before surgery (expose patient to risks of transfusion).

Urgent or emergency surgery

According to the INR, give vitamin K (phytomenadione) with prothrombin complex concentrate (factors II, VII, IX, X) or FFP as in Table 12.2.

Restarting warfarin

- Check: does the patient still need warfarin?
- Resume oral anticoagulants as soon as the patient can take tablets.
- If vitamin K has been given, there will be further 48–72h delay in achieving therapeutic anticoagulation on top of slow warfarin action due to accumulated clotting factors.
- Standard loading regimen is 10mg for 2 days, this needs to be adjusted taking into account the patient's usual warfarin dosage: a patient taking 1mg of warfarin daily will need much lower loading dose, maybe 4mg twice, a patient on 10mg warfarin daily may need 20mg twice.

Table 12.2 Recommendations for management of bleeding and excessive anticoagulation (British Society for Haematology)

INR 3.0–6.0, target 2.5	Reduce or stop warfarin
INR 4.0–6.0, target 3.5	Restart warfarin when INR <5.0
INR 6.0–8.0, no bleeding	Stop warfarin Restart when INR <5.0
INR >8.0, no bleeding	Stop warfarin Restart warfarin when INR <5.0 If other risk factors for bleeding, give vitamin K 5mg PO or 0.5mg IV
Major bleeding or emergency surgery, INR >2.5	Stop warfarin Give prothrombin complex concentrate 50U/kg or FFP 15mL/kg Give vitamin K 5–10mg IV

Heparin

Key facts

- Unfractionated heparin binds and potentiates action of anti-thrombin III, as well as inactivating activated factors XII, Xi, IX, and X.
- LMWH acts more predictably to inactivate factor Xa.
- Unfractionated heparin acts immediately, and if stopped, effects wear off in around 6h depending on liver and renal function.
- Uncommon but important side-effects: thrombocytopaenia (onset 5–10 days, ↓platelets >50%, paradoxical thrombosis), hyperkalaemia.

Thromboprophylaxis

- Low- and medium-risk patients need thrombo-prophylaxis once the INR is <2.0. This is usually SC unfractionated heparin 5000U bd, but weight-adjusted LMWH is more predictable in its anti-thrombotic effect and has an equally low risk of bleeding complications. SC heparin can be started preoperatively.
- For patients at high risk of thromboembolism (e.g. mechanical heart valve), a continuous infusion of heparin can be given, with a loading dose of 5000U followed by a continuous infusion of 18U/kg/h adjusted according to the APTT 4h after start and each dose adjustment (check local lab for target range).
- Certain surgical procedures (e.g. neurosurgery) demand very low or no anticoagulant activity. Even with mechanical heart valves, the risk of thrombosis is very low even if warfarin is stopped for up to 7 days.
- Previous DVT or PE puts the patient at ↑risk of recurrence during surgery. The factors known to further increase the likelihood of a DVT are given in Table 12.3.
- Prophylaxis should be given to those at high risk. This is discussed further on 📖 p. 61.

Table 12.3 Factors predisposing to DVT

Endothelial injury	Hypercoagulability	Stasis
Indwelling venous lines	Malignancy	Prolonged bed rest during chronic illness before surgery
Irritant injection	Oral contraception	Hip surgery
Sepsis	Dehydration	Gynaecological surgery
Thrombophlebitis obliterans	Hereditary thrombophilia	Obesity
	Blood dyscrasia	Post partum
	Idiopathic	Varicose thrombophlebitis

Starting heparin infusion
- Give a bolus of 5000U heparin IV.
- Start a heparin infusion at a rate of 2000U/h (25,000 IVL heparin in 50mL NS IV, at a rate of 4mL/h, titrate to APTT/APTR).
- Measure APTT 6-hourly and adjust the rate of heparin infusion according to Table 12.4.
- Target range for APTT is 70–90, for APTR 1.5–2.5.
- Give heparin until the INR is in the target range.

Table 12.4 Adjustment of heparin infusion rate according to APTT ratio

APTT	Change in heparin dose
>150	Stop heparin for 2h and recheck at 2h If bleeding consider 2U FFP or protamine 25mg IV
120–150	Reduce by 1000U/h
90–120	Reduce by 500U/h
70–90	No change
50–70	Increase by 500U/h
30–50	Increase by 1000U/h
<30	Give bolus 2000U and increase infusion by 2000U/h

Table 12.5 Investigation of common causes of postoperative bleeding

Condition	History and examination	APTT	PT	INR	Plts	Hb	TEG	FDP	DD	Other
Heparin	Check drug history with patient and carer, check drug chart	↑↑	↑	↑	→	→	↑R	→	→	↑Heparin level
Coumadin		↑↑	↑↑	↑↑	→	→	↑R	→	→	
Clopidogrel		→	→	→	→	→	↑K↓ MA	→	→	↓↓ Plt function studies
Haemophilia	Long Hx bruising etc.	↑↑	→	→	→	↓	↑R	→	→	↓ Factor VIII or IX
Massive transfusion	Recent Tx >8u	↑	↑	→	↓	↓/→	↑R&K↓ MA	→/↑	→/↑	Fibrinogen low
DIC	Sepsis, CPB	↑	↑	↑	↓	↓/→	↑↑ R&K↓ MA	↑↑	↑↑	Fibrinogen low
Thrombo-cytopenia	Spleno-megaly	→	→	→	↓↓	→	↑R&K↓ MA	→	→	
HIT	Heparin	→	→	→	↓↓	→	↑R&K↓ MA	→	→	Heparin antibodies
Surgical bleeding	No other bleeding site	Any of these tests may be mildly deranged, but usually normal								
Artefact	Heparin in sample (wrong tube), sample taken proximal to infusion, long delay until testing									

Example ECGs

Normal sinus rhythm

Electrocardiograph

<u>Normal ECG</u>

PR interval   120 - 200ms
QRS interval   <120ms
QT interval   350-430ms
PR and QT intervals vary with heart rate

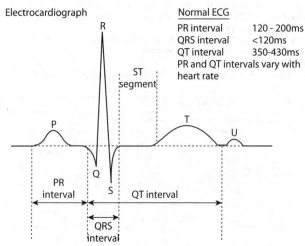

Fig. 12.1 Normal sinus rhythm. Reproduced with permission from Sanders S, Dawson J, Datta S, and Eccles S (2005). *Oxford Handbook for the Foundation Programme*, Oxford University Press, Oxford.

Atrial fibrillation

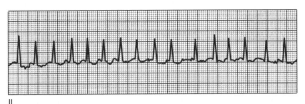

II

Fig 12.2 Atrial fibrillation. Note: irregularly irregular rhythm (QRS) and assent p-waves. Reproduced with permission from Chikwe J, Beddow E, and Glenville B (2006). *Cardiothoracic Surgery*, Oxford University Press, Oxford.

Acute anterior MI

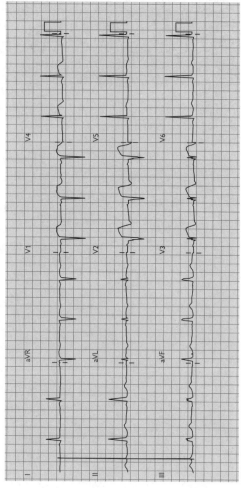

Fig. 12.3 Acute anterior MI. Note: ST segment elevation in anterior leads (V_2, V_3) with lateral ischaemia (ST segment depression) in lateral leads (II, III, aVL, V_5, V_6). Reproduced with permission from Sanders S, Dawson J, Datta S, and Eccles S (2005). *Oxford Handbook for the Foundation Programme*, Oxford University Press, Oxford.

Acute inferior MI

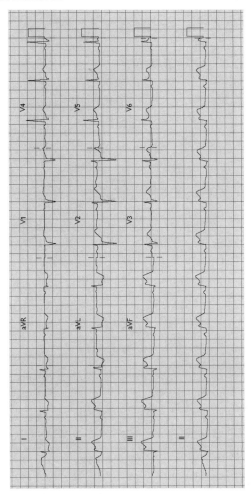

Fig. 12.4 Acute inferior MI. Note: ST segment elevation in inferior leads (II, III, aVF) and reciprocal changes in aVL/aVR. The latter do not represent ischaemia but rather are the mirror of the inferior leads. Reproduced with permission from Sanders S, Dawson J, Datta S, and Eccles S (2005). *Oxford Handbook for the Foundation Programme*, Oxford University Press, Oxford.

Myocardial ischaemia

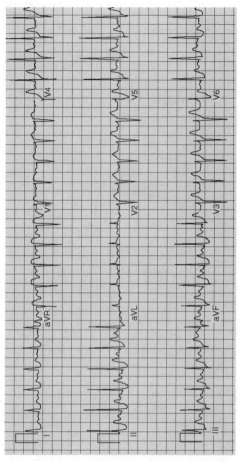

Fig. 12.5 Myocardial ischaemia. Note: wide spread ST segment depression indicating (nees) global ischaemia. The ST elevation in aVR is reciprocal and does not represent a right ventricular MI. Reproduced with permission from Sanders S, Dawson J, Datta S, and Eccles S (2005). *Oxford Handbook for the Foundation Programme*, Oxford University Press, Oxford.

Right bundle branch block

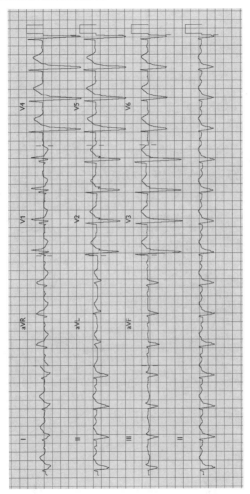

Fig. 12.6 Right bundle branch block. Note: wide QRS complex, right axis devia-
tion and RSR, in V₁. NB: RBBB allows assessment of ST segment for ischaemia.
Reproduced with permission from Sanders S, Dawson J, Datta S, and Eccles S (2005).
Oxford Handbook for the Foundation Programme, Oxford University Press, Oxford.

Left bundle branch block

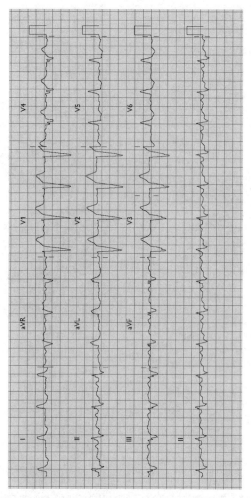

Fig. 12.7 Left bundle branch block. Note: very broad, notched QRS and inverted T waves. The latter are no ischaemia indicator of and cannot be interpreted in the context of ischaemic chest pain. In patients with a good classical presentation of ischaemic chest pain. However, new LBBB is an indication for thrombolysis. If ↑ Heart block and LBBB (trifasciculer block) CBH is likely, refer to cardiology. Reproduced with permission from Sanders S, Dawson J, Datta S, and Eccles S (2005). *Oxford Handbook for the Foundation Programme*, Oxford University Press, Oxford.

Lethal dysrhythmias

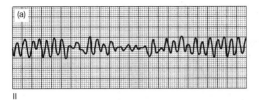

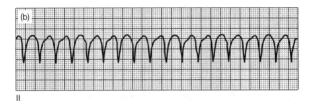

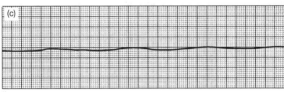

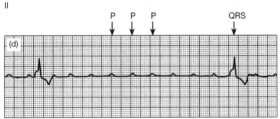

Fig 12.8 Lethal dysrhythmias. (a) Ventricular fibrillation; (b) ventricular tachycardia; (c) asystole; (d) complete heart block. Reproduced with permission from Chikwe J, Beddow E, and Glenville B (2006). *Cardiothoracic Surgery*, Oxford University Press, Oxford.

Hyperkalaemia

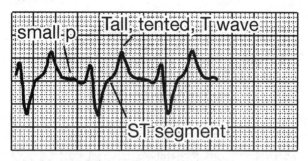

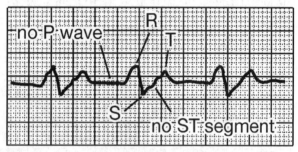

Fig 12.9 EGC changes in hyperkalaemia. Note: also the wide QRS complex.
Reproduced with permission from Chikwe J, Beddow E, and Glenville B (2006).
Cardiothoracic Surgery, Oxford University Press, Oxford.

Ventricular tachycardia

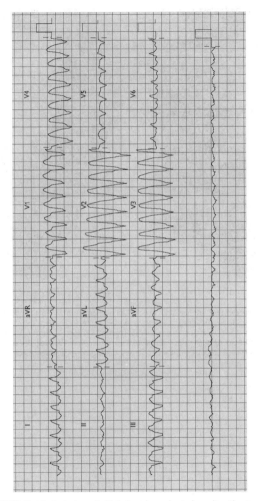

Fig. 12.10 Ventricular tachycardia. Note: broad complex tachycardia without obvious p-waves. This differentiates VT from LBBB (broad complex) with atrial flutter (discernable P-wave). Reproduced with permission from Sanders S, Dawson J, Datta S, and Eccles S (2005). *Oxford Handbook for the Foundation Programme*, Oxford University Press, Oxford.

Normal PA CXR

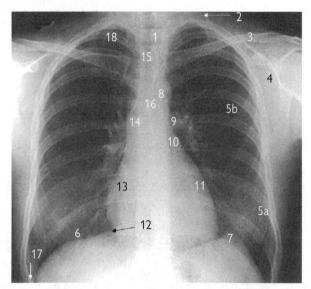

Fig. 12.11(a) Normal PA CXR. Plain PA chest X-ray. 1. Spinous process of T1 2. 1st left rib 3. Left clavicle 4. Body of left scapula 5a: 9th rib posteriorly (left) 5b: 3rd rib anteriorly (left) 6. Right hemidiaphragm 7. Left hemidiaphragm 8. Aortic knuckle 9. Pulmonary trunk 10. Left atrial appendage 11. Left ventricle 12. Inferior vena cava 13. Right atrium 14. Superior vena cava 15. Trachea 16. Carina 17. Right costophrenic angle 18. Apex right lung. Reproduced with permission from Chikwe J, Beddow E, and Glenville B (2006). *Cardiothoracic Surgery*, Oxford University Press, Oxford.

Plain left lateral chest X-ray

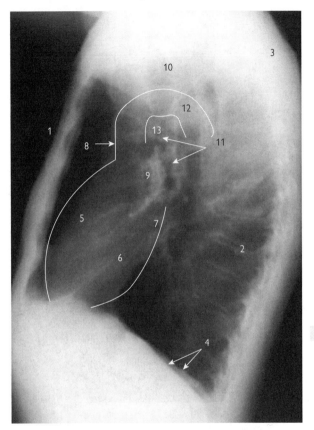

Fig. 12.11(b) Plain left lateral chest X-ray. 1. Manubriosternal junction 2. Body of thoracic vertebrae 3. Body of scapula 4. Right and left hemidiaphragms 5. Right ventricle 6. Left ventricle 7. Left atrium 8. Ascending aorta 9. Pulmonary trunk 10. Proximal trachea 11. Distal trachea 12. Distal arch of aorta 13. Aortopulmonary window. Reproduced with permission from Chikwe J, Beddow E, and Glenville B (2006). *Cardiothoracic Surgery*, Oxford University Press, Oxford.

Normal AXR

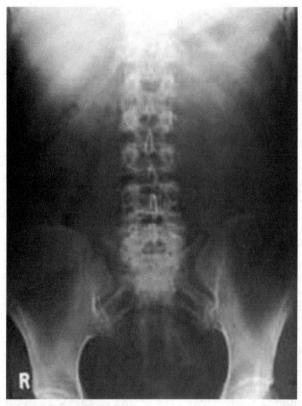

Fig 12.12 Normal abdominal plain film.

Table 12.6 Large bowel vs small bowel obstruction

	Small intestine	Large intestine
Number of loops	Lots	Few
Distribution of loops	Central	Peripheral
Diameter of loops	>2.5cm	>6cm
Haustrae[1]	No	Yes
Valvulae conniventes[2]	Yes	No
Faeces present	Nil	Yes

1 Haustrae folds which do not completely cross the bowel lumen wall.

2 Valvulae conniventes folds which do completely cross the bowel lumen wall.

Reproduced with permission from Sanders S, Dawson J, Datta S, and Eccles S (2005). *Oxford Handbook for the Foundation Programme*, Oxford University Press, Oxford.

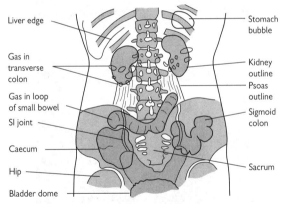

Fig. 12.13 Main features of the abdominal X-ray. Reproduced with permission from Sanders S, Dawson J, Datta S, and Eccles S, (2005). *Oxford Handbook for the Foundation Programme*, Oxford University Press, Oxford.

Normal CT chest

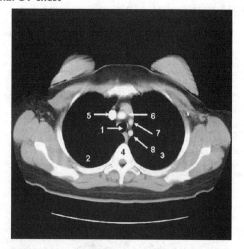

(a)

(b)

Fig. 12.14 (a–b) Normal CT chest 1. Trachea 2. Right lung 3. Left lung 4. Body of T3 5. SVC full of contrast 6. Brachiocephalic artery 7. Left common carotid 8. Left subclavian 9. Aortic arch 10. Oesophagus 11. Pulmonary trunk 12. Ascending aorta 13. Descending aorta 14. Carina 15. Hemiazygous vein 16. Left atrium 17. Right atrium 18. Right ventricle.. Reproduced with permission from Chikwe J, Beddow E, and Glenville B (2006). *Cardiothoracic Surgery*, Oxford University Press, Oxford.

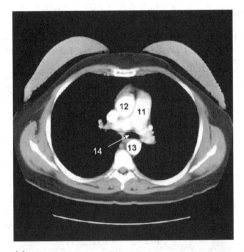

(c)

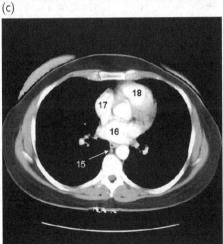

(d)

Fig. 12.14 (c–d) *(contd.)* Normal CT chest 1. Trachea 2. Right lung 3. Left lung 4. Body of T3 5. SVC full of contrast 6. Brachiocephalic artery 7. Left common carotid 8. Left subclavian 9. Aortic arch 10. Oesophagus 11. Pulmonary trunk 12. Ascending aorta 13. Descending aorta 14. Carina 15. Hemiazygous vein 16. Left atrium 17. Right atrium 18. Right ventricle.. Reproduced with permission from Chikwe J, Beddow E, and Glenville B (2006). *Cardiothoracic Surgery*, Oxford University Press, Oxford.

Conversion charts

Table 12.7 Height conversion chart. Adapted with permission from Sanders S, Dawson J, Datta S, and Eccles S (2005). *Oxford Handbook for the Foundation Programme*, Oxford University Press, Oxford.

m	inch	feet	inch	m	inch	feet	inch
1.36	53.5	4	5.5	1.67	66	5	6
1.37	54	4	6	1.69	66.5	5	6.5
1.38	54.5	4	6.5	1.70	67	5	7
1.40	55	4	7	1.71	67.5	5	7.5
1.41	55.5	4	7.5	1.73	68	5	8
1.42	56	4	8	1.74	68.5	5	8.5
1.43	56.5	4	8.5	1.75	69	5	9
1.45	57	4	9	1.76	69.5	5	9.5
1.46	57.5	4	9.5	1.78	70	5	10
1.47	58	4	10	1.79	70.5	5	10.5
1.48	58.5	4	10.5	1.80	71	5	11
1.50	59	4	11	1.81	71.5	5	11.5
1.51	59.5	4	11.5	1.83	72	6	0
1.52	60	5	0	1.84	72.5	6	0.5
1.54	60.5	5	0.5	1.85	73	6	1
1.55	61	5	1	1.87	73.5	6	1.5
1.56	61.5	5	1.5	1.88	74	6	2
1.57	62	5	2	1.89	74.5	6	2.5
1.59	62.5	5	2.5	1.90	75	6	3
1.60	63	5	3	1.92	75.5	6	3.5
1.61	63.5	5	3.5	1.93	76	6	4
1.62	64	5	4	1.94	76.5	6	4.5
1.64	64.5	5	4.5	1.95	77	6	5
1.65	65	5	5	1.97	77.5	6	5.5
1.66	65.5	5	5.5	1.98	78	6	6

Table 12.8 Weight conversion chart

kg	St	lbs	kg	St	lbs	kg	15St	lbs
1	0	2.2	34	5	5	67	10	8
2	0	4.4	35	5	7	68	10	10
3	0	6.6	36	5	9	69	10	12
4	0	8.8	37	5	12	70	11	0
5	0	11	38	5	14	71	11	3
6	0	13	39	6	2	72	11	5
7	1	1	40	6	4	73	11	7
8	1	4	41	6	6	74	11	9
9	1	6	42	6	9	75	11	11
10	1	8	43	6	11	76	11	14
11	1	10	44	6	13	77	12	2
12	1	12	45	7	1	78	12	4
13	2	1	46	7	3	79	12	6
14	2	3	47	7	6	80	12	8
15	2	5	48	7	8	81	12	11
16	2	7	49	7	10	82	12	13
17	2	9	50	7	12	83	13	1
18	2	12	51	8	0	84	13	3
19	3	14	52	8	3	85	13	5
20	3	2	53	8	5	86	13	8
21	3	4	54	8	7	87	13	10
22	3	7	55	8	9	88	13	12
23	3	9	56	8	11	89	14	0
24	3	11	57	8	14	90	14	2
25	3	13	58	9	2	91	14	5
26	4	1	59	9	4	92	14	7
27	4	4	60	9	6	93	14	9
28	4	6	61	9	8	94	14	11
29	4	8	62	9	11	95	14	13
30	4	10	63	9	13	96	15	2
31	4	12	64	10	1	97	15	4
32	5	1	65	10	3	98	15	6
33	5	3	66	10	6	99	15	8

(Continued)

Table 12.8 Weight conversion chart (*continued*)

kg	St	lbs	kg	St	lbs	kg	St	lbs
100	15	10	117	18	6	134	21	1
101	15	13	118	18	8	135	21	4
102	16	1	119	18	10	136	21	6
103	16	3	120	18	13	137	21	8
104	16	5	121	19	1	138	21	10
105	16	7	122	19	3	139	21	12
106	16	10	123	19	5	140	22	1
107	16	12	124	19	7	141	22	3
108	17	0	125	19	10	142	22	5
109	17	2	126	19	12	143	22	7
110	17	5	127	19	14	144	22	9
111	17	7	128	20	2	145	22	12
112	17	9	129	20	4	146	22	14
113	17	11	130	20	7	147	23	2
114	17	13	131	20	9	148	23	4
115	18	2	132	20	11	149	23	6
116	18	4	133	20	13	150	23	9

Dermatomes

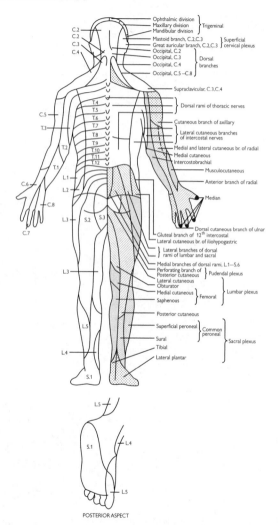

Fig. 12.15 Dorsal. Reproduced with permission from Collier M, Longmore M, and Brinsden M (2006). *Oxford Handbook of Clinical Specialties* 7e, Oxford University Press, Oxford.

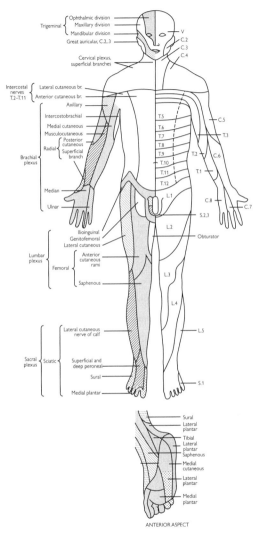

Fig. 12.16 Ventral. Reproduced with permission from Collier M, Longmore M, and Brinsden M (2006). *Oxford Handbook of Clinical Specialties* 7e, Oxford University Press, Oxford.

Index

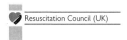
Adult Advanced Life Support Algorithm

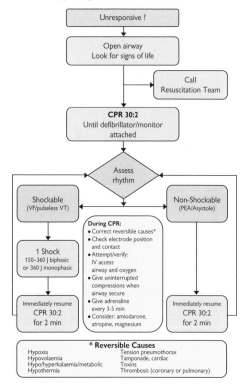

Unresponsive ?

↓

Open airway
Look for signs of life

→ Call Resuscitation Team

↓

CPR 30:2
Until defibrillator/monitor attached

↓

Assess rhythm

Shockable (VF/pulseless VT) ← → Non-Shockable (PEA/Asystole)

During CPR:
- Correct reversible causes*
- Check electrode position and contact
- Attempt/verify:
  IV access
  airway and oxygen
- Give uninterrupted compressions when airway secure
- Give adrenaline every 3-5 min
- Consider: amiodarone, atropine, magnesium

1 Shock
150–360 J biphasic
or 360 J monophasic

↓

Immediately resume CPR 30:2 for 2 min

Immediately resume CPR 30:2 for 2 min

* Reversible Causes

Hypoxia	Tension pneumothorax
Hypovolaemia	Tamponade, cardiac
Hypo/hyperkalaemia/metabolic	Toxins
Hypothermia	Thrombosis (coronary or pulmonary)

Key ALS and emergency drug doses

Drugs

Adrenaline	1mg IV as soon as IV access, repeat every 3-5 mins (This is one whole syringe – 10mls of 1:10,000)
Amiodarone	300mg bolus, repeat 150mg, infusion 900mg / 24h
Atropine sulphate	3mg IV once only
Bicarbonate	50mmol if K+>5.5mmol/l (one 50ml syringe)
Calcium chloride 10%	10mL IV
Lidocaine	1mg/kg (not if amiodarone already given)

Reproduced with permission,© UK Resuscitation Council, 2005.